Clinical Epidemiology of Chronic Liver Diseases

Robert J. Wong • Robert G. Gish
Editors

Clinical Epidemiology of Chronic Liver Diseases

Springer

Editors
Robert J. Wong
Division of Gastroenterology
and Hepatology
Alameda Health System Highland Hospital
Oakland, CA
USA

Robert G. Gish
Robert G. Gish Consultants LLC
Hepatitis B Foundation
Stanford Health Care
San Diego, CA
USA

ISBN 978-3-319-94354-1 ISBN 978-3-319-94355-8 (eBook)
https://doi.org/10.1007/978-3-319-94355-8

Library of Congress Control Number: 2018956812

This Springer imprint is published by the registered company Springer Nature Switzerland AG
The registered company address is: Gewerbestrasse 11, 6330 Cham, Switzerland

Preface

Chronic liver disease is a major cause of morbidity and mortality worldwide. In the United States, chronic liver disease is the 12th leading cause of death among adults, and worldwide hepatocellular carcinoma (HCC) is the second leading cause of cancer-related deaths. Furthermore, chronic liver disease secondary to viral hepatitis is a major contributor to morbidity and mortality, both among western countries as well as African and Asia-Pacific regions. Recent concerning trends in obesity and metabolic syndrome prevalence worldwide have generated much interest in the associated hepatic manifestation of metabolic syndrome—nonalcoholic fatty liver disease (NAFLD). The emergence of NAFLD as a leading cause of chronic liver disease is particularly concerning, given the large estimated burden of NAFLD worldwide and the significant hepatic and cardiovascular morbidity and mortality associated with this condition.

The changing epidemiology of chronic liver disease has been fueled by several major developments. The emergence of and implementation of vaccination programs for chronic hepatitis B virus in many countries has led to declining incidence of new infections particularly in highly endemic regions. Furthermore, early preventative screening and implementation of antiviral therapies and hepatitis B immunoglobulin together with vaccination has further reduced rates of vertical transmission. The recent improvements and increasing availability of safer and more effective antiviral therapies for treatment of chronic hepatitis C virus has worked hand in hand with increased screening efforts to bring the field closer to eradication of hepatitis C virus. However, the incidence of chronic hepatitis C infection worldwide may also be affected by increasing prevalence of intravenous drug use, changes in narcotic laws, and restrictions on needle exchanges in different parts of the world. Furthermore, increased awareness and implementation of screening for HCC among at risk individuals together with improvements in treatment options have translated into improvements in HCC survival. Many other improvements in the field of chronic liver disease, both in areas of diagnostics as well as therapeutics have continued to improve outcomes among patients affected by these diseases.

The current publication aims to provide an updated review of the epidemiology of chronic liver disease worldwide. We draw from the expertise of leading clinicians and clinical researchers in the field. In particular, the unique aspects of this publication include a breadth of expertise from various world regions as well as a specific emphasis on the study design and methodology of included studies. We first introduce the reader to key concepts and principles in clinical epidemiology and use these concepts to highlight and dissect some of the landmark studies in each of the topic chapters. As you will see, at the conclusion of each topic chapter, a table of landmark studies will be provided to summarize the major publications with key results and major limitations of each study. We hope that this compilation of expertise will provide the reader with an updated worldwide perspective of chronic liver disease clinical epidemiology.

Oakland, CA Robert J. Wong
San Diego, CA Robert G. Gish

Contents

Principles of Clinical Epidemiology

1

Rita Popat and Julia Simard

Abstract

Broadly, epidemiology studies the distribution and determinants of health (or disease)-related states at the population-level. This chapter introduces readers to key concepts in clinical epidemiology, applying epidemiologic reasoning and methods to clinical medicine. This includes the role of descriptive epidemiology in medicine and important methods in analytic epidemiology such as common study designs, principles of defining exposures and outcomes, an overview of measures, and sources of bias that can threaten internal validity. Not only does this chapter cover principles that are important whether one is designing a study involving prospective data collection or utilizing existing data, but will also aid in the interpretation of existing research and the published medical and scientific literature.

Keywords

Population · Bias · Confounding · Exposure · Outcome · Generalizability

Epidemiology is the study of the distribution and determinants of health-related states in populations. Information regarding disease frequency helps identify segments of the population that are at highest risk and where preventive efforts should be focused. Information regarding risk factors (determinants) helps develop preventive and treatment strategies that are then evaluated for efficacy before implementation. While descriptive epidemiology studies the distribution of disease by

R. Popat (✉) · J. Simard
Division of Epidemiology, Department of Health Research and Policy,
Stanford University School of Medicine, Stanford, CA, USA
e-mail: rpopat@stanford.edu

R. J. Wong, R. G. Gish (eds.), *Clinical Epidemiology of Chronic Liver Diseases*,
https://doi.org/10.1007/978-3-319-94355-8_1

person (who), place (where), and time (when), analytic epidemiology studies the determinants (risk factors) of disease.

Epidemiologic principles inform how to design, conduct, analyze, and interpret research studies. For example, to evaluate whether a risk factor is associated with the risk of developing a disease, consideration is given to select the best study design to evaluate this research question, identify a representative sample of the population to study, and utilize accurate measurements for ascertaining the exposure and outcomes. Analytic approaches used to quantify the exposure-outcome relationship are informed by the study design and measurements. Interpretation of the results need to account for whether biases and random error were adequately addressed in the design, conduct, and analysis of the study.

Clinical epidemiology applies epidemiologic methods to address problems encountered in clinical medicine. For example, descriptive epidemiology helps the clinician consider which diseases to look for in the patient. Knowledge of who is at risk helps identify patients who would benefit from screening. In patients diagnosed with a disease, knowledge about risk factors can help identify disease etiology, inform prognosis, and assist with treatment decisions. Therefore, clinical epidemiology can play an integral role in evidence based medicine and clinical decision making (Fig. 1.1).

In this chapter we introduce important principles of clinical epidemiology beginning with how to define a study population, exposures, and outcomes. We will discuss the role of descriptive epidemiology in medicine and present important methods in analytic epidemiology that include common study designs, measures of association, and study biases.

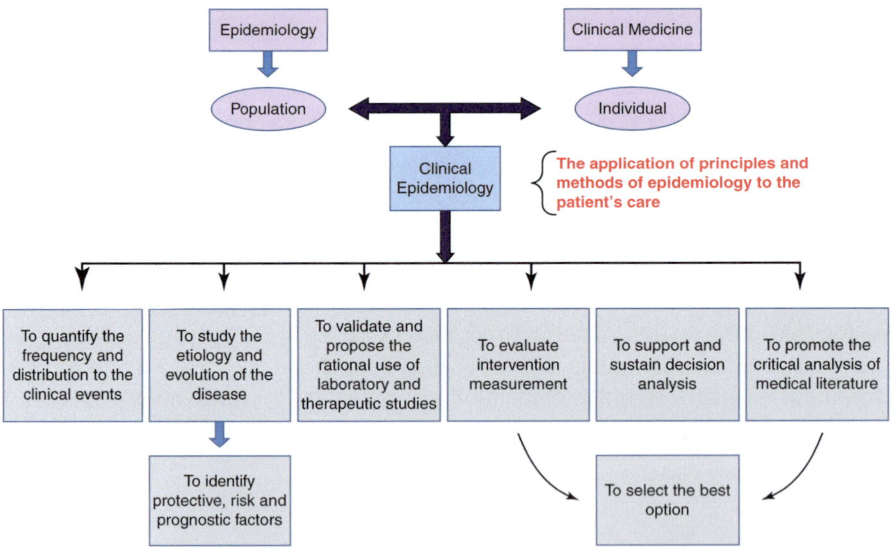

Fig. 1.1 Uses of clinical epidemiology (source: Díaz-Vélez C et al. (2013). Clinical Epidemiology and Its Relevance for Public Health in Developing Countries. In: Rodriguez-Morales (ed) Current Topics in Public Health, InTech, Chapter 12; https://doi.org/10.5772/54901)

1.1 Defining a Population for Clinical Epidemiology Studies

It is not feasible to study the entire population to evaluate an exposure-outcome relationship. Therefore, we select a sample from the target population of interest to evaluate our research question. When the sample studied is representative of the target population, inferences based on the sample are considered generalizable to the target population of interest. Clinical epidemiology studies focus on patients rather than the general population, so the target population is generally defined based on subjects having a certain disease of interest, for example, patients with cirrhosis of the liver. We identify a source population from which we can identify a sample of patients with cirrhosis. The source population could be a tertiary referral based hospital, a community clinic, or a pre-paid health care organization. If we are interested in studying patients that represent the entire disease spectrum (mild to severe), it is important that patients in the source population are representative of this target population. Cirrhosis patients at a tertiary referral center may be sicker compared to patients from a community clinic and not representative of the target population, thereby compromising generalizability. Once the source population is identified, eligible patients who meet pre-specified inclusion and exclusion criteria are approached to participate in the study. To ensure internal validity of the study, patients who participate in the study (sample) should be representative of eligible patients in the source population.

1.2 Defining Exposure

An "exposure" is any factor that may be associated with an outcome of interest. For example, if we want to study whether diabetes mellitus increases the risk of chronic nonalcoholic fatty liver disease, diabetes is the primary exposure variable of interest. We would want to make sure that the method for ascertaining diabetes is reliable and accurate. For example, if we are using medical record data and relying on ICD-9 codes to ascertain this information, then we would want to ensure that presence of this code correctly identifies diabetes. When defining exposure, it is also important to carefully consider time in relation to onset of the outcome. In the case of chronic liver disease (CLD), there is likely to be a protracted preclinical period, that is, a lag between disease onset and clinical detection. As a result, it may be difficult to capture the "etiologically relevant time window" when ascertaining the exposure. Once the symptoms are present, one could argue that the exposure has had its impact and that exposures captured between symptom onset and diagnosis are less relevant to disease etiology. In addition to looking at the right time, the format or definition of the exposure is important. For example, a study examining disease risk associated with smoking might initially consider ever exposure to cigarette smoke. If the etiologically relevant exposure is current or recent exposure to cigarette smoke, it may be difficult to observe the exposure-outcome relationship because former and current smokers will be combined in the ever smoker group.

1.3 Defining Outcome

Etiologic research studies will generally define some disease diagnosis as the outcome and this information could be obtained from a medical record or laboratory test. Studies evaluating prognosis or treatment efficacy will generally use health related outcomes (e.g., mortality, complications, quality of life) ascertained from medical records, interviews, or other records. Similar to exposure variables, outcome variables should also be measured reliably and accurately. Since the risk factors, treatment and prognosis of CLD depends on the etiology, it is important to make sure that the outcome is defined to include an etiologically homogeneous group, otherwise it may be challenging to observe an exposure-outcome relationship. For example, diabetes may be an important risk factor only for non-alcoholic and non-infectious CLD and we may miss an association if we include all etiologic types of CLD when defining the outcome.

1.4 Descriptive Epidemiology

Descriptive epidemiology provides information about the distribution of disease by person, place, and time. It can help clinicians decide which diseases to look for in their patients and in some cases also help with etiology. For example, a patient from sub-Saharan Africa is more likely to have hepatitis B as the cause of liver cirrhosis compared to a patient from North America [1].

The two measures of disease frequency are prevalence and incidence. *Prevalence* is a proportion and defined as the number of people with the disease (numerator) in the population of interest (denominator). Because prevalence estimates existing cases, it provides information regarding disease burden in the population and helps health agencies identify priorities for allocating resources as well as research.

Incidence represents occurrence of new disease. Cumulative incidence or risk is a proportion and defined as the number of new cases (numerator) among those at risk for developing the disease (denominator) over a specified time period. Incidence rate is the number of new cases out of the total person-time contributed by the study population at risk of becoming a case. Incidence and prevalence are closely related. Prevalence is proportional to the number of new cases (incidence) and the average duration of disease. More information on incidence and prevalence is covered in Chap. 4.

Deciding whether to include prevalent or incident cases in a clinical research study is important as risk factors associated with risk of developing the disease may differ from those associated with surviving with the disease. Therefore, if the interest is in evaluating exposures that increase the risk of disease, one should include incident cases in the sample.

Descriptive epidemiology is also useful for surveillance purposes and can help generate hypotheses for etiologic research. For example, the incidence of hepatocellular carcinoma (HCC) has been increasing in the U.S population since

1973. However, Njei et al. reported that the rate of increase has slowed down from 2006 to 2011 [2], which could be explained by an improvement in primary prevention strategies (e.g., hepatitis B vaccination programs) as well as advances in treatment of chronic hepatitis, which can reduce the risk of progression to cirrhosis and HCC.

1.5 Analytic Epidemiology

The goals of analytic epidemiology involve evaluation of factors associated with disease risk or prognosis, as well as evaluating preventive and treatment strategies. Analytic studies generally involve a comparison group and fall into two categories: experimental and observational.

In an *experimental study*, the investigator randomly assigns the exposure for each eligible individual and follows them over time to evaluate the effects of the exposure. For example, in a clinical trial to evaluate the efficacy of lamivudine, patients with chronic hepatitis B with histologically confirmed cirrhosis were randomly assigned to receive lamivudine (100 mg/day) or placebo for five years [3]. The primary outcome was time to disease progression, where progression was operationally defined as a composite outcome (e.g., hepatic decompensation, hepatocellular carcinoma, or death, etc.).

While new treatments are required to be evaluated using an experimental design, it is often unethical or not possible to randomize exposures. In these cases the researcher relies on observational methods. In *observational* studies, the investigator observes who has the exposure generally based on self-reported information or from medical records. The three common observational study designs include cohort, case-control, and cross-sectional studies.

In a *cohort study*, individuals in the study population are selected based on their exposure status and then their outcome is determined. For example, to evaluate whether obesity increases the risk of cirrhosis in alcoholic liver disease, eligible individuals with alcoholic liver disease (but without cirrhosis) will be identified and their obesity status (yes or no) will be recorded. All individuals, obese and not obese, will be followed up for five years to determine the risk of developing cirrhosis. This type of cohort study is *prospective* in nature because the outcome has not yet occurred at the time the study begins and follow-up of all participants is required to ascertain the outcome. The longer the follow-up time, the higher the probability that some subjects may withdraw, die, or be lost to follow-up. *Censoring* is a term used to describe this type of loss—the investigator no longer knows when or whether an individual develops the outcome so that individual stops contributing follow-up time and information. Using person-time data and estimating rates is one approach that allows the investigator to account for this.

An alternative type of cohort study is a *retrospective cohort study*. In this type of study, the outcome has already occurred at the time the study starts, however, it is possible to identify an eligible sample of participants and determine their exposure from information collected in the past, that is, before the outcome occurred. The risk or rate of developing the outcome is estimated from that time forward, similar to a prospective study. While retrospective cohort studies can be more time efficient compared to prospective cohort studies, they are only feasible when relevant exposure and outcome information can be obtained in an objective manner. For example, in the obesity-cirrhosis example, if obesity is defined based on body-mass-index (BMI), this information is likely to be present in the medical record. However, if obesity is operationally defined based on hip-to-waist ratio or triceps fold, then it is unlikely to be recorded in the medical record because these measurements are not part of routine care.

In a well-designed cohort study, prospective or retrospective, exposure temporally precedes outcome. This enables us to estimate the risk or rate of developing the outcome and also satisfies an important criterion for inferring whether an exposure is causally associated with the outcome.

In a *case-control study*, individuals are selected based on the outcome of interest and we define those with the outcome as cases and those without the outcome as controls. Then, investigators determine the distribution or frequency of exposure in these cases and controls. Case-control designs are often retrospective in nature because information about exposure is generally ascertained after the outcome has already developed. Therefore, exposure information is often subject to recall bias or other misclassification. However, concerns regarding the quality of exposure measurements depend on the exposure of interest and how this information is ascertained. For example, going back to the obesity-cirrhosis question, asking cases (with cirrhosis) and controls (without cirrhosis) to recall their BMI prior to diagnosis date for cases and an index data for controls may lead to bias, particularly if the exposure, obesity, is perceived by cases to be related to the disease. However, if the investigators could get this information for cases and controls from another source, such as the medical record before the outcome occurred, then the potential for recall bias is reduced. Identifying appropriate controls for a case-control study is also difficult, and inappropriate controls can lead to selection bias (more on this in Sect. 1.8) [4]. Despite these challenges, if done correctly case-control studies can be an efficient way to answer a research question. Instead of collecting exposure and outcome information on the whole population of interest, a sample of cases and controls can be obtained and results can be equivalent to those from a cohort study.

A *nested case-control study* is a type of case-control study that selects its cases and controls from a cohort population that has been followed for a period of time. Nested case-control studies are particularly useful when it is either too costly or not feasible to perform additional biomarker analyses on an entire cohort. Since exposure data is collected before the onset of the disease, the potential for recall bias and temporal ambiguity is reduced in nested case-control studies.

In a *cross-sectional study*, information on exposure, outcome, and additional covariates of interest are collected at the same time. This allows for estimation of prevalence and can also be used to estimate the relationship between the prevalence of exposure with the outcome. The association between aspirin use and liver fibrosis among adults with suspected chronic liver disease was reported using the data from the National Health and Nutrition Examination Survey III, a cross-sectional survey of a nationally representative sample of US adults [5]. Information on aspirin use in NHANES III was limited to the month prior to the entry of study. Although aspirin use was associated with a significantly lower composite liver fibrosis index, there was insufficient information to establish temporality—when did they start taking aspirin? How does aspirin use relate to the onset of fibrosis? This is particularly important since any potential protection against liver fibrosis likely requires long-term aspirin use.

We have described the traditional study designs that typically examine groups of people on the basis of an exposure or outcome. In some alternative study designs, individuals act as both the exposed and unexposed (case-crossover [6]) or only those with the outcome are included (case-only [7]). There are also study designs that investigate not at the level of the individual but at the level of a group or population (ecological studies [8]) or studies (systematic review and meta-analysis [9]).

1.6 Measures of Association

A measure of disease frequency quantifies how often the disease outcome has occurred in a group of interest. Some measures include proportion, risk, and rate as described earlier (Sect. 1.4). For example, prevalence and cumulative incidence or risk are proportions. These measures are unit-less and range from 0 to 1 (or 0–100%). In contrast, an incidence rate has units (person-time) and can range from 0 to infinity. Another measure of frequency is odds, which is most frequently used in case-control studies.

In analytic studies the goal is to quantify the exposure-outcome association by comparing the relevant measures of disease frequency between two groups. There are relative and absolute measures of association (also known as effect measure). The *risk difference,* an absolute effect measure, is the risk in the exposed minus the risk in the unexposed. The *relative risk* is a generic term used for ratio based measures. For example, the *risk ratio* is calculated by dividing the risk in the exposed by the risk in the unexposed. Similarly, one could calculate a prevalence ratio, incidence rate ratio or an odds ratio. The *hazard ratio*, which is estimated by Cox proportional hazards models in survival analysis, is similar to an incidence rate ratio (for more details see Chap. 5 on Survival Analysis). The choice of measure of disease frequency and effect measure depends on the study design used and the goal of the research study.

In the example below, we use data from a prospective study by Yang et al. [10] to illustrate how effect measures are computed.

Example 1.6: Computing Effect Measures

Yang et al. conducted a prospective cohort study to determine the relation between positivity for hepatitis B surface antigen (HBsAg) and hepatitis B envelope antigen (HBeAg) and the development of HCC [10]. The table below shows the incidence of HCC during the follow up.

Incidence of hepatocellular carcinoma during follow-up[a]

Results of HBV[a] antigen tests	Person-years of follow-up	No. of men	No. of cases of hepatocellular carcinoma	Incidence rate (IR) Cases/100,000 person-yr (95% Confidence interval)
HBsAg− and HBeAg−	74,205	9532	29	39.1 (26.2–56.1)
HBsAg+ and HBeAg−	15,418	1991	50	324.3 (240.7–427.5)
HBsAg+ and HBeAg+	2,736	370	32	1169.4 (799.9–1650.9)

[a]*HBV* hepatitis B virus, *HBsAg* hepatitis B surface antigen, HBeAg hepatitis B e antigen

Using the information above we can compute the following effect measures (*IR* Incidence rate, *R* Risk):

(1) Incidence rate ratio[a]	$= IR_{exposed}/IR_{unexposed} = IR_{HBsAg+,\ HBeAg+}/IR_{HBsAg-,\ HBeAg-}$
	= 1169.4 per 10^5 p-yr/39.1 per 10^5 p-yr = **29.9**
(2) Risk ratio[a]	$= R_{exposed}/R_{unexposed} = R_{HBsAg+,\ HBeAg+}/R_{HBsAg-,\ HBeAg-}$
	= (32/370)/(29/9532) = (0.0865)/(0.003) = **28.8**
(3) Odds ratio[a]	$= Odds_{outcome\ in\ exposed}/Odds_{outcome\ in\ unexposed}$
	$= [R_{exposed}/(1 - R_{exposed})]/[R_{unexposed}/(1 - R_{unexposed})]$
	= [0.0865/0.9135]/[0.003/0.997] = **31.5**
(4) Rate difference[b]	$= IR_{exposed} - IR_{unexposed} = IR_{HBsAg+,\ HBeAg+} - IR_{HBsAg-,\ HBeAg-}$
	= 1169.4 per 10^5 p-yr − 39.1 per 10^5 p-yr = 1130.3 per 100,000 p-yr

[a]Relative effect measures
[b]Absolute effect measure

1.7 Some Notes About Statistical Inference (p-Values and Confidence Intervals)

In example 1.6, the unadjusted (or crude) incidence rate ratio was 29.9. This relative risk (RR) suggests that the risk of HCC was approximately 30-fold higher among those who were seropositive for HBsAg and HBeAg as compared with men who were negative for both. However, due to inherent statistical randomness associated with sampling, in order to make the correct inference we would want more information. For example, we would like to know the probability (p-value) of observing a RR of 30 or more extreme if there was no association between seropositivity and HCC (the null hypothesis). In addition, we would also like to know something about the precision around this point estimate by estimating the 95% confidence interval. While p-values and confidence intervals provide important information, they are frequently misinterpreted [11] and overemphasized. The interpretation of a study's results should not just focus on statistical significance but take all the evidence into account, including the direction and magnitude of the association (i.e., clinical significance), and consider whether the findings are likely to be affected by bias or chance.

1.8 Bias

For an analytic study to produce a valid estimate of an exposure-outcome association, the study must be designed, conducted, analyzed, and interpreted in ways that reduces the potential of generating biased results. Systematic errors introduced by the investigator in sampling, collecting, or interpreting data can introduce bias thereby threatening the internal validity of the study. Random errors can also affect study results by producing imprecise estimates. However, careful consideration of sample size and power during the planning phase can help address these concerns. In this section we will discuss the three primary sources of bias that can affect the internal validity of a study: confounding, selection bias, and misclassification (or information bias).

1.8.1 Confounding

A confounder is defined as a variable that is independently associated with the outcome and exposure, and is not the causal pathway between the exposure and outcome. When the distribution of a potential confounder is unequal between the groups being compared, it can result in biased estimates of the exposure-outcome relationship. In experimental studies, randomization can help control for confounding because both measured and unmeasured confounders tend to get distributed equally (i.e., balanced) between the experimental and control group (thereby removing the independent association between confounders and the exposure). To preserve the benefits of randomization, it is also important to use intention-to-treat analysis where subjects are analyzed based on the group they were initially assigned to, irrespective of adherence.

In observational studies, randomization is not possible, so investigators use approaches in the design or analysis phase to control for confounding. In the design phase of observational studies, *restriction* or *matching* can minimize confounding. When using the restriction approach, we remove the association between the exposure and the confounder by restricting the sample to one level of the confounder. For example, sex is an important confounder of most exposure-outcome relationships. By restricting the study to include only males, there is no longer a way for exposure and disease to be influenced by sex. In matching, the study population is chosen to have a similar distribution of the confounding variable. Matching can be quite powerful, but needs to be carefully considered particularly in case-control studies where it may inadvertently introduce confounding or bias the association towards the null [12].

The traditional approaches of restriction and matching can only help address a few confounders. The ability to handle several confounders requires analytic

Table 1.1 Associations between composite fibrosis index and aspirin use among individuals with chronic liver disease using NHANES III data (Jiang et al. [5])

	Coefficient[a]	95% CI	p-value
Unadjusted	−0.17	−0.41 to 0.07	0.2
Model 1[b]	−0.27	−0.47 to −0.07	0.008
Model 2[c]	-0.24	−0.42 to −0.06	0.009

There were 520 aspirin users and 1336 non-users

[a]Beta coefficients for the composite fibrosis index measured in the unit of standard deviation associated with aspirin/ibuprofen use using sampling weights in NHANES III to allow inference of the US civilian population

[b]Model 1 was calculated by multivariable regression adjusted for age

[c]Model 2 was calculated by the multivariable regression adjusted for age, gender, ethnicity, BMI, smoking, alcohol history, income poverty index, level of education, type of insurance, histories of coronary artery disease, stroke, diabetes, hypertension, arrhythmia, number of daily medications and the use of lipid-lowering medication or acetaminophen

approaches such as statistical adjustment using a multivariable regression model. Stratifying results by the confounding factor is also a reasonable approach, but not very efficient when multiple confounders need to be considered and when confounders include continuous variables.

For example, in the cross-sectional study of aspirin use and liver fibrosis described earlier [5], the unadjusted results showed a modest inverse association in patients with chronic liver disease that was not statistically significant at the alpha = 0.05 level (Coefficient −0.17, 95% CI −0.41 to 0.07; p-value 0.2; see Table 1.1). Since aspirin use was not randomized, several potential confounders needed to be considered. For example, compared to non-users, aspirin users were older and had a higher prevalence of comorbidities such as arrhythmia, hypertension, and coronary artery disease. In fact, *confounding by indication* is a well-known type of confounding where an association (e.g., aspirin-liver fibrosis) is influenced by the underlying indication for exposure or treatment. Subjects who have coronary heart disease or are older are more likely to take aspirin and may be more likely to develop liver fibrosis as well, thereby obscuring a potential protective effect of aspirin use. Researchers used a linear regression model to account for potential confounders. Interestingly, in this study, age was the most important confounder and after adjusting for age, the inverse association between aspirin use and liver fibrosis was strengthened (Coefficient −0.27, 95% CI −0.47 to −0.07; p-value 0.008). Further adjustment for comorbidities did not change the association by much (Coefficient −0.24, 95% CI −0.42 to −0.06; p-value 0.009). There can still be *residual confounding* if there are unmeasured confounders or confounders are not measured correctly or properly specified (for example, adjusting for age using a binary variable [<60 vs. ≥60] instead of age as a continuous variable, could result in residual confounding).

Other methods to control for confounding in observational studies include propensity scores [13] when we have measured confounders and instrumental variables [14] or external adjustment [15] when there are unmeasured confounders.

1.8.2 Selection Bias

Selection bias is a form of sampling bias due to *systematic differences* between those who are selected for a study (or agree to participate) and those who are not selected (or refuse to participate). Selection bias can arise from procedures used to select subjects, factors that influence study participation, or factors that influence participant attrition.

In a case-control study, selection bias occurs when the exposure of interest is associated with the selection of cases, controls or both. A hospital-based case-control study was performed to examine the association of coffee consumption with pancreatic cancer [16]. Cases included subjects with a confirmed diagnosis of pancreatic cancer. Controls were selected from inpatients hospitalized by the attending physicians who had hospitalized the cases, so that the selection process of cases and controls were similar. Cases reported a higher prevalence of coffee consumption compared to controls (94.5% vs. 86%, respectively). However, the prevalence of coffee drinking in the hospital-based controls was much *lower* than the target population of general adults because the controls had gastrointestinal disorders (like gastritis, peptic ulcers) and had reduced coffee consumption. The less than ideal choice of a control group may have led to the spurious association between coffee intake and pancreatic cancer that has not been subsequently confirmed [17].

In cohort studies and randomized clinical trials, selection bias can result from differential loss-to-follow-up or *informative censoring*. In this situation, people who remain in the study to be analyzed no longer represent the original study population. For example, in a trial comparing two treatments, subjects on treatment A are more likely to experience side effects and drop out of the study. The individuals remaining in the treatment A group are only those who have not experienced the side effect and may appear healthier than those on treatment B. Comparing the two groups may lead to the incorrect conclusion that treatment A is associated with better outcomes. Therefore, it is important for investigators conducting prospective studies to minimize loss-to-follow-up (gold standard is considered to be 80% follow-up of the inception cohort).

Investigators can use the following strategies to minimize the potential for selection bias: (1) ensure that participation in the study is not impacted by the exposure or the outcome (e.g., blind subjects to study hypothesis); (2) attempt to recruit all cases within the source population; (3) ensure controls and cases are selected from the *same* target population; (4) minimize non-response and refusals; and (5) minimize loss to follow-up (in cohort studies and RCTs).

1.8.3 Misclassification

Misclassification, also known an information bias or broadly measurement error, occurs when we erroneously classify an individual's exposure or outcome status. Misclassification results when the methods used for ascertaining measurements

Table 1.2 Measures of accuracy

		True classification of outcome/exposure status (gold standard)		
		Present	Absent	
Method used in study to classify outcome/exposure status	Present	True positives A	False positives B	A + B
	Absent	False negatives C	True negatives D	C + D
		Sensitivity = A/(A+C)	Specificity = D/(B+D)	

lack accuracy. Sensitivity and specificity are commonly used measures of accuracy when a reference or gold-standard is available for ascertaining the outcome or exposure (see Table 1.2). For disease classification, *sensitivity* is the proportion of cases who truly have the disease and *specificity* is the proportion of subjects who truly do not have the disease.

Liver biopsy is considered the gold standard method for diagnosis of cirrhosis. However, non-invasive techniques based on serum or imaging markers may be used in studies. Utilization of non-invasive measures, while more convenient and economical, are likely to result in some misclassification of disease status because these measures are not 100% sensitive or specific. When disease misclassification is independent of exposure status (i.e., similar misclassification in exposed and unexposed groups), this is referred to as *non-differential misclassification*, which tends to bias associations towards the null (i.e. underestimates the association). In contrast, *differential misclassification* occurs when the degree of disease misclassification depends on exposure status. For example, in a randomized clinical trial, if all subjects in the treatment arm received a biopsy but subjects in the control arm only received non-invasive tests, then this would result in differential misclassification, which may overestimate or underestimate the association.

Exposure misclassification can also bias the exposure-outcome association in a manner similar to disease misclassification. For example, in a case-control study of alcohol consumption and the risk of HCC, suppose both the cases and controls were to underreport exposure to alcohol. This situation would result in non-differential misclassification that would bias the association towards the null. *Recall bias* is an example of differential misclassification of the exposure in which cases recall their exposure differently than controls.

Investigators can use the following strategies to minimize the potential for misclassification bias: (1) choose objective measures (e.g., pharmacy records vs. self-report use of medications) and hard outcomes (e.g. mortality); (2) test reliability and validity of instruments used to determine outcome and exposure; (3) train and blind interviewers to outcome status and study hypothesis; (4) blind subjects to study hypothesis; (5) use similar methods for determining outcome and exposure in all study subjects (reduces potential for differential misclassification); and (6) use incident cases in case-control studies, not prevalent cases. Table 1.3 [18] summarizes the features, advantages, and limitations and sources of bias of traditional study designs.

Table 1.3 Summary of study designs

Study design	Description	Advantages	Limitations and biases
Observational			
Cross-sectional	Measures prevalence of risk factors (e.g., interventions, exposures) and outcomes at one time point	Relatively inexpensive, easy, and quick; often generalizable: provides valid estimates of prevalence for risk factors and outcomes	Cannot determine whether risk factors preceded outcomes; may uncover risk factors associated with duration (or survival) rather than cause of outcome; inefficient for rare risk factors and outcomes; may be subject to nonresponse bias, recall bias, and confounding
Case-control	Selects participants based on outcome status (case or control) and asks them about past risk factors	Efficient for rare outcomes; relatively inexpensive, easy, and quick	Getting comparable control subjects is often tricky; temporal relationship between risk factors and the outcome may be uncertain; inefficient for rare risk factors; cannot be used to estimate rates or risks of the outcome or risk ratios; may be subject to recall bias and confounding
Prospective cohort	Measures risk factors in an outcome-free cohort and observes them until they develop the outcome	Temporality is certain: risk factors preceded outcomes; prevents bias that may occur after a person develops an outcome; provides valid estimates of rates and risks of outcomes; can be used to study multiple outcomes	Can be lengthy and costly; inefficient for rare outcomes: may be affected by loss to follow-up and confounding
Retrospective cohort	Similar to a prospective cohort study, but the cohort is assembled after outcomes have already occurred, by using stored records	Similar benefits as a prospective cohort study but also faster and cheaper	Risk factor data were not collected specifically for the study, and thus certain variables and confounders may be unavailable; data quality may be low; requires stored or electronic records; may be affected by loss to follow-up (may not be able to get outcome information on everyone in the retrospectively assembled cohort) and confounding

(continued)

Table 1.3 (continued)

Study design	Description	Advantages	Limitations and biases
Experimental			
Randomized controlled trial	Participants are randomly assigned to interventions and then followed up over time	Criterion standard for showing cause-and-effect relationships; randomization minimizes confounding; blinding and placebos help minimize bias	Expensive; not practical for showing long-term effects; not always generalizable; not always ethical or feasible

Source: Sainani KL, Popat RA (2011) Understanding study design. PM & R 3(6): 573–7

1.9 Generalizability

If the results of a study are expected to be similar in another population, the study is said to be generalizable to that other population, or have external validity. It makes sense to consider external validity only when a study has internal validity. To determine generalizability, the eligibility criteria and the composition of the study population should be taken into account. To determine whether a study has external validity, one can ask the question "Would we expect the results seen in study population X to be the same in population Y?" If there is a plausible biological difference between population X and Y that would cause the association to be different, generalizability may be limited, for example if population X was all male and population Y was all female.

Acknowledgments We would like to thank Renee Miller for her editorial assistance with this book chapter.

References

1. Tsochatzis E, Bosch J, Burroughs A. Liver cirrhosis. Lancet. 2014;383(9930):1749–61.
2. Njei B, Rotman Y, Ditah I, Lim J. Emerging trends in hepatocellular carcinoma incidence and mortality. Hepatology. 2015;61(1):191–9.
3. Liaw Y, Sung J, Chow W, Farrell G, Lee C, Yuen H, et al. Lamivudine for patients with chronic hepatitis B and advanced liver disease. N Engl J Med. 2004;351(15):1521–31.
4. Wacholder S, McLaughlin J, Silverman D, Mandel J. Selection of controls in case-control studies. Am J Epidemiol. 1992;135(9):1019–28.
5. Jiang Z, Feldbrügge L, Tapper E, Popov Y, Ghaziani T, Afdhal N, et al. Aspirin use is associated with lower indices of liver fibrosis among adults in the United States. Aliment Pharmacol Ther. 2016;43(6):734–43.
6. Maclure M, Mittleman A. Should we use a case-crossover design? Annu Rev Public Health. 2000;21(1):193–221.
7. Gatto N. Further development of the case-only design for assessing gene-environment interaction: evaluation of and adjustment for bias. Int J Epidemiol. 2004;33(5):1014–24.
8. Sitas F, Thompson M. A role for the ecological study in the developing world. S Afr Med J. 1993;83:753–6.

9. Moher D, Liberati A, Tetzlaff J. Preferred reporting items for systematic reviews and meta-analyses: the PRISMA statement. Ann Intern Med. 2009;151(4):264–9. W64.
10. Yang H, Lu S, Liaw Y, You S, Sun C, Wang L, et al. Hepatitis B e antigen and the risk of hepatocellular carcinoma. N Engl J Med. 2002;347(3):168–74.
11. Greenland S, Senn S, Rothman K, Carlin J, Poole C, Goodman S, et al. Statistical tests, P values, confidence intervals, and power: a guide to misinterpretations. Eur J Epidemiol. 2016;31(4):337–50.
12. Szklo M, Nieto F. Epidemiology: beyond the basics. 3rd ed. Burlington, MA: Jones & Bartlett Learning; 2014.
13. Sainani K. Propensity scores: uses and limitations. PM&R. 2012;4(9):693–7.
14. Baiocchi M, Cheng J, Small D. Instrumental variable methods for causal inference. Stat Med. 2014;33(13):2297–340.
15. Schneeweiss S. Sensitivity analysis and external adjustment for unmeasured confounders in epidemiologic database studies of therapeutics. Pharmacoepidemiol Drug Saf. 2006;15(5):291–303.
16. MacMahon B, Yen S, Trichopoulos D, Warren K, Nardi G. Coffee and cancer of the pancreas. N Engl J Med. 1981;304(11):630–3.
17. Feinstein A, Horwitz R, Spitzer W, Battista R. Coffee and pancreatic cancer. The problems of etiologic science and epidemiologic case-control research. JAMA. 1981;246(9):957–61.
18. Sainani K, Popat R. Understanding study design. PM&R. 2011;3(6):573–7.

Understanding Study Design for Clinical Epidemiology Studies

2

Jenny Krause Cohen and Irene H. Yen

2.1 Overview of Chapter

This chapter presents information about three types of study designs commonly used for liver disease research. Each section provides a set of terms used when presenting research using the given design, an overview of the design, key aspects of the methods used, strengths and limits of the design, and a clinical vignette which draws from relevant research on a liver disease and highlights key aspects of the design.

2.2 Case Control Study

Terms:

- Case
- Control
- Confounder
- Matching
- Odds Ratio

J. K. Cohen
Division of Primary Care, Department of Medicine, Highland Hospital, Oakland, CA, USA

I. H. Yen (✉)
University of California, San Francisco, San Francisco, CA, USA
e-mail: iyen@ucmerced.edu

R. J. Wong, R. G. Gish (eds.), *Clinical Epidemiology of Chronic Liver Diseases*,
https://doi.org/10.1007/978-3-319-94355-8_2

2.2.1 Overview

A case-control study is one that compares patients who have a disease or outcome of interest (*cases*) with patients who do not have the disease or outcome (*controls*) and compares how frequently the exposure to a risk factor is present in each group to determine if an association exists between the risk factor and the disease. Most case-control studies are retrospective, in that the exposure is assessed by looking back in time ***after*** identifying the cases (diseased) and the controls (non-diseased). A prospective study identifies the cases and controls as subjects are recruited, based on disease status.

Case control studies are *observational* because no intervention is attempted and no attempt is made to alter the course of the disease. As such, causality cannot be concluded from the statistical analyses, but rather associations can be detected. The goal is to retrospectively determine the exposure to the risk factor of interest from each of the two groups of individuals: cases and controls. These studies are designed to estimate *odds ratios*. An odds ratio (OR) is a measure of association between an exposure and an outcome. The OR represents the odds that an outcome will occur given a particular exposure, compared to the odds of the outcome occurring in the absence of that exposure.

- OR = 1 Exposure does not affect odds of outcome
- OR > 1 Exposure associated with higher odds of outcome
- OR < 1 Exposure associated with lower odds of outcome

Usually the OR is reported with a 95% confidence interval (CI), which provides a range of OR that could occur if the same study were repeated in the same population. The 95% CI is affected by the sample size of the study cohort as well as the precision of the calculated OR values. A large CI indicates a low level of precision of the OR, whereas a small CI indicates a higher precision of the OR. Szumilas provides a good review and systematic explanation of the concept and calculation of OR [1].

When reading a paper which features a case-control study, things to assess are:

- What is the definition of the *case*?
  - How was the disease diagnosis ascertained: self-report, laboratory measure, chart review?

    If the disease diagnosis is based on self-report, this introduces potential biases. People with the disease who have more access to medical care are more likely to be diagnosed and know their diagnosis. People who have the disease who are not diagnosed could be incorrectly identified as a control. This would tend

  to make it more difficult to find that the exposure is associated with the disease, a bias toward the null hypothesis (i.e. there is no association between outcome and exposure).
  - What are the inclusion and exclusion criteria: age range, co-morbid conditions, language?
- What is the definition of *control*?
- Did the authors identify potential *confounders*?
  When a non-casual association is observed between a given exposure and outcome is a result of the influence of a third variable, it is termed confounding, with the third variable termed a confounding variable. A confounding variable is causally associated with the outcome of interest, and non-causally or causally associated with the exposure, but is not an intermediate variable in the causal pathway between exposure and outcome [2].
- Were controls matched to cases?
  - *Matching* is intended to reduce *confounding*. For example, matching on age can be helpful in minimizing potential confounding based on age. Matching would be carried out in a way that when a case is identified, the control would be identified matching on age, within a certain range (e.g. a 45-year-old case would be matched with a 43-47-year old control). These matched pairs are analyzed together, to see if either or both was exposed. In some cases more than one control is matched, e.g. 2:1 or 3:1, in order to increase statistical power.
    If matching is done on a characteristic that is not a known confounder, this can lead to bias. The matched characteristic cannot be studied as a risk factor as the process of matching takes the characteristic out of the analysis (evenly distributes it across cases and controls). Rose and van der Laan provide a more in-depth discussion regarding the concept of matching in study designs [3].
- How was the exposure ascertained? Self-report? Chart review?
  If people are asked about exposures, people who have the disease may report exposures that are potential causes because they attribute cause to those exposures, which could lead to a bias away from the null hypothesis and overestimate the potential association between outcome and exposure.

When a non-casual association is observed between a given exposure and outcome is a result of the influence of a third variable, it is termed confounding, with the third variable termed a confounding variable. A confounding variable is causally associated with the outcome of interest, and non-causally or causally associated with the exposure, but is not an intermediate variable in the causal pathway between exposure and outcome [2].

Clinical Vignette

Six weeks ago, you started one of your primary care patients on a proton pump inhibitor (PPI) for presumed gastro esophageal reflux (GERD) after she complained of mid epigastric pain at night worse when laying down and after eating heavy meals. She has a history of chronic hepatitis C virus infection complicated by cirrhosis with a most recent Childs-Pugh-Turcotte (CPT) class B given her bilirubin of 1.5 mg/dL, albumin of 2.9 g/dL, INR of 1.5, small volume ascites, and lack of encephalopathy. Today in follow-up, she is febrile, tachycardic, and has new abdominal pain, but does note resolution of her GERD symptoms. She denies melena or hematochezia and notes no changes in her bowel habits, but given your concern for community-acquired spontaneous bacterial peritonitis (SBP), you decide to send her to the Emergency Department for further evaluation and treatment. She did not have a history of SBP, prior paracentesis, or history of esophageal or gastric varices. As you consider her case, you wonder if the recent initiation of PPIs could be related to her SBP and you do a quick literature search. You are able to find three large retrospective case-control studies looking at patients with cirrhosis and comparing those with and without SBP all of which showed in multivariate analyses that PPIs increased the risk for SBP [4–6]. Most recently Ratelle, *et al.* conducted a case control study in which they matched each case of SBP to two controls and showed in their multivariate analysis that PPIs were independently associated with increased odds of SBP [7].

Ratelle *et al.* found that those on PPIs were independently associated with SBP with an odds ratio of 2.09 [7]. You worry that perhaps the patients with SBP represented an older and sicker population than the control group, however, the authors matched age and CPT class to control for this potential confounding. Similarly, the authors matched on year of hospital admission to control for possible changes in PPI prescribing habits.

Based on the strength of their data, you decide to stop your patient's PPI and be more cautions in the future about prescribing PPIs in patients with cirrhosis who are at risk for SBP.

2.3 Randomized Controlled Trial

Terms:

- Random/randomization
- Confounder/confounding
- Blind/Blinded/Blinding
- Sensitivity
- Specificity
- Positive predictive value

- Negative predictive value
- Number needed to treat
- Absolute risk reduction

2.3.1 Overview

Randomized Controlled Trial (RCT)—A study design that randomly assigns participants into an experimental group or a control group. The experimental group receives a new treatment, e.g. medication or combination therapy or intervention. The control group receives standard of care or a placebo. The outcomes for the two groups are compared, e.g. death, hospitalization, re-admission, laboratory test measure. Placebo can be chosen for the RCT control group when there is no recognized gold standard of care. The RCT is testing the new treatment against no treatment. A placebo is provided, e.g. sugar pill, because studies have shown that people may respond to treatment simply because attention is being paid to them or because there is regression to the mean, a shift from a more extreme state to a less extreme state.

Variations of the RCT design. A *blinded* design means that people administering the treatment (whether it is the experimental one or the control) do not know which group the participating patient is in.

Common pitfalls: An RCT should be a study of one population only. Was the randomization actually "*random*," or are there really two populations being studied? For example, let's say that morning patients are assigned to the experimental group and afternoon patients are assigned to control. Perhaps schedulers give patients who need more time to get to the office the afternoon appointments. Are there other characteristics about needing more time that will affect how they respond to the treatment? In most published RCTs, Table 1 provides the demographics of the study cohort, and can provide valuable information to determine whether the comparator groups are truly similar.

If the RCT is tracking disease incidence, the results can be used to calculate:

Sensitivity or true positive rate—the proportion of patients diagnosed with the condition who are correctly identified to have the condition.

Specificity or true negative rate—the proportion of patients who do not have the condition who are correctly identified not to have the condition.

Positive predictive value (PPV)—the probability that the patients with a positive screening test have the disease (e.g. patients who get a positive mammogram who have breast cancer).

Number needed to treat (NNT)—the average number of patients who need to be treated to prevent one additional bad outcome (e.g. the number of patients that need to be treated for one to benefit compared with a control). For example, if a treatment has an NNT of 10, it means you have to treat 10 people with the drug to prevent one additional bad outcome. To calculate the NNT, you need to know the *Absolute Risk Reduction (ARR);* the NNT is the inverse of the ARR:

$$\mathrm{NNT} = 1/\mathrm{ARR}$$

Where ARR = CER (Control Event Rate) – EER (Experimental Event Rate).

NNTs are always rounded up to the nearest whole number. Often times, authors will also present the Number needed to harm (NNH). Comparing the NNT to the NNH can give clinicians insight into the cost benefit of the intervention in question.

Clinical Vignette

You are called by the Emergency Department attending to admit a 34 year-old man who reports two days of vomiting coffee-ground emesis. He endorses drinking 12 beers daily for the last five years and occasionally drinking a pint of scotch; his last drink was around midnight. This is his first time interacting with the medical system since he was a teenager and denies any past medical history. Review of systems is negative for diarrhea, fevers, chills, shortness of breath, or chest pain. His triage vitals are notable for a heart rate of 110 beats/min and blood pressure of 95/60 mmHg. On exam he has spider angiomas and a palpable sleep tip, but no ascites nor scleral icterus. His initial labs included a serum creatinine of 2.0 mg/dL , alanine aminotransferase (ALT) of 100 U/L, aspartate aminotransferase (AST) of 200 U/L, total bilirubin 9.0 mg/dL, a hemoglobin of 6.5 mg/dL, platelet count of 135,000/mL, and prothrombin time of 31 s (reference range 11–14 s). He is negative for hepatitis virus A, B, and C. Initially he is given one unit of packed red blood cells, started on a proton pump inhibitor infusion, and admitted to the intensive care unit. The next day, upper endoscopy reveals esophageal varices with a large bleeding vessel that are amenable to band ligation and ceftriaxone is added to his treatment regimen. He remains hemodynamicaly stable, but on hospital day two his liver function tests continue to worsen and you calculate his discriminate function to be over 32. You are ambivalent about starting prednisolone or pentoxifylline and recall a recently published paper on the topic.

Based on your understanding of Thursz *et al.*'s 2015 NEJM publication [8], you decide not to give prednisolone or pentoxifylline given that neither drug showed 90-day or one-year mortality benefit. You feel this is a reasonable conclusion to draw because your patient's presenting clinical picture mirrored that of the study's inclusion criteria (thus the study population was generalizable to your patient). You are also aware that factors such as age, encephalopathy, leukocytosis, synthetic function, and degree of renal failure all can influence mortality and after looking at the author's multivariate logistic-regression model in which these variables were adjusted for, the effect of prednisolone on mortality at 90 days as well as at one year was non-significant.

2.4 Cohort Study

Terms:

- Cohort
- Observational
- Exposure

- Selection bias
- Confounding/confounder
- Information or measurement bias

2.4.1 Overview

The word "cohort" has been adopted into epidemiology to define a set of people followed over a period of time. An outcome or disease-free study population is identified by an exposure or event of interest and followed in time until the disease or outcome of interest occurs.

Exposure is defined at the beginning of the study. This feature is a strength of the cohort study, as the design allows for the ability to establish causality. The design also allows for the study of rare exposures.

There are a number of potential biases that can occur for cohort studies, and readers need to be cognizant of these potential biases when assessing the quality of studies. Selection bias could occur if the exposed or unexpected subjects were identified in a manner or through a factor that is also connected to the outcome of interest. Not taking into consideration confounding could also lead to biased results. A confounder is a factor associated with exposure of interest and possibly also a cause of the outcome of interest. Finally, information bias also known as measurement bias occurs with inaccurate measurement of key study variables. Measurement bias can lead to misclassification. For example, an unexposed could be classified as exposed or vice versa. If the error is random, then the misclassification is random and should not affect the interpretation of the data. If the error is non-random, this may bias the study results.

Clinical Vignette

You receive a letter from a patient's lawyer informing you that your patient, a 56-year-old man who was recently diagnosed with hepatocellular carcinoma (HCC), is suing his employer, a manufacturer of polyvinyl chloride (PVC) pipes. The patient is worried that his exposure to vinyl chloride, an organochloride used to make the PVC pipes, caused his illness and his lawyer contacts you for more information about the link between vinyl chloride and HCC. You are aware that angiosarcomas are associated with vinyl chloride, but are unsure of the association between vinyl chloride and HCC. You find two cohort studies, but they have slightly conflicting conclusions. In Ward *et al.*'s publication based on 12,700 European men with occupational vinyl chloride exposures followed for 8 years, the authors described an exposure-response trend between duration of exposure and the 10 verified cases of HCC that occurred within their cohort during the study period [9]. A US study by Mundt *et al.* followed 10,109 men with occupational vinyl exposures for at least 1 year between 1942 and 1972 and found a link between vinyl chloride and excess mortality risk from cancer of the liver and biliary tract, but this link seemed mostly to be driven by angiosarcoma and they were unable to draw conclusions about a link between vinyl chloride and HCC [10]. You have a difficult time deciding how to compare the data from these studies as each used a different cohort, a different end-point, and you are concerned that there could have been misclassification of HCC and angioscarcomas in the American study.

Upon further searching, you find a meta-analysis by Boffetta et al. that evaluated both Ward *et al.* and Mundt *et al.* in addition to six other studies [11]. The authors of the meta-analysis used random-effects models in cases that lacked heterogeneity and concluded that there was an increased meta-standardized mortality ratio (SMR) for both angiosarcoma and HCC. Based on these data, you decide that there likely is enough evidence to argue that your patient's occupational exposure contributed to his cancer.

References

1. Szumilas M. Explaining odds ratios. J Can Acad Child Adolesc Psychiatry. 2010;19:227–9.
2. Szklo M, Nieto J. Epidemiology: beyond the basics. Burlington, MA: Jones and Bartlett Learning; 2007.
3. Rose S, Laan MJ. Why match? Investigating matched case-control study designs with causal effect estimation. Int J Biostat. 2009;5:1.
4. de Vos M, De Vroey B, Garcia BG, Roy C, Kidd F, Henrion J, Deltenre P. Role of proton pump inhibitors in the occurrence and the prognosis of spontaneous bacterial peritonitis in cirrhotic patients with ascites. Liver Int. 2013;33:1316–23.
5. Goel GA, Deshpande A, Lopez R, Hall GS, van Duin D, Carey WD. Increased rate of spontaneous bacterial peritonitis among cirrhotic patients receiving pharmacologic acid suppression. Clin Gastroenterol Hepatol. 2012;10:422–7.
6. Choi EJ, Lee HJ, Kim KO, Lee SH, Eun JR, Jang BI, Kim TN. Association between acid suppressive therapy and spontaneous bacterial peritonitis in cirrhotic patients with ascites. Scand J Gastroenterol. 2011;46:616–20.
7. Ratelle M, Perreault S, Villeneuve JP, Tremblay L. Association between proton pump inhibitor use and spontaneous bacterial peritonitis in cirrhotic patients with ascites. Can J Gastroenterol Hepatol. 2014;28:330–4.
8. Thursz MR, Forrest EH, Ryder S, investigators S. Prednisolone or pentoxifylline for alcoholic hepatitis. N Engl J Med. 2015;373:282–3.
9. Ward E, Boffetta P, Andersen A, Colin D, Comba P, Deddens JA, De Santis M, et al. Update of the follow-up of mortality and cancer incidence among European workers employed in the vinyl chloride industry. Epidemiology. 2001;12:710–8.
10. Mundt KA, Dell LD, Austin RP, Luippold RS, Noess R, Bigelow C. Historical cohort study of 10 109 men in the North American vinyl chloride industry, 1942–72: update of cancer mortality to 31 December 1995. Occup Environ Med. 2000;57:774–81.
11. Boffetta P, Matisane L, Mundt KA, Dell LD. Meta-analysis of studies of occupational exposure to vinyl chloride in relation to cancer mortality. Scand J Work Environ Health. 2003;29:220–9.

3 Understanding the Interpretation of Disease Incidence and Prevalence

Ehsan Chitsaz and Sheila Kumar

Abstract

One of the main goals in epidemiology is to describe the disease of interest, quantify the frequency of the disease, and study the risk factors and potential causes of the disease. "Measures of occurrence," which are used to describe frequency of diseases, are the descriptive values in clinical epidemiology that describe events or outcomes, such as mortality or morbidity. Two of the main measures of occurrence that are used in the field of epidemiology are "incidence" and "prevalence." These types of measures of occurrence are used in different ways by experts from various backgrounds. Clinicians can use incidence and prevalence in direct patient care to describe the frequency of a disease of interest, to help predict the course of a patient, and to estimate an individual's risk for a disease and its complications. Public health professionals can use incidence and prevalence to describe the conditions and burden of a disease of interest, to identify the areas/conditions/disease where resources should be directed, and to compare between patients, subgroups of population, and finally, health care systems. Finally, researchers can use incidence and prevalence to compare diseases and define clinical outcomes in studies. In this chapter, we will discuss the basics of incidence and prevalence, which are essential to the comprehension and interpretation of different indices of disease frequency.

Keywords

Incidence · Prevalence · Frequency data · Measures of occurrence

---

E. Chitsaz · S. Kumar (✉)
Digestive Diseases Branch, National Institutes of Diabetes and Digestive and Kidney Diseases, National Institutes of Health, Bethesda, MD, USA
e-mail: sheila.kumar@nih.gov

R. J. Wong, R. G. Gish (eds.), *Clinical Epidemiology of Chronic Liver Diseases*,
https://doi.org/10.1007/978-3-319-94355-8_3

3.1 Frequency Data

The ability to describe frequencies and rate of disease states is integral to the understanding of epidemiology. We will begin with frequency data, which is generally expressed as one of two major forms: "Count" and "Ratio". "Ratio" can further be subdivided to include "Proportion" and "Rate". These variables will help us to eventually understand incidence and prevalence.

Count: The crude number of individuals or subjects who meet the case definition.

Example: There are currently 4,200 patients with the diagnosis of colon cancer in the state of Maryland.

Thus, a "count" refers to a numeric value that describes the number of individuals with the disease, or condition, of interest. This way to measure frequency data has implications in terms of assessment of individual cases within a community/population, which may ultimately have implications in such public health measure as resource allocation. However, a count does not provide any information about the occurrence of cases in relation to the size of total population. This is where "ratio," "proportion," and "rate" are of use.

Ratio: The fraction of one entity (the numerator- which generally represents individuals with the disease of interest) relative to another entity (the denominator).

Example: There are 2.7 cases of colon cancer for every 1 gastroenterologist.

Thus, a "ratio" describes the relationship of the numerator to the denominator, and be subdivided into "proportions" and "ratios," where the denominator comprises either the total population or is a function of time, respectively. Of note, as seen in the example above, the numerator and denominator in a ratio do not have to have the same units of expression.

Proportion: A type of ratio where the numerator (individuals with the disease of interest) is a subgroup of the denominator; thus, the two values have similar units.

Example: Of all adults undergoing screening colonoscopy, 20% are found to have polyps.

It is important here to pay attention to the specific qualities of the proportion. The numerator identifies the number of cases and is a subgroup of the denominator. The denominator identifies the total population—both the individual cases, as well as those who do not meet the case definition. Therefore, by definition, the numerator and denominator must have similar units.

Rate: A type of ratio where time is expressed, or implied, in the denominator and the numerator again expressed the number of individual cases. Therefore, rate essentially describes the rapidity of change in the number of cases over time.

Example: There are 135,430 of new cases of colon cancer per year (2016).

Understanding these four measures of frequency data is central to understanding "incidence" and "prevalence." Refer to Table 3.1 for characteristics of these measures.

Table 3.1 Frequency data

Measure	Description	Numerical expression	Example	Epidemiology indices
Count	Number of occurrences	A	Number of patients with colorectal cancer in a given community	Frequency
Ratio	Fraction of two values (may not have similar units)	A/B	Number of patients with colorectal cancer relative to the number of gastroenterologists	Incidence odds, prevalence odds
Proportion	A type of ratio where numerator is always a part of the denominator	A/A + B	Number of new diagnoses of colorectal cancer among total number of colonoscopies	Cumulative incidence, point prevalence
Rate	A type of ratio where denominator implies time	A/time	Number of new diagnosis of colon cancer per year	Incidence density, period prevalence

3.2 Incidence

"Incidence" describes the number of new individuals who meet the case definition (for example, the disease of interest), within a defined period, among the total at-risk population. In other words, the numerator is the incident (or new) cases that occur during the observation period. The denominator includes the at-risk population, and hence excludes both those individuals who already have the diagnosis (and by this virtue, cannot develop the condition), as well as individuals who are incapable of experiencing the disease due to biologic reasons. For example, men cannot develop ovarian cancer and thus would be excluded from the at-risk population in a study for incidence of ovarian cancer.

Incidence is calculated as the number of new cases of condition X, divided by the total number of individuals in the population who are at risk for condition X.

Incidence may be further subdivided into three measures: cumulative incidence (or incidence proportion), incidence density (or incidence rate), and incidence odds.

3.2.1 Cumulative Incidence (Incidence Proportion)

The most commonly used approach to estimate incidence is the "cumulative incidence." In this measure, the population of interest is fixed in size. In other words, each new case enters the study at the same time, and subsequently, each individual is followed for the entire observation period. The numerator thus comprises any new cases accumulated throughout the entire study period, while the denominator encompasses all at-risk individuals within the target population throughout the entire study period. Since the numerator is a subset of the denominator, and thus qualifies as a proportion, the cumulative incidence is also called the incidence proportion.

$$\text{Cumulative incidence (or incidence proportion)} \\ = \frac{\#\,\text{new cases during entire study period}}{\text{total at-risk population at beginning of study period}}$$

3.2.2 Incidence Density (Incidence Rate)

In "incidence density," the population is again fixed in size, and each new case enters the study at the same time, similar to what is seen when using the cumulative incidence. However, each individual is not observed for equal amounts of time. Thus, each individual case will contribute in a manner that is relative to the time they have been observed. This is most useful in studies when the population is ever-changing. The numerator remains the number of new cases during the observation period. However the denominator is the time each individual was observed, totaled for all individuals—also called person-time. Since the denominator is a function of time, incidence density is also called "incidence rate".

$$\text{Incidence density (or incidence rate)} = \frac{\#\,\text{new cases during entire study period}}{\text{total person-time}}$$

Of note, it can be difficult to actually measure person-time. Say one individual develops the disease of interest after 5 years, such that they would contribute 4.5 person-years to the denominator (it is generally assumed that a disease-free individual who then develops the disease contributes half of the last time period used when still disease-free), while another individual remained disease free for 10 years and would thus contribute 10 person-years to the denominator. These two individuals would thus contribute a total of 14.5 person-years to the denominator. As one can imagine, this calculation can be fairly tedious when doing large clinical studies.

Another caveat to be aware of, when using incidence density, is the assumption, inherent to this measure, that the probability of developing the disease remains constant over the study period- this may not be true for diseases that become more common with age.

3.2.3 Incidence Odds

"Incidence odds" is a less commonly used incidence measure. Here, the numerator again is the number of new cases during the observation period. However, the denominator in this measure is the number of individuals who do not develop the disease during that period.

$$\text{Incidence odds} = \frac{\#\,\text{new cases of disease during entire study period}}{\#\,\text{disease-free individuals at the start of the study period}}$$

Of note, the incidence odds approximate the cumulative incidence if the event rate is low. For example, let's say that among 1000 patients undergoing screening colonoscopy in the month of June, 10 patients developed a delayed post-polypectomy bleed. The incidence odds of delayed post-polypectomy bleed in the month of June would be 10/(1000 – 10), or 0.0101. Meanwhile, the cumulative incidence would be 10/1000 = 0.0100. Conversely, cumulative incidence and incidence odds begin to diverge when the event rate is high. For example, if 400 patients out of 1000 developed a delayed post-polypectomy bleed after undergoing screening colonoscopy in the month of June, the incidence odds would be 400/(1000 – 400), or 0.67, whereas the cumulative incidence would be 400/1000, or 0.40.

3.3 Prevalence

"Prevalence" refers to the total number of individuals who meet the case definition at any given point in time, during the study period, among the at-risk total population. Thus, in contrast to incidence, where only new cases are of interest, prevalence counts both new and existing cases in the numerator. Please refer to Table 3.2.

Prevalence is calculated as the number of new and existing cases of condition X, divided by the total number of individuals in the population who are at risk for condition X.

Prevalence may also be further subdivided into three measures: point prevalence, period prevalence, and prevalence odds.

3.3.1 Point Prevalence

"Point prevalence" represents the prevalence of the disease in a "snapshot" of a population at a specific time point, and is the most common use of prevalence. The numerator in this measure is the number of cases at a specific time point (both existing and new), while the denominator is the total population at that same point in time. Because the numerator is a subset of denominator, point prevalence is a proportion.

Table 3.2 Incidence versus prevalence

	Incidence	Prevalence
Numerator	New cases identified during a given time period	All cases (i.e., existing and new) in a population during a given time period
Denominator	*At-risk* population	*At-risk* population

$$\text{Point prevalence} = \frac{\#\,\text{cases of disease}\left(\text{new and existing}\right)\text{at a specific time-point}}{\#\,\text{total population at the same specific time-point}}$$

3.3.2 Period Prevalence

While point prevalence describes the prevalence at a single point in time, "period prevalence" refers to prevalence within a defined period. Period prevalence refers to the number of cases (both existing and new) at any point of time from the beginning of the defined period until the end of the period. In other words, period prevalence counts both cases that existed at the onset of the study period, as well as any new cases that developed at any time throughout the study period. Again, since the numerator is a subset of denominator, point prevalence is a proportion.

$$\text{Period prevalence} = \frac{\#\,\text{cases of disease}\left(\text{new and existing}\right)\text{during a specific time period}}{\#\,\text{total population during the same time period}}$$

Although point prevalence is more generally reported, period prevalence can be useful, since it can be thought of as the sum of point prevalence when measured at the onset of the observation period, plus the cumulative incidence of disease during the defined observation period. Thus, this measure can be useful when looking at the life-time prevalence of a condition.

3.3.3 Prevalence Odds

"Prevalence odds" refers to the ratio of the number of individuals with the disease (existing and new cases) at a specific time point, in relation to the individuals who do not have that disease at that specified time point.

$$\text{Prevalence odds} = \frac{\#\,\text{all cases of disease at a specific time-point}}{\#\,\text{disease-free individuals at that specific time-point}}$$

3.4 The Relationship Between Incidence and Prevalence

Although incidence and prevalence are two different measures of occurrence, they do have an inherent relationship. Incidence represents "new" cases diagnosed within an observation period, while prevalence represents total number of cases ("existing" and "new") observed at a point in time or over a period of time. Thus, prevalence can be thought of as a "pool," where the subjects with the disease at any given instant are in the pool, including both "old" and "new" cases. New cases are constantly entering the pool- the rate at which this occurs is represented by incidence. Meanwhile, the time that cases spend in the "pool" prior to leaving is reflected in the "duration of the disease," which is directly dependent on the biological nature of the disease/ natural history, likelihood of cure/recovery time, and the morbidity of the disease. In a steady state (where incidence is fairly constant), the relationship between prevalence and incidence can be expressed thusly:

$$\text{Prevalence} = \text{Incidence} \times \text{Duration of Disease}$$

Thus, duration of disease will affect how much time each case spends in the "pool," and whether incidence or prevalence is affected. For example, numerous chronic conditions have a long duration of disease- patients live several decades after diagnosis, there are no definitive cures, and morbidity is low. An example of this type of disease would be osteoarthritis. Therefore, most patients with osteoarthritis will remain in the "pool", and while the incidence may be low because there are not many "new" cases, the existing cases will continue to contribute to the prevalence.

Another way of looking at this relationship is that high prevalence may indicate high incidence or long duration of disease, whereas low prevalence may indicate low incidence or short duration of disease, whether this is because a cure exists or because there is high morbidity and mortality from the disease.

3.5 Reporting Incidence and Prevalence

Thus far, we have discussed how to calculate and interpret incidence and prevalence. Like any other statistical measures, incidence and prevalence provide the "point estimate" of the measure. In reality, incidence and prevalence are usually determined in a study population which is a sample of the entire population. Since the study population is subject to sampling error, where it may not entirely represent or resemble the general population, it is important to report "interval estimates" in addition to "point estimates". Therefore, incidence and prevalence are usually reported as their point estimates as well as the confidence interval.

References

1. Coggon D, et al. Epidemiology for the uninitiated. New York: John Wiley & Sons; 2009.
2. Fletcher R, et al. Clinical epidemiology. The essentials. Baltimore, MD: Victor Graphics Inc.; 1996.
3. Gertsman BB. Epidemiology kept simple. An introduction to traditional and modern epidemiology. Hoboken, NJ: Wiley-Liss; 2003.
4. Gordis L. Epidemiology, vol. 308. New York, NY: WB Saunders Company, A Harcourt Health Sciences Company; 2009. p. 6.
5. Oleckno WA. Epidemiology: concepts and methods. Long Grove, IL: Waveland Press; 2008.
6. Wassertheil-Smoller S. Biostatistics and epidemiology. New York: Springer; 2003.

Understanding Survival Analyses

4

Somasundaram Subramaniam

Keywords
Survival analysis · Overall survival · Censoring · Kaplan–Meier survival estimate · Cox proportional hazards · Log-rank test

4.1 Introduction

4.1.1 What is Survival Analysis?

Survival analysis uses statistical methods to calculate and describe the "time-to" occurrence of a particular event. These techniques are widely employed in medical and epidemiological studies. As the term survival analysis indicates, the time-to-event of interest is often death, but these methods are frequently used to analyse other intervals, like time-to relapse of a disease or time-to recurrence of a cancer.

The usual statistical methods cannot be used in time-to-event analysis because not all events may have occurred by the time that the data is being analysed. In order to overcome this issue, *censored observations* are used in survival analysis. Furthermore, the occurrence of events does not follow a normal distribution. These unique features of survival analysis require specialized techniques.

There are some similarities in methods used in survival analysis and in standard statistics to compare survival times in two or more groups and to account for the presence of other variables (continuous, binary or categorical) such as age, disease stage (TNM group), etc. Regression models can be applied to account for the impact of some of these variables by calculating the hazard function.

S. Subramaniam
Swedish Cancer Institute, Seattle, WA, USA
e-mail: Somasundaram.Subramaniam@swedish.org

R. J. Wong, R. G. Gish (eds.), *Clinical Epidemiology of Chronic Liver Diseases*,
https://doi.org/10.1007/978-3-319-94355-8_4

Survival analyses techniques which will be discussed include survival curves, hazard function, Kaplan–Meier estimators [1], and Cox proportional hazards calculations [2].

4.1.2 Why Measure Survival Analysis?

Survival analysis is the basis on which treatments are recommended, compared against each other, and approved by regulatory agencies. Thus, it is extraordinarily useful in the practice of clinical medicine.

Survival analysis is widely used in epidemiological studies to measure the impact of a certain intervention on the long-term outcomes of the study population. Survival analysis is employed in almost all Phase III and most Phase II clinical trials to provide information about the efficacy of the medication, device or procedure being studied.

Survival data, which include censored time points, provides investigators with objective information which can be used to guide treatment and policy decisions. For example, the finding that sorafenib extends median survival in patients with hepatocellular carcinoma, led to the drug being approved for treatment by the Food and Drug Administration in the United States and European Medicines Agency in Europe.

Similarly, when physicians recommend medications, they rely heavily on survival analytics from clinical trials to determine a medication's efficacy for the patient population being treated. This information helps inform patients about their prognosis, likelihood of response, and duration of benefit.

4.2 Basics and Definitions

4.2.1 Censoring

Censoring is a process to account for the subjects who have not yet experienced the event of interest, and those who have dropped out of the study for other reasons [3]. The survival time for a censored subject is assumed to be at least as long as the time of the last observation.

If all subjects in a clinical trial experience the event of interest, then there are no censored observations. Investigators can calculate exact survival time for each patient. However, in clinical trials, it is unusual that complete survival times will be available when the analysis is being carried out because subjects may not have experienced the outcome of interest or may be lost to follow-up and the occurrence of the event of interest is therefore unknown.

For example, studies commonly report survival data at arbitrarily chosen time points, like 5 years from enrolment of the subjects. Some subjects may have died over the 5 years and their survival can be calculated exactly; other subjects may still be alive at 5 years so the actual duration of survival for this group is unknown – it is only known that they have survived at least 5 years. Similarly if a subject is lost-to-follow up before 5 years, it is unknown to the investigator if the subject is still alive or if they died after being lost to follow-up. To overcome this missing data, the subject is censored at the time of the last visit as that is the last time point in which it is certain that the subject was alive. In summary, censoring is used to overcome the challenge of unknown survival times for a subset of the study group.

4.2.2 Distribution of Survival Data

Standard statistical tests, like Student's *t*-tests or analysis of variance (ANOVA), which compare observations, rely on an underlying normal (or bell-shaped) distribution of events. Time-to-event distributions, however, do not follow a predictable pattern and often have a skewed distribution. Therefore, standard statistical tests cannot be applied to survival data.

4.2.3 Survival Probability and Hazard Function

In survival analysis, the concept of survival probability is helpful in gauging the utility of an intervention. S*urvival probability (or survival function)* is the likelihood of surviving a certain period of time. This probability is easily displayed on a survival curve.

The *hazard function* is a related probability that quantifies the likelihood of the event of interest taking place at a particular point in time. The hazard function captures the incident event rate.

4.2.4 Univariate Vs. Multivariate Models

The univariate approach in survival analysis means that we study an impact of only one variable at a time, for example, treatment, on the survival time. The typical approach here is to perform a Kaplan–Meier estimate and use the log-rank test to compare groups, for example those who were treated with new drug vs. those who were treated with a placebo.

Multivariate approach requires regression modelling to account for, as the name suggests, multiple variables. The most common technique for this purpose is the Cox proportional hazards model. Multivariate models allow for incorporation of additional relevant variables to estimate the impact of this on the primary variable being studied [4]. For example, in a clinical study examining survival after an intervention, covariates may include age, stage of disease and baseline health characteristics.

4.2.5 Collecting the Data

To apply these survival analysis statistical tools, in addition to the usual descriptive patient data, relevant time points need to be collected. For each patient, the typical time points required are the time from which survival time is calculated, for example, the time of first diagnosis or time at enrolment into a study, and, the date of the event of interest if such an event occurred (the date of death for example). If the event of interest did not occur, the date of the last observation (for example, last appointment) would be used. For each patient, survival time is computed using the starting date and the ending date, and a binary variable is assigned to denote the occurrence of an event (1) or censored observation (0).

Additionally, other patient and disease factors, which do not change with time, are also gathered such as age at the beginning of the study, gender, type of therapy, co-morbidities, etc. It is important to note that the accuracy of the analysis depends on the data available at the time of analysis, specifically with regards to censored data. For accurate survival analysis, updated data is required.

4.3 Methods

4.3.1 Kaplan–Meier Estimator

The most widely used tool to estimate the survival probabilities is the *Kaplan–Meier* estimator. Kaplan–Meier is a statistical measure that helps deal with censoring observations and estimate survival probabilities.

Its usage is usually illustrated via *survival curve* (Fig. 4.1).

The survival curves are the step functions and they illustrate probability of surviving a specific period of time. Each step symbolizes the occurrence of an event. From a survival curve plot we can estimate the median survival and also the

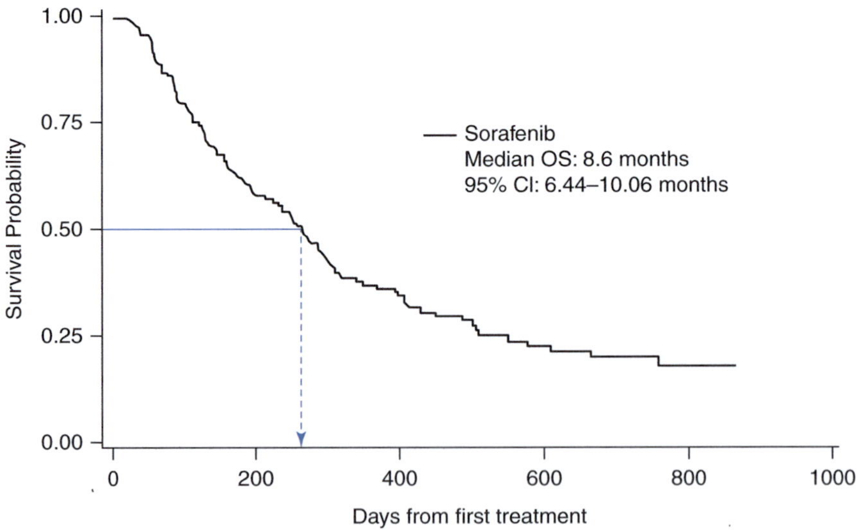

Fig. 4.1 Survival curve evaluating overall survival in patients treated with sorafenib [5]

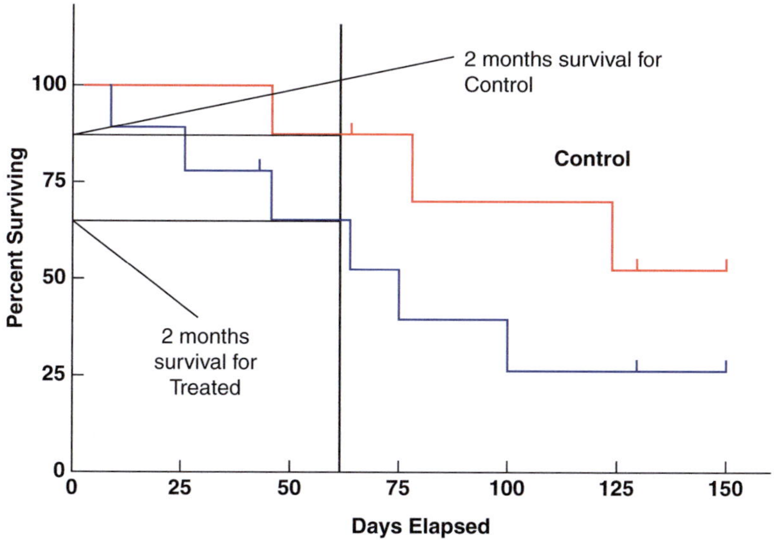

Fig. 4.2 Hypothetical example of survival analysis comparing treated patients and control patients

probability of surviving a specific period of time. For example, from the curve above we can observe that the median overall survival (survival for the 50th percentile of patients) is 258 days (8.6 months) (Fig. 4.1).

In this second hypothetical example (Fig. 4.2), vertical markings on the survival lines denote the censored observations. From a survival curve plot we can estimate probability of surviving a specific period for a specific group. In the above graph, the 2-months survival probability for the Control group (red line) is 80% whereas for the Treated group (blue line) it is only 70% (Fig. 4.2).

4.3.2 Log-Rank Test

The log-rank test is a widely-used method to compare survival curves in order to determine if the differences between the curves are due to chance alone or if there is a real difference in outcomes. This helps to decide if results can be generalized for the population at large.

The log-rank test compares the expected and observed differences between curves with the null hypothesis that there is no difference between the curves. The log-rank test statistic is compared against a chi-square distribution table. Thus, a *p*-value can be calculated to determine if there is a statistical difference between the survival curves. However, the *p*-value does not provide information on the actual size of the effect, only its statistical significance.

It may be necessary to compare more than two survival curves at a time. In this situation, a log-rank test reports the overall comparison results, meaning that if the *p*-value is less than 0.05, it is not implied that all curves are significantly different from each other. Therefore, pairwise comparisons should be carried out for each pair of survival curves. A stratified log-rank test can be used to account for baseline differences in risk between different strata, or groups. Each stratum must be defined by a categorical variable, for example, gender or stage of disease.

4.3.3 Life Tables

Life tables, also known as actuarial tables, are used in reporting on very large samples, such as those in population studies. This allows the specific survival times to be read quickly and exactly.

4.3.4 Cox Model

The limitation of the log-rank test or any other test comparing the survival curves is the fact that it can be applied only to compare rather small number of survival curves. A large number of survival curves would require an unwieldy number of pair wise comparisons. Also, there may be a preference to classify certain variables, like age, as a continuous variable in order to examine the impact on survival time. For these situations, a multivariate statistical model can be employed.

The Cox proportional hazards model is the most popular survival model and is similar to multivariate regression models as it contains response variables and continuous or categorical predictors [6]. The Cox survival model actually graphs the hazard function. This function describes the number of events per unit time, or the risk of an event occurring. An important feature of the model is the *baseline hazard function,* which is the hazard when all covariates equal zero. Another notable feature of a Cox model is that it is not a linear function with respect to time, which means that the hazard function can, and probably will, change over time.

A great advantage of a Cox model is that the baseline hazard function does not need to be specified and any continuous or categorical covariates can be included in the model as predictors. These covariates have to be time-fixed, gathered before the starting date of the follow-up. Cox models produce a *hazard ratio (HR)* for each variable. This is a ratio of the two hazards (two risks of events), for the two patients having different characteristics. Therefore, the model cannot estimate a specific risk of an event occurring for a patient with a given characteristics, such as age, tumor stage, etc.; it can only estimate which risk is higher or lower for the two patients. Therefore, the model states how the risk of an event occurring changes if we change one predictor while keeping the other predictors fixed. A hazard ratio of 1 indicates an equal chance of an event occurring; a HR of greater than 1 suggests that the risk of an event (for example, death) is more likely and a HR of less than 1 suggests an event is less likely to occur.

4.3.5 Cox Model Assumptions

Before applying a Cox model, it is important to be aware of some assumptions underlying the model. Firstly, it is assumed that the censoring mechanism should not be related to the event occurrence, which is known as *non-informative censoring*. For example, the continuation of follow-up is not dependent on a patient's condition. The second assumption is the proportionality of hazards, which states that the survival curves for two examined groups should have hazard functions that are proportional over time. The Cox model is sometimes referred to as *Cox Proportional Hazards Model* (Cox PH model).

References

1. Kaplan EL, Meier P. Nonparametric estimation from incomplete observations. J Am Stat Assoc. 1958;53:457–81.
2. Cox DR, Oakes D. Analysis of survival data. Monographs on statistics and applied probability. London/New York: Chapman and Hall; 1984.
3. Clark TG, Bradburn MJ, Love SB, et al. Survival analysis part I: basic concepts and first analyses. Br J Cancer. 2003;89:232–8.
4. Bradburn MJ, Clark TG, Love SB, et al. Survival analysis part II: multivariate data analysis—an introduction to concepts and methods. Br J Cancer. 2003;89:431–6.
5. Lin SM, Lu SN, Chen PT, et al. HATT: a phase IV, single-arm, open-label study of sorafenib in Taiwanese patients with advanced hepatocellular carcinoma. Hepatol Int. 2017;11:199–208.
6. Vittinghoff E. Regression methods in biostatistics: linear, logistic, survival, and repeated measures models. 2nd ed. Statistics for biology and health. New York: Springer; 2012.

Global Epidemiology of Chronic Liver Disease

5

Nimzing Gwamzhi Ladep, Sheikh Mohammad Fazle Akbar, and Mamun Al Mahtab

Abstract

This chapter provides a global summary of the epidemiology of chronic liver disease. The synopsis presented here regards the pattern of chronic liver disease in sub-Saharan Africa, Asia, Europe and Latin America.

Electronic search engines were employed and papers published in the English language were reviewed during the write up process. The search words included: "rates" AND "prevalence" AND "epidemiology" AND "liver diseases" OR "HBV" OR "HCV". Data were summarised in maps and tables for ease of understanding and landmark papers used during the review process were highlighted in a table.

Whereas alcohol is the most important factor associated with chronic liver disease in most developed industrialised countries of the world, viral hepatitis B (HBV) is the most common factor in sub-Saharan Africa and Asia. Eastern European countries have recorded high rates of HBV infection as well. Of the viral factors, hepatitis C virus (HCV) is the most common cause of chronic liver

N. G. Ladep (✉)
Arrowe Park Hospital, Wirral University Teaching Hospital NHS Foundation Trust, Upton, UK

Imperial College London, London, UK

Jos University Teaching Hospital, Jos, Nigeria

University of Jos, Jos, Nigeria
e-mail: n.ladep@imperial.ac.uk

S. M. F. Akbar
Toshiba General Hospital, Higashi Oi 6-3-22, Shinagawa, Tokyo, Japan
e-mail: sheikh.akbar@toshiba.co.jp

M. Al Mahtab
Department of Hepatology, Bangabandhu Sheikh Mujib Medical University, Shanbagh, Dhaka, Bangladesh
e-mail: shwapnil@agni.com

R. J. Wong, R. G. Gish (eds.), *Clinical Epidemiology of Chronic Liver Diseases*,
https://doi.org/10.1007/978-3-319-94355-8_5

disease in Europe, although, the prevalence of HCV in some developing countries have been recorded to be higher than obtainable in Europe. Non-alcoholic fatty liver disease is increasingly being implicated as the cause of chronic liver disease in all regions of the world.

5.1 Introduction

The definition and other aspects of chronic liver disease have been elaborated elsewhere in this book. Indeed, chronic liver disease is a spectrum and constitutes several entities; from inflammation caused by infections by viruses, lasting for about six or more months and culminating in complications, such as cirrhosis and hepatocellular carcinoma. Owing to socioeconomic, genetic as well as environmental factors, the epidemiology of the chronic liver disease is variable across different regions of the world. We shall discuss in broad terms, the global epidemiology of chronic liver disease by regions.

5.2 Chronic Liver Disease in Africa

5.2.1 Epidemiology of Chronic HCV Infection in Africa

The prevalence of hepatitis C in Africa is estimated at between 2.5% and 9.9%. As history of intravenous drug use (IDU) is not routinely volunteered by patients in Africa owing to stigmatisation, the contribution of IDU in the transmission of HCV is largely unknown. Most cases of HCV are thought to have been acquired via receipt of unscreened blood products and use of unsterile needles/syringes [1].

The distribution of HCV infection in Africa varies by regions. Central and West African regions have the highest prevalence of HCV infection. Southern and East African countries have relatively lower rates of HCV infection (Fig. 5.1).

5.2.2 Epidemiology of Chronic HBV Infection in Africa

Chronic hepatitis B infection rate in Africa, as determined by HBsAg is approximately 8–20%. Most HBV transmission in Africa is postulated to be via the horizontal route—occurring largely in early childhood. About 80% of people with chronic HBV in Africa are presumed to have become infected by the age of 10. Studies of the prevalence of HBV in Africa have so far been mostly cross-sectional, with data primarily drawn from blood donors (Table 5.1). These studies observed rates of HBV infection ranging between 1% and 22% in blood donors.

Population surveys observed 4.4% and 17.6% HBV rates in African countries. Whereas West Africa has the highest prevalence of HBV, regions of Central and southern Africa have relatively lower rates of HBV infection. Apart from a single

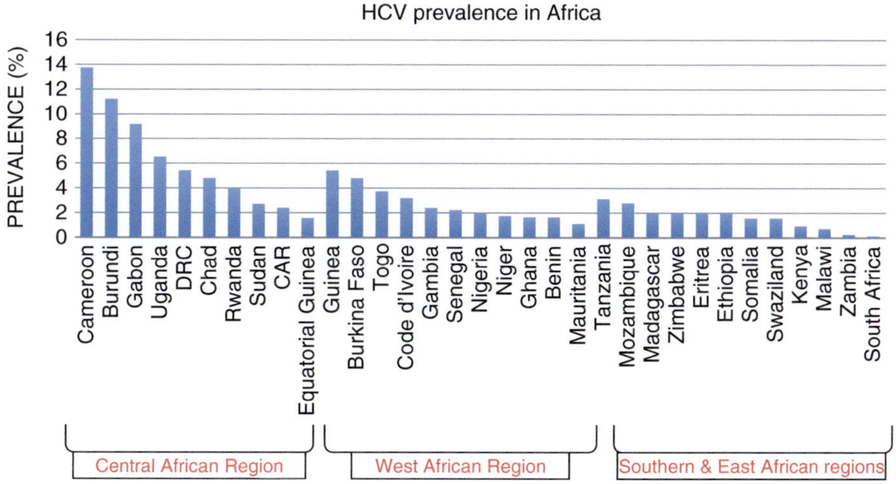

Fig. 5.1 Prevalence of hepatitis C infection by countries displayed by region of African countries

Table 5.1 Prevalence of hepatitis B viral infection by countries in sub-Saharan countries

Country	Setting	Sample size	Prevalence/ rate (%)	Year of study
Ghana [3]	Systematic review	105,435	12.3	2016
Southwest Nigeria [4]	Cross-sectional	130	10	2015
Rwanda [5]	HCW cross-sectional	378	2.9	2015
Southwest Ethiopia [2]	CLD retrospective records	578	22.3	2014
Northern Uganda [6]	Population survey	790	17.6	2013
Democratic Republic of Congo [7]	Blood donors	3292	3.7	2013
Angola	Cross-sectional	431	9.3	2013
Cameroon [8]	Blood donors	543	10.1	2013
Kenya [9]	Cross-sectional	100	3.0	2012
South Sudan [10]	Blood donors	400 men	6.25	2009
Southwestern Nigeria [11]	Blood donors	33,682	13.2	2008
Mozambique	Blood donors	1578	1.0	2007
Kenya [12]	Cross-sectional pregnant women	2241	9.3	2006
Uganda [13]	Cross-sectional (medical students)	182	11.0	2005
Ethiopia [14]	Population survey	4736	7.0	2003
Northcentral Nigeria [15]	Cross-sectional	524	10.3	2002
South Africa [16]	Population survey	400	6.8	1995
Tanzania [17]	Population survey	1004	4.4	1994
Northwest Nigeria [18]	Blood donors/pregnant women	287/224	22.0/11.6	1994
Namibia [19]	Children	248	7.3	1994

study from Northern Uganda, in which was found a prevalence of 17.6%, East African populations have an intermediate rate of HBV infection. Studies of the contribution of HBV to chronic liver disease found that HBsAg was positive in 22.3% in 578 patients in Ethiopia [2].

5.2.3 Epidemiology of Alcoholic Liver Disease in Africa

Alcohol consumption in Africa is often viewed as antisocial behaviour and patients tend to under report the amount of alcohol consumed. Moreover, a large proportion of the locally brewed fermented drinks have unknown quantity of ethanol and therefore in some cases, even small amounts may portend significant damage to the liver. Additionally, the containers in which these beverages are brewed are postulated to release excess iron leading to higher than normal values (iron overload syndromes)—further damaging the already inflamed liver.

There is paucity of data from Africa specifically implicating alcohol as the sole aetiologic agent for chronic liver disease in patients from this region. A study from Uganda in 2013 used the "CAGE" symptoms to attribute alcohol as the cause of liver disease in 46.8% of 380 chronic liver disease patients. Of those, only 10% had cirrhosis of the liver, most of who were men [20]. Ndububa et al. reported the fact that 35.2% of a sample population of 145 Nigerian patients being managed for chronic liver disease drank alcohol "significantly" [21]. Another study in a different geographical region on Nigeria (West Africa), dedicated to studying 51 patients with cirrhosis observed that 76% of the patients had reported significant alcohol consumption [22]. The criterion used in the definition of significant was, however, not clearly defined in the research methods of these studies from Nigeria.

5.2.3.1 Epidemiology of Non-Alcoholic Fatty Liver Disease in Africa

There are not many data exploring the burden of non-alcoholic fatty liver disease (NAFLD) in sub-Saharan Africa. Four studies carried out in three countries, including South Africa, Sudan and Nigeria have documented the fact that NAFLD is not a rare problem in Africa. The studies were done between 2010 and 2015, all in hospital settings. In Sudan, NAFLD was found to be present in 50.3% of 167 patients with type 2 diabetes mellitus [23]. Earlier, the same authors had reported NAFLD in 20% of 100 relatives of patients accompanying them to hospital in Sudan [24].

In South Africa, 111 (47.6%) of 233 patients were found to have NAFLD by ultrasound (US); 36% of who had nonalcoholic steatohepatitis, while 17% had advanced cirrhosis. The rate of NAFLD was rather low in a single hospital-based study from Southwest Nigeria. Onyekwere et al. reported 8.7% and 4.5% rates of NAFLD in diabetics and non-diabetics respectively, in a hospital sample of 150 persons [25].

Population-based studies would best provide the optimal estimate of the true representation of this global problem in the African setting. Infrastructural challenges as well as personnel would however pose a real challenge in this regard in the foreseeable period.

5.3 Epidemiology of Chronic Liver Disease in Asia

5.3.1 Epidemiology of Chronic HBV and HCV in Asia

The two major hepatotrophic viruses causing chronic liver disease, HBV and HCV, are highly prevalent in most Asian countries. It is assumed that about 240–370 million people of the world are chronically infected with HBV [26] and about 150 million people are infected with the HCV [27]. Considerable numbers of both chronic HBV and HCV infected persons live in Asian countries and they exhibit a wide spectrum of chronic liver diseases, such as chronic hepatitis B (CHB) and chronic hepatitis C (CHC), cirrhosis of liver (LC), and hepatocellular carcinoma (HCC). HBV infection is assessed by the presence of hepatitis B surface antigen (HBsAg) in the sera, however, several other virological, immunological and biochemical parameters are checked for assessing the state of pathological conditions of these patients. On the other hand, HCV infection can be confirmed by presence of anti-HCV antibodies as well as by HCV RNA and evaluation of other parameters allow assessing the nature and state of liver diseases. In spite of above mentioned pathological features, chronic HBV and HCV infection may have an uneventful course. In particular, chronic HBV infection passes through various phases of pathological processes in which the extent and nature of liver diseases remain mainly elusive.

In the context of epidemiology of HBV in Asian countries, the prevalence of HBsAg, a marker of ongoing HBV replication, among general population shows considerable variations in different countries and even in different parts of the same country. It appears that about 97 million people of China (roughly 7%) are chronically infected with HBV and about 20 million of them have been suffering from active chronic HBV infection or their complications [28] However, there is a reduction of HBsAg carrier rate in China from 9.8% in 1992 to 7.2% in 2006. HBsAg carrier rates have also been reduced in China among children (<10 years old) due to implementation of HBV vaccination [29]. Another country with a population of more than 1 billion in Asia is India, and HBV prevalence in India seems to be about 3.1% in the non-tribal population and 11.85% in tribal populations with wide geographical variations within this subcontinent due to differences in socioeconomic status, religion, culture and tribal practices [30]. In other countries of Asia, HBV prevalence varies from 1% to 14% based on population group and age variability.

In addition to HBsAg positivity, the positivity of anti-HBc (HBV core antibody) may be as high as 40% in many Asian countries. Thus, utmost cautions should be applied during blood transfusion and organ transplantation. However, due to various unavoidable social and economic factors, these problems have not been properly addressed by the majority of countries in Asia. Molecular epidemiology of HBV also shows several important facts. HBV has several genotypes and most of these are found in Asian countries. In the Pacific belt, the common genotypes are HBV genotype B and C, whereas genotypes A and D are more common in Western parts of Asia. Some countries like India and Bangladesh harbour genotypes A, C and D. Although still unclear, it appears that HBV genotype C is associated with a more severe type of liver diseases in Japan and other countries with high prevalence of HBV genotype C.

Recent data show that about 92–150 million people in the world are estimated to be HCV-specific antibody positive. The HCV prevalence ranges from 0.3% in some parts of Malaysia to 13.1% in Uzbekistan [31]. The rate of HCV viraemic patients also ranges from 40% to 80% of anti-HCV positive patients. Although the total numbers of HCV-infected patients are highest in China (about 14 million), the ratio of HCV-infected people among total population is extremely high in Mongolia and Uzbekistan. Regarding HCV genotype, 1 and 2 are most prevalent in most countries of Asia; however, genotype 3 is seen in Pakistan, Malaysia, South Korea, Armenia, Georgia, Uzbekistan, Sri Lanka and Thailand. HCV genotype 6 is also commonly seen in Southeast Asian countries.

In the course of time some patients with chronic HBV and chronic HCV develop progressive liver diseases like liver cirrhosis and liver cancer, specifically HCC.

- Chronic HBV and HCV infection is highly prevalent in Asia.
- In spite of introduction of vaccination against HBV, new cases of HBV infection are also common in Asia. This may be attributable to Asia-specific social and economic factors. Also, interruption of proper vaccination due to natural calamity, famine, and political unrest may be responsible for new cases of HBV in Asia.
- Most of the chronic HBV- and HCV-infected patients are unaware of their illness.
- HBV and HCV free blood transfusion is yet to be established in many regions of Asia.
- Little is known about epidemiology of HBV and HCV-related liver cirrhosis in Asia
- HBV patients with anti-HBe (HBV envelope antibody positive) and progressive liver damage is not rare in Asia, rather these may be the main proportions of patients in Asia.

5.3.2 Epidemiology of NAFLD in Asia

NAFLD is linked with obesity and type 2 diabetes mellitus (T2DM). NAFLD progresses from simple steatosis (NAFLD), to non-alcoholic steatohepatitis (NASH), cirrhosis and cirrhosis-related complications such as HCC. NASH is a more advanced stage of NAFLD, such that about 20% of NASH patients progress to liver cirrhosis or even some patients with NASH show HCC with or without liver cirrhosis [32]. Both patients with NAFLD and NASH are on the rise in Asia. Over the last two decades, the prevalence of patients who are overweight or obese increased remarkably among 7- to 18-year-old students in China [33]. The age- and sex-adjusted rates of overall obesity and central obesity in the Chinese adult population were 7.5% and 12.3%, respectively. The age-standardized prevalence of metabolic syndrome was 9.8% (95% CI 9.0–10.6%) in men and 17.8% (16.6–19.0%) in women in China. For children ≥10 years, the prevalence of metabolic syndrome was 32.3% in the obese group and 8.4% in the overweight group [34].

In fact, patients with NAFLD and NASH have been detected in considerable numbers in almost all countries of Asia. Many studies have demonstrated the high prevalence of NAFLD and NASH in Japan, but well-designed epidemiological studies are yet to be accomplished in many developing and resource-constrained countries of Asia.

5.4 Epidemiology of Chronic Liver Disease in Europe

5.4.1 Epidemiology of Alcoholic Liver Disease in Europe

Alcohol, by far is the most common cause of chronic liver disease in Europe; either as a stand-alone or in combination with other aetiological factors. Alcohol is consumed heavily in Europe, more than in any other region of the world (World Health Organization, European status report on alcohol and health, 2010). Data examining 24 European countries during 2000–2005 showed a varied range of standardised mortality rates for alcohol-related liver diseases between 3 and 47 per 100,000 men. The highest rate was in Hungary, and the lowest was in Latvia. Recent data has confirmed that 69% of HCC in France was due to alcohol consumption [35]. Increasing incidence of alcohol-related cirrhosis has also been reported during the last 10 years in Denmark and Estonia [36, 37].

5.4.2 Epidemiology of Chronic Hepatitis C in Europe

Hepatitis C virus is the most common cause of chronic viral hepatitis in Europe, showing varied rates for studied countries. Using anti-HCV antibody, the prevalence of chronic HCV was reported to range from 0.13% to 3.26%. The lowest rate was found in Belgium whilst the highest was in Romania [38, 39]. Current or previous intravenous drug users account for majority of cases of chronic HCV in Europe; with rates of 50% and 59.8% in Cyprus and France, respectively [40, 41].

Although available data are considered inconclusive, an estimated 8 million people are infected with HCV, representing a prevalence range of 1.1–1.3% in 22 countries of Europe [42]. The World Health Organisation data highlight a prevalence rate of >1.2% in southern and eastern Europe; relative to a rate of <0.1% in northern Europe.

Prior to screening of blood and blood products before transfusion, the most common route of HCV transmission was via blood transfusion. Intravenous drug use (IDU) is by far the most common route of HCV transmission in Europe currently, with an estimated prevalence of 15–90% among people who use drugs [43]. Nosocomial transmission is an important route of transmission reported in Eastern Europe.

5.4.3 Epidemiology of Chronic Hepatitis B in Europe

Recent World Health Organization data indicate that approximately 13.3 million people living in the European region have chronic hepatitis B infection, representing

1.8% of the adult population. Eastern Europe harbours the largest share of HBV population in Europe. The incidence of HBV infection is 1.49 per 100,000 population, significantly lower than 8.7 per 100,000 for HCV infection. Latvia, Austria and Bulgaria have recorded incidence rates of 7.2, 7.8 and 9.8 per 100,000 population, respectively. Indeed the highest incidence of HBV is in Iceland (15 per 100,000) [44].

5.4.4 Epidemiology of Hepatitis D Infection in Europe

Hepatitis D virus is an RNA virus that often requires co-infection with HBV to infect an individual. HDV (delta virus) occurs worldwide. In industrialised countries of the world, including Europe, it is important among immigrant populations from endemic HDV areas as well as IDUs. HDV has been reported to be on the increase in Europe [45]. Although the temporal prevalence of HDV varies widely in most of Europe, the endemicity of the delta virus remains constant in Eastern Europe and Turkey; ranging between 7% and 33% of chronic liver disease patients. Outbreaks of severe and fulminant liver disease during the last two decades have been reported in Mongolia [46], Greenland [47] and Russia [48].

5.4.5 Epidemiology of Hepatitis E Infection in Europe

Hepatitis E virus (HEV) causes acute infections in most cases. Chronic hepatitis E infection is extremely rare and important in immunosuppressed individuals; for example, among patients taking immunosuppressant medications following organ transplantation. HEV was thought to be rare in industrialised countries but recent data proves otherwise. Traditionally, HEV is transmitted via fecal-oral route. In Europe however, zoonotic transmission has been recognised through uncertain means. It is postulated that this could be via eating undercooked or raw meats of pigs, deer, rabbits or rats (https://www.britishlivertrust.org.uk/liver-information/liver-conditions/hepatitis-e/; accessed online on 31/01/2017).

5.5 Epidemiology of Non-Alcoholic Fatty Liver Disease in Europe

The worldwide emergence of "globesity" has seen an increasing incidence of chronic liver disease attributable to NAFLD. The true prevalence of NAFLD in Europe is not known and what we document as the contribution of NAFLD to chronic liver disease may be a "tip of the iceberg" phenomenon. With availability of effective drugs for viral hepatitis, NAFLD has emerged as the leading cause of chronic liver disease in Europe. With a wide variation in the prevalence of this metabolic disorder, the median prevalence of NAFLD for Europe is placed at 25–26%. The most robust data involving 14 European countries found a prevalence of 33% when the Fatty Liver Index was used to identify cases [49]. The prevalence is higher in diabetic patients when abdominal ultrasound was used to identify cases—70% and 46% in Italy [50] and UK [51], respectively. The clinical significance of NAFLD is due to the fact that it predisposes to NASH and not uncommonly, HCC. Indeed, a recent study has confirmed the fact that NAFLD contributed significantly to the rate of HCC in the northern region of England [52].

5.5.1 Genetic Disorders (Haemochromatosis, Alpha-1-Antitrypsin Deficiency & Wilson's Disease)

Hereditary haemochromatosis (HH) is the most common recessive genetic disorder in Caucasians associated with iron overload syndrome. The disease is most common (about 80%) in those with homozygosity for C282Y genetic deficiency. Compound heterozygotes such as C282Y/H63D do present with clinically significant disease as well. The prevalence of HH is about 0.5% in people of northern European descent. As it has variable penetrance, not all with the disorder present with clinically important disease. If left untreated, the chronic complications include cirrhosis as well as HCC. The impact of chronic viral hepatitis as well as alcohol consumption on progression of liver damage in patients with HH is exponential rather than additive. Only a third of patients with severe form of alpha-1-antitrypsin (A1AT) deficiency, a metabolic disorder, go on to develop chronic liver disease, including cirrhosis and HCC. Although A1AT deficiency is encountered in almost all countries of Europe, this condition is most commonly encountered in Scandinavian countries [53].

5.5.2 Autoimmune Hepatitis

Owing to misclassification and/or misdiagnosis, the true prevalence of autoimmune hepatitis (AIH) is not known. Of the two types of AIH, type 1 constitutes 80% of cases and affects females more than males by a ratio of 3:1. AIH has a bimodal peak age at presentation; the first, in childhood and the second, by age 40. In Europe, the estimated point prevalence is 10–15 per 100,000 population [54]. Type 2 AIH is less common and presents often in a fulminant manner, associated with high fatality.

5.6 Chronic Liver Disease in Latin America

Chronic liver diseases of various types are prevalent in almost all countries of Latin America. However, robust evidence-based data are lacking from most of these countries.

5.6.1 Epidemiology of Chronic HBV Infection in Latin America

It is estimated that 7–12 million Latin Americans are chronically infected with HBV. However, there is considerable heterogeneity regarding HBsAg prevalence among different countries of Latin America and even among different parts of the same country of this region. This may be attributable to the diverse nature of human migration and adaptation of HBV in Latin America. Although Latin America may be divided into Central America, Caribbean and South America, this chapter would describe epidemiology of chronic liver diseases on the basis of data of individual countries.

HBsAg prevalence exhibits a heterogeneous distribution in Latin America. Mexico, Honduras, Nicaragua, Costa Rica, Panama, Cuba, Paraguay, Uruguay, Chile, Argentina, Peru and north Colombia are regarded as countries with low prevalence of HBV (<2.0% HBsAg seroprevalence), whereas, Guatemala, Belize, El Salvador, Honduras, Haiti, and the Dominican Republic, Puerto Rico, Ecuador, Venezuela, Guyana, Surinam, French Guyana and the south of Brazil are regarded as areas with intermediate HBV prevalence (HBsAg prevalence of 2–8%). On the other hand, Peru, southern Colombia, northern Bolivia and northern Brazil are known for their high HBsAg seroprevalence (HBsAg >8%) [55–58].

Recent studies have shown that some countries of Latin America such as Panama, Columbia and Venezuela have shifted from intermediate to low prevalence areas. However, most of these countries show high prevalence of anti-HBc that may be indicative of past infection and controlled present HBV infection [59, 60]. Thus, further nation-wide studies are warranted to combat HBV in these countries.

The molecular epidemiology of HBV in Latin America is not only diverse and interesting, but it also provides interesting data on bridging between human migration and HBV genotype adaptation. Both HBV genotypes F and H are detected in most parts of Latin America. HBV genotype F has been found as the predominant genotype in Central America, and this genotype is prevalent among the HBV-infected Amerindians in all countries of South America, such as Venezuela, Colombia, Peru, Bolivia, Argentina, and Brazil [61]. It should be noted that HBV genotype F is also predominantly seen among Alaskans and this indicative of migration of human race from north to south in the American continent. HBV genotype H has been predominantly isolated from both Amerindians and mestizos in Mexico that can be further divided into sub-genotypes and/or sub-clusters [58]. In addition to HBV genotypes F and H, HBV genotypes D and A, as well as genotypes B and C are also found in Latin American countries. The prevalence of HBV genotypes D and A among white people of Mexico and Argentina indicate their origin in European countries. On the other hand, prevalence of HBV genotypes B and C among Asian migrants also provide a scientific basis of diverse HBV genotype distribution in Latin America. Genotype G represents a minor HBV genotype in Latin America [62].

It also appears that HBV genotype has an influence on HBV-related complications such as occurrence of HCC. HBx gene mutations have been detected in HCC patients with HBV genotype F [63]. Taken together, molecular epidemiology of HBV in Latin America may provide valuable information that may be used as references for global HBV epidemics.

5.6.2 Epidemiology of HCV Infection in Latin America

Some estimates about HCV epidemiology in Latin America have been published in the literature. However, it is difficult to assess real epidemiological picture of HCV in Latin America due to scarcity of convincing data. The prevalence of HCV ranges from 1.3% to 1.7% in Argentina, whereas it ranges from 0.9% to 1.9% in Brazil among the general population. However, it is slightly lower among blood donors. Some estimates of HCV infection in some other Latin American countries are available. However, most of these studies have been accomplished in blood donors. This may not accurately represent the true estimates of HCV in those countries. Overall, it seems that HCV prevalence is about 1–2% in most Latin American countries [64].

HCV genotype 1 is the most prevalent HCV genotype in most countries of Latin America. HCV genotypes 2 and 3 are also prevalent in Argentina, whereas HCV genotype 3 is seen in Brazil in moderate prevalence (about 10%). Intravenous drug users (IDU) represent a major source of HCV infection in Latin America and studies have shown that HCV infection prevail among 54.6% IV IDU Argentines [64].

5.7 Epidemiology of Non-Alcoholic Fatty Liver Disease in Latin America

The worldwide prevalence of NAFLD has been estimated at 20–30%, but the prevalence is unknown in the Latin Americas because of a lack of epidemiological studies. The prevalence of NAFLD is increasing globally, and it is set to become the predominant cause of chronic liver disease in many parts of the world. The prevalence of NAFLD varies among ethnic/racial groups, with the Latin American population being affected disproportionately. The severity of NAFLD also may be greater in the Latino population. The increased prevalence and severity of NAFLD in Latino Americans likely is related to the interplay between issues such as genetic factors, access to health care, or the prevalence of chronic diseases such as metabolic syndrome or diabetes. Data on prevalence of NAFLD are sparse and not provided due to lack of evidence-based studies in Latin America. However, prevalence of NAFLD has reached a world-wide pandemic in most parts of the world and Latin America is not an exception to this.

Conclusions

Chronic liver disease is a major global health burden. The prevalence of predisposing factors varies widely across different regions of the world and could account for the differential patterns of chronic liver disease. Lifestyle, healthcare practices, as well as socioeconomic factors play vital roles in the epidemiology of chronic liver diseases worldwide. Whereas alcohol is the most important factor associated with chronic liver disease in most developed industrialised countries of the world, HBV is the most common factor in sub-Saharan Africa and Asia. Eastern European countries have recorded high rates of HBV infection as well. Of the viral factors, HCV is the most common cause of chronic liver disease in Europe, although the prevalence of HCV in some developing countries have been recorded to be higher than in Europe. NAFLD is increasingly being implicated as the cause of chronic liver disease in all regions of the world. There is urgent need to determine the long-term clinical significance of metabolic factors in the aetiology of chronic liver disease globally.

Summary Table of Landmark Literature

Study title and authors	Study design	Summary results	Main limitations
Karoney MJ & Siika AM. Hepatitis C virus infection in Africa: a review. Pan African Medical. 2013;14:44. https://doi.org/10.11604/pamj.2013.14.44.2199	Narrative review article on HCV epidemiology in Africa involving articles published from 1995-onwards	• HCV prevalence of 5.3% for Africa • Genotypes 1, 4 & 5 are the most commonly encountered	• Studies were based on anti-HCV antibody in sera • Not all countries were included • Mostly hospital-based samples
Muhlberger N, et al. HCV-related burden of disease in Europe: a systematic assessment of incidence, prevalence, morbidity, and mortality. BMC Public Health. 2009;9:1471–2459	Systematic review of data for the WHO European region with emphasis on 22 countries.	• Prevalence of HCV ranges from 1.1% to 1.3% in the 22 focus countries • Estimated 7.3–8.8 million people are infected	• Data on burden of HCV in Europe are scarce • WHO data used is not currently considered to be the most comprehensive source and need updating
Blachier M, et al. The burden of liver disease in Europe: A review of available epidemiological data. J Hepatol. 2013;58:593–608	Systematic review, using MEDLINE, EMBASE, and the Cochrane Library with MeSH terms: "liver" and ["disease" or "epidemiology"]	• Chronic hepatitis B affects 0.5–0.7% • HCV rate was 0.13–3.26% • NAFLD ranged 2–44%	
Wang F, et al. The global burden of liver disease: the major impact of China. Hepatology. 2014;60:2099–2108	Review article	• Over 300 million people in China suffer from liver disease, HBV being the most common • Prevention efforts has led to decrease in HBV-related morbidities	

References

1. Ladep NG, Lesi OA, Mark P, Lemoine M, Onyekwere C, Afihene M, et al. Problem of hepatocellular carcinoma in West Africa. World J Hepatol. 2014;6(11):783–92.
2. Taye S, Abdulkerim A, Hussen M. Prevalence of hepatitis B and C virus infections among patients with chronic hepatitis at Bereka Medical Center, Southeast Ethiopia: a retrospective study. BMC Res Notes. 2014;7:272.
3. Ofori-Asenso R, Agyeman AA. Hepatitis B in Ghana: a systematic review & meta-analysis of prevalence studies (1995–2015). BMC Infect Dis. 2016;16:130.
4. Motayo BO, Faneye AO, Udo UA, Olusola BA, Ezeani I, Ogiogwa JI. Seroprevalence of transfusion transmissible infections (TTI), in first time blood donors in Abeokuta, Nigeria. Afr Health Sci. 2015;15(1):19–24.
5. Kateera F, Walker TD, Mutesa L, Mutabazi V, Musabeyesu E, Mukabatsinda C, et al. Hepatitis B and C seroprevalence among health care workers in a tertiary hospital in Rwanda. Trans R Soc Trop Med Hyg. 2015;109(3):203–8.
6. Ochola E, Ocama P, Orach CG, Nankinga ZK, Kalyango JN, McFarland W, et al. High burden of hepatitis B infection in Northern Uganda: results of a population-based survey. BMC Public Health. 2013;13:727.
7. Namululi BA, Guerrieri C, Dramaix MW. Prevalence and incidence of HIV and hepatitis B among blood donors and estimated residual risk of transmission of HIV and HBV virus by blood transfusion. A study at the Provincial General Referee Hospital Bukavu, Democratic Republic of the Congo. Rev Epidemiol Sante Publique. 2013;61(2):139–44.
8. Noubiap JJ, Joko WY, Nansseu JR, Tene UG, Siaka C. Sero-epidemiology of human immunodeficiency virus, hepatitis B and C viruses, and syphilis infections among first-time blood donors in Edea, Cameroon. Int J Infect Dis. 2013;17(10):e832–7.
9. Muchiri I, Okoth FA, Ngaira J, Tuei S. Seroprevalence of Hav, Hbv, Hcv, and Hev among acute hepatitis patients at Kenyatta National Hospital in Nairobi, Kenya. East Afr Med J. 2012;89(6):199–205.
10. Abou MA, Eltahir YM, Ali AS. Seroprevalence of hepatitis B virus and hepatitis C virus among blood donors in Nyala, South Dar Fur, Sudan. Virol J. 2009;6:146.
11. Fasola FA, Kotila TR, Akinyemi JO. Trends in transfusion-transmitted viral infections from 2001 to 2006 in Ibadan, Nigeria. Intervirology. 2008;51(6):427–31.
12. Okoth F, Mbuthia J, Gatheru Z, Murila F, Kanyingi F, Mugo F, et al. Seroprevalence of hepatitis B markers in pregnant women in Kenya. East Afr Med J. 2006;83(9):485–93.
13. Pido B, Kagimu M. Prevalence of hepatitis B virus (HBV) infection among Makerere University medical students. Afr Health Sci. 2005;5(2):93–8.
14. Abebe A, Nokes DJ, Dejene A, Enquselassie F, Messele T, Cutts FT. Seroepidemiology of hepatitis B virus in Addis Ababa, Ethiopia: transmission patterns and vaccine control. Epidemiol Infect. 2003;131(1):757–70.
15. Sirisena ND, Njoku MO, Idoko JA, Isamade E, Barau C, Jelpe D, et al. Carriage rate of hepatitis-B surface antigen (HBsAg) in an urban community in Jos, Plateau State, Nigeria. Niger Postgrad Med J. 2002;9(1):7–10.
16. Gaobepe M, Aspinall S, Bos P. Hepatitis B viral markers in Bushmen at Schmidtsdrift, South Africa: baseline studies for immunisation. East Afr Med J. 1995;72(7):421–3.
17. Pellizzer G, Ble C, Zamperetti N, Stroffolini T, Upunda G, Rapicetta M, et al. Serological survey of hepatitis B infection in Tanzania. Public Health. 1994;108(6):427–31.
18. Harry TO, Bajani MD, Moses AE. Hepatitis B virus infection among blood donors and pregnant women in Maiduguri, Nigeria. East Afr Med J. 1994;71(9):596–7.
19. Aspinall S, Joubert JJ, Evans AC, Joseph S, Steele AD, Lecatsas G. Prevalence of hepatitis B in !Kung (San) children from Bushmanland, Namibia. Ann Trop Paediatr. 1994;14(2):163–7.
20. Opio CK, Seremba E, Ocama P, Lalitha R, Kagimu M, Lee WM. Diagnosis of alcohol misuse and alcoholic liver disease among patients in the medical emergency admission service of a large urban hospital in Sub-Saharan Africa; a cross sectional study. Pan Afr Med J. 2013;15:23.

21. Ndububa DA, Ojo OS, Adetiloye VA, Aladegbaiye AO, Adebayo RA, Adekanle O. The contribution of alcohol to chronic liver disease in patients from South-west Nigeria. Niger J Clin Pract. 2010;13(4):360–4.
22. Okeke EN, Malu AO, Obafunwa JO, Nwana EJ. Aetiological significance of alcohol in liver cirrhosis on the Jos Plateau. West Afr J Med. 2002;21(1):12–4.
23. Almobarak AO, Barakat S, Suliman EA, Elmadhoun WM, Mohamed NA, Abobaker IO, et al. Prevalence of and predictive factors for nonalcoholic fatty liver disease in Sudanese individuals with type 2 diabetes: Is metabolic syndrome the culprit? Arab J Gastroenterol. 2015;16(2):54–8.
24. Almobarak AO, Barakat S, Khalifa MH, Elhoweris MH, Elhassan TM, Ahmed MH. Non alcoholic fatty liver disease (NAFLD) in a Sudanese population: What is the prevalence and risk factors? Arab J Gastroenterol. 2014;15(1):12–5.
25. Onyekwere CA, Ogbera AO, Balogun BO. Non-alcoholic fatty liver disease and the metabolic syndrome in an urban hospital serving an African community. Ann Hepatol. 2011;10(2):119–24.
26. Ott JJ, Stevens GA, Groeger J, Wiersma ST. Global epidemiology of hepatitis B virus infection: new estimates of age-specific HBsAg seroprevalence and endemicity. Vaccine. 2012;30(12):2212–9.
27. Wang FS, Fan JG, Zhang Z, Gao B, Wang HY. The global burden of liver disease: the major impact of China. Hepatology. 2014;60(6):2099–108.
28. Cui Y, Jia J. Update on epidemiology of hepatitis B and C in China. J Gastroenterol Hepatol. 2013;28(Suppl 1):7–10.
29. Luo Z, Li L, Ruan B. Impact of the implementation of a vaccination strategy on hepatitis B virus infections in China over a 20-year period. Int J Infect Dis. 2012;16(2):e82–8.
30. Batham A, Gupta MA, Rastogi P, Garg S, Sreenivas V, Puliyel JM. Calculating prevalence of hepatitis B in India: using population weights to look for publication bias in conventional meta-analysis. Indian J Pediatr. 2009;76(12):1247–57.
31. Gower E, Estes C, Blach S, Razavi-Shearer K, Razavi H. Global epidemiology and genotype distribution of the hepatitis C virus infection. J Hepatol. 2014;61(1 Suppl):S45–57.
32. Bellentani S, Scaglioni F, Marino M, Bedogni G. Epidemiology of non-alcoholic fatty liver disease. Dig Dis. 2010;28(1):155–61.
33. Gu D, Reynolds K, Wu X, Chen J, Duan X, Reynolds RF, et al. Prevalence of the metabolic syndrome and overweight among adults in China. Lancet. 2005;365(9468):1398–405.
34. Fan JG, Zhu J, Li XJ, Chen L, Lu YS, Li L, et al. Fatty liver and the metabolic syndrome among Shanghai adults. J Gastroenterol Hepatol. 2005;20(12):1825–32.
35. Borie F, Tretarre B, Bouvier AM, Faivre J, Binder F, Launoy G, et al. Primitive liver cancers: epidemiology and geographical study in France. Eur J Gastroenterol Hepatol. 2009;21(9):984–9.
36. Parna K, Rahu K. Dramatic increase in alcoholic liver cirrhosis mortality in Estonia in 1992-2008. Alcohol Alcohol. 2010;45(6):548–51.
37. Jepsen P, Vilstrup H, Andersen PK, Lash TL, Sorensen HT. Comorbidity and survival of Danish cirrhosis patients: a nationwide population-based cohort study. Hepatology. 2008;48(1):214–20.
38. Quoilin S, Hutse V, Vandenberghe H, Claeys F, Verhaegen E, De Cock L, et al. A population-based prevalence study of hepatitis A, B and C virus using oral fluid in Flanders, Belgium. Eur J Epidemiol. 2007;22(3):195–202.
39. Gheorghe L, Iacob S, Csiki IE. Prevalence of hepatitis C in Romania: different from European rates? J Hepatol. 2008;49(4):661–2. author reply 663
40. Demetriou VL, van de Vijver DA, Hezka J, Kostrikis LG, Cyprus IVDU Network, Kostrikis LG. Hepatitis C infection among intravenous drug users attending therapy programs in Cyprus. J Med Virol. 2010;82(2):263–70.
41. Jauffret-Roustide M, Le Strat Y, Couturier E, Thierry D, Rondy M, Quaglia M, et al. A national cross-sectional study among drug-users in France: epidemiology of HCV and highlight on practical and statistical aspects of the design. BMC Infect Dis. 2009;9:113.
42. Muhlberger N, Schwarzer R, Lettmeier B, Sroczynski G, Zeuzem S, Siebert U. HCV-related burden of disease in Europe: a systematic assessment of incidence, prevalence, morbidity, and mortality. BMC Public Health. 2009;9:34.

43. Esteban JI, Sauleda S, Quer J. The changing epidemiology of hepatitis C virus infection in Europe. J Hepatol. 2008;48(1):148–62.
44. WHO. 2017. http://ecdc.europa.eu/en/publications/Publications/101012_TER_HepBandC_survey.pdf. Accessed Feb 2017.
45. Rizzetto M. Hepatitis D: thirty years after. J Hepatol. 2009;50(5):1043–50.
46. Tsatsralt-Od B, Takahashi M, Endo K, Buyankhuu O, Baatarkhuu O, Nishizawa T, et al. Infection with hepatitis A, B, C, and delta viruses among patients with acute hepatitis in Mongolia. J Med Virol. 2006;78(5):542–50.
47. Borresen ML, Olsen OR, Ladefoged K, McMahon BJ, Hjuler T, Panum I, et al. Hepatitis D outbreak among children in a hepatitis B hyper-endemic settlement in Greenland. J Viral Hepat. 2010;17(3):162–70.
48. Flodgren E, Bengtsson S, Knutsson M, Strebkova EA, Kidd AH, Alexeyev OA, et al. Recent high incidence of fulminant hepatitis in Samara, Russia: molecular analysis of prevailing hepatitis B and D virus strains. J Clin Microbiol. 2000;38(9):3311–6.
49. Gastaldelli A, Kozakova M, Hojlund K, Flyvbjerg A, Favuzzi A, Mitrakou A, et al. Fatty liver is associated with insulin resistance, risk of coronary heart disease, and early atherosclerosis in a large European population. Hepatology. 2009;49(5):1537–44.
50. Targher G, Bertolini L, Padovani R, Rodella S, Tessari R, Zenari L, et al. Prevalence of nonalcoholic fatty liver disease and its association with cardiovascular disease among type 2 diabetic patients. Diabetes Care. 2007;30(5):1212–8.
51. Williamson RM, Price JF, Hayes PC, Glancy S, Frier BM, Johnston GI, et al. Prevalence and markers of advanced liver disease in type 2 diabetes. QJM. 2012;105(5):425–32.
52. Dyson J, Jaques B, Chattopadyhay D, Lochan R, Graham J, Das D, et al. Hepatocellular cancer: the impact of obesity, type 2 diabetes and a multidisciplinary team. J Hepatol. 2014;60(1):110–7.
53. Fairbanks KD, Tavill AS. Liver disease in alpha 1-antitrypsin deficiency: a review. Am J Gastroenterol. 2008;103(8):2136–41. quiz 2142
54. Francque S, Vonghia L, Ramon A, Michielsen P. Epidemiology and treatment of autoimmune hepatitis. Hepat Med. 2012;4:1–10.
55. Alvarado-Mora MV, Pinho JR. Epidemiological update of hepatitis B, C and delta in Latin America. Antivir Ther. 2013;18(3 Pt B):429–33.
56. Zampino R, Boemio A, Sagnelli C, Alessio L, Adinolfi LE, Sagnelli E, et al. Hepatitis B virus burden in developing countries. World J Gastroenterol. 2015;21(42):11,941–53.
57. Tanaka J. Hepatitis B epidemiology in Latin America. Vaccine. 2000;18(Suppl 1):S17–9.
58. Roman S, Jose-Abrego A, Fierro NA, Escobedo-Melendez G, Ojeda-Granados C, Martinez-Lopez E, et al. Hepatitis B virus infection in Latin America: a genomic medicine approach. World J Gastroenterol. 2014;20(23):7181–96.
59. Roman S, Panduro A, Aguilar-Gutierrez Y, Maldonado M, Vazquez-Vandyck M, Martinez-Lopez E, et al. A low steady HBsAg seroprevalence is associated with a low incidence of HBV-related liver cirrhosis and hepatocellular carcinoma in Mexico: a systematic review. Hepatol Int. 2009;3(2):343–55.
60. Roman S, Tanaka Y, Khan A, Kurbanov F, Kato H, Mizokami M, et al. Occult hepatitis B in the genotype H-infected Nahuas and Huichol native Mexican population. J Med Virol. 2010;82(9):1527–36.
61. Livingston SE, Simonetti JP, McMahon BJ, Bulkow LR, Hurlburt KJ, Homan CE, et al. Hepatitis B virus genotypes in Alaska Native people with hepatocellular carcinoma: preponderance of genotype F. J Infect Dis. 2007;195(1):5–11.
62. Roman S, Panduro A. HBV endemicity in Mexico is associated with HBV genotypes H and G. World J Gastroenterol. 2013;19(33):5446–53.
63. Leon B, Taylor L, Vargas M, Luftig RB, Albertazzi F, Herrero L, et al. HBx M130K and V131I (T-A) mutations in HBV genotype F during a follow-up study in chronic carriers. Virol J. 2005;2:60.
64. Weissenbacher M, Rossi D, Radulich G, Sosa-Estani S, Vila M, Vivas E, et al. High seroprevalence of bloodborne viruses among street-recruited injection drug users from Buenos Aires, Argentina. Clin Infect Dis. 2003;37(Suppl 5):S348–52.

Epidemiology of Chronic Liver Disease in the United States

6

Yihan Yang, Jeffrey Luk, and Andre N. Sofair

Abstract

Chronic liver disease is a common cause of morbidity and mortality in the United States. The most common causes of liver disease include non-alcoholic fatty liver disease (NAFLD), chronic hepatitis C virus infection, alcoholic liver disease, and chronic hepatitis B virus infection. Through a discussion of various surveillance methods as well as their strengths and weaknesses, we review the epidemiology, risk factors, and natural history of each of these diseases and discuss prevention measures that have been effective in decreasing incidence rates.

Keywords

Incidence · Prevalence · Epidemiology · Liver diseases · Non-alcoholic fatty liver disease · Hepatitis b · Hepatitis c · Liver diseases · Alcoholic

6.1 Introduction

An understanding of accurate disease burden forms the foundation of appropriate public health and clinical care policy and resource allocation. Disease frequency may be determined from the pool of existing cases (prevalence) or from the contribution of new cases (incidence) [1]. Because liver disease is often insidious, it is difficult to ascertain an accurate picture of the burden of disease.

Population-based studies of liver disease are important in ascertaining the epidemiology of disease and to determine the contribution from various etiologies. Where data come from is also important in determining the accuracy of the information. Liver disease is disproportionately seen in urban centers so surveillance in these

Y. Yang · J. Luk · A. N. Sofair (✉)
Department of Medicine, Yale University School of Medicine, New Haven, CT, USA
e-mail: andre.sofair@yale.edu

R. J. Wong, R. G. Gish (eds.), *Clinical Epidemiology of Chronic Liver Diseases*,
https://doi.org/10.1007/978-3-319-94355-8_6

sites would give a different picture than state-wide surveillance [2]. Surveillance in referral gastroenterology or hepatology practices compared with surveillance in primary care practices or in the general population could lead to referral bias in the types of cases ascertained [3–5].

6.2 General Epidemiology and Burden of Disease

The National Health and Nutrition Examination Surveys (NHANES) are a series of cross-sectional national surveys designed to provide representative health measures and conditions among civilian non-institutionalized individuals in the United States. Approximately 5000 people aged 6 and older are sampled annually utilizing standardized interviews, physical examinations, and collection of biologic samples. Using these data, the prevalence rates for chronic liver disease (CLD) were 11.8% from 1988 to 1994, 15.7% from 1999 to 2004 and 14.8% from 2005 to 2008. The prevalence due to chronic hepatitis C virus infection (HCV) (1.95%, 1.97%, 1.68%) and alcohol liver disease (1.38%, 2.21%, 2.05%) remained generally stable over these three time periods. However, the prevalence of NAFLD increased from 5.5% to 9.8% to 11.0% in this short time frame [6]. The prevalence of obesity, diabetes, and insulin resistance all increased over this time period [6]. It is worth noting that individuals with higher prevalence rates of liver disease, such as immigrants, the homeless, hospitalized persons, and those in prison, are underrepresented in the NHANES data.

Based on work in three sentinel sites in the United States for instance [3], we determined an incidence rate of 63.9 cases per 100,000 population diagnosed with chronic liver disease referred to a gastroenterologist or hepatologist between 1999 and 2001. Of these cases, 42% were related to HCV, 22% to HCV and alcohol, 9% related to NAFLD, 8% from alcohol alone, and 3% to chronic hepatitis B virus infection (Fig. 6.1). Of these, 18% presented with cirrhosis. In a small retrospective surveillance primary care practice study in one town in Connecticut, we found NAFLD to be the most common cause of CLD, accounting for 30% of cases. HCV accounted for 25%. In this study, the overall prevalence of CLD was 3.7% (95% CI 2.8–4.7%) [4]. These site-specific differences highlight the challenge of ascertaining accurate burden of disease given that health care utilization may be based on the availability of treatment in different settings.

In 2004, total U.S. hospital discharges for CLD were 759,000 [7]. According to the American Gastroenterology Association (AGA) in 1998, the direct cost of liver disease in the United States was 9.1 billion dollars with indirect costs of 655 million dollars for a total cost of 9.77 billion dollars [1]. In 2014, chronic liver disease and cirrhosis was the 12th leading cause of death in the United States [8]. As the current cohort of patients with chronic hepatitis C ages, those with cirrhosis and hepatocellular carcinoma will increase in the coming decades, as will liver-related deaths and overall cost [9]. As noted in one report, the determination of liver-disease related deaths uses one ICD-9 code (571; chronic liver disease and cirrhosis) to code for liver diseases. Using this number, the rate of death has been relatively stable (25,000

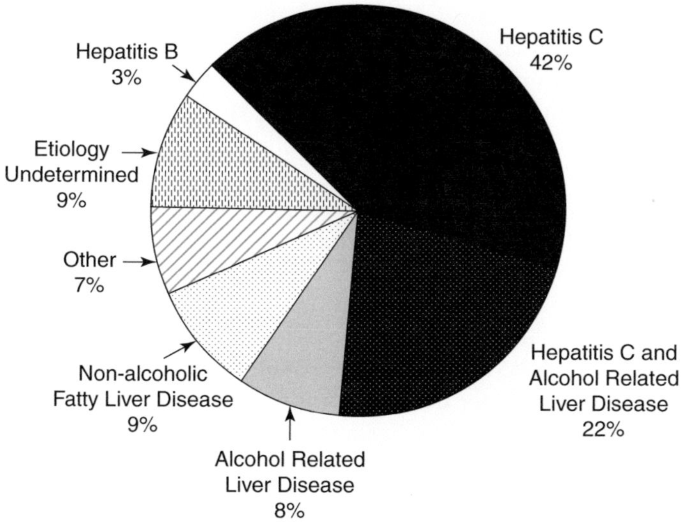

Fig. 6.1 Underlying etiologies in patients newly diagnosed with chronic liver disease. Chronic liver disease surveillance network. 1999–2001, $n = 1040$. From Bell BP et al. American Journal of Gastroenterology. 2008;103(11):2727–36

per year) for the past two decades. If one uses a broader list of codes (i.e. viral hepatitis, primary liver cancer, intrahepatic bile duct cancer, esophageal varices, fulminant liver disease, hepatic coma, portal hypertension, hepatorenal syndrome and others), the number almost doubles to 44,677 [1]. Both African Americans (hazard ratio, 1.9; 95% CI: 1.4–2.6) and Hispanics (hazard ratio, 2.0; 95% CI: 1.3–2.9) had an almost twofold risk of death from liver cirrhosis compared to whites [3]. At its peak in 1973, the mortality rate was 35.3 per 100,000 for African American men, 19.2 per 100,000 for white men, 18.4 per 100,000 for African American women, and 8.7 per 100,000 for white women [2, 10].

6.3 Non-alcoholic Fatty Liver Disease (NAFLD)

NAFLD is characterized by hepatic lipid accumulation seen either by imaging or by biopsy that may manifest as non-alcoholic fatty liver (NAFL) or non-alcoholic steatohepatitis (NASH), depending on the presence of associated inflammation. It is typically seen in the absence of significant ethanol intake (less than 14 drinks per week) or another cause of hepatic steatosis and is typically considered to be a manifestation of the metabolic syndrome (hypertriglyceridemia, low HDL cholesterol, central obesity, insulin resistance, and hypertension). Other conditions associated with NAFLD include polycystic ovarian syndrome, hypothyroidism, HCV, starvation, hyperalimentation, obstructive sleep apnea, hypopituitarism, Wilson disease, hypogonadism, medications (amiodarone, antiretroviral medications, methotrexate, tamoxifen, corticosteroids, valproate), and inborn errors of metabolism [6, 11].

In the general U.S. population, NAFLD is believed to be the most common form of liver disease. It is estimated that the prevalence of ultrasound-ascertained NAFLD is 19% corresponding to an estimate of 28.8 (95% confidence interval: 26.6, 31.2) million adults with NAFLD nationwide [5]. Men, Hispanics (and more specifically Mexican-Americans), those with diabetes, insulin resistance without diabetes, with dyslipidemia, and with obesity are disproportionately affected [5, 12].

Of individuals with chronic liver disease (CLD), NAFLD accounted for 47% of cases from 1988 to 1994, 62.8% in 1999 to 2004 and 75.1% from 2005 to 2008. In patients with obesity undergoing bariatric surgery, the prevalence of NAFLD is as high as 90% and up to 5% of patients have cirrhosis [13–15]. NAFLD is believed to be the most common cause of cryptogenic cirrhosis [11, 16] . These patients commonly have the metabolic risk factors for NAFLD and the histologic features of steatosis are often lost with the development of cirrhosis [1, 11].

Williams et al. reported on the ethnic distribution of biopsy-proven NAFLD in a cohort of patients with abnormal liver ultrasounds. Similar to previous reports, Hispanic persons had the highest prevalence of NAFLD (58.3%), followed by Caucasian (44.4%), and African American (35.1%) persons [10, 17]. In this same study [17], Hispanics were found to have a higher prevalence of NASH compared with Caucasians (19.4% vs. 9.8%; $p = .03$).

The natural history of fatty liver tends to be dichotomous; NAFLD is generally benign whereas NASH can progress to cirrhosis, liver failure, and hepatocellular cancer. The long-term outcomes of patients with NAFLD and NASH have been reported in several studies. Generally, (a) patients with NAFLD have increased overall mortality compared to matched control populations, (b) the most common cause of death in patients with NAFLD, NAFL and NASH is cardiovascular disease likely owing to similar risk factors, and (c) patients with NASH (but not NAFL) have an increased liver-related mortality rate [11, 18–25].

6.4 Hepatitis C

The hepatitis C virus (HCV) was discovered in 1989, and tests for it soon followed. Most prior cases of non-A, non-B hepatitis are believed to have been viral hepatitis C. Starting in the late 1980s, NHANES has included HCV antibody and retrospective confirmatory HCV RNA testing. Analysis of over 20,000 serum samples from NHANES participants between 1988 and 1994 suggested that an extrapolated 2.7 million people in the United States had chronic HCV infection [26]. Between 1999 and 2002, analysis of over 15,000 samples showed an estimate of 3.2 million people with chronic HCV [27]. A more recent analysis of 2003 through 2010 data of over 20,000 participants showed a prevalence of 1%, which extrapolates to approximately 2.7 million people with chronic HCV [26].

As already mentioned, a particular criticism of the NHANES cohorts has been its exclusion of several high-risk populations, leading to an underestimate of the true prevalence of HCV in the United States. Edlin et al. conducted a systematic review of studies that incorporated subgroups of individuals excluded from NHANES, particularly those who were hospitalized, residing in nursing homes, active-duty

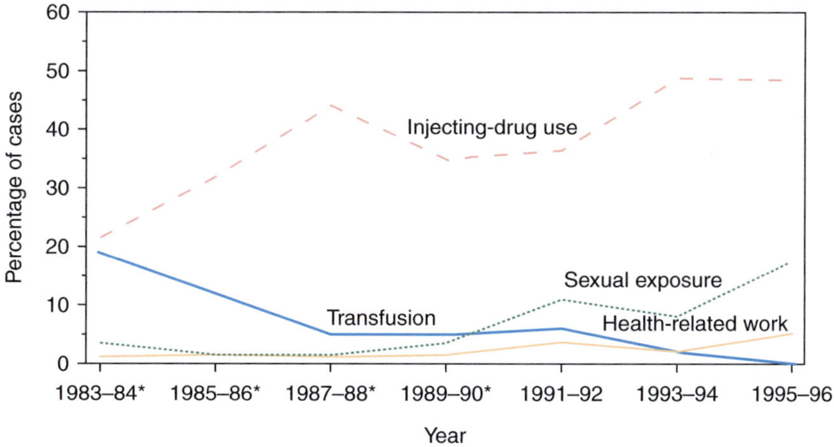

*Data presented for non-A, non-B hepatitis.
Source: Centers for Disease Control and Prevention.

Fig. 6.2 Reported cases of acute hepatitis C by selected risk factors—United States, 1983–1996

military, homeless, incarcerated, and Native Americans residing in reservations. The authors estimated that approximately 1 million individuals excluded from NHANES had a positive HCV antibody test, of which 0.8 million had chronic HCV infection. This brings the estimated total number of individuals in the United States with chronic HCV to at least 3.5 million, a prevalence of approximately 1.3% [28].

As a blood-borne pathogen, HCV infection is most common in individuals with percutaneous blood exposure (Fig. 6.2) [29]. Through logistic regression models of individuals aged 20–59, NHANES identified that individuals who were illicit drug users and recipients of blood transfusions before 1992 were more likely to be infected with HCV [26]. Specifically, the prevalence of HCV virus infection was highest in persons with hemophilia requiring transfusions before 1987 at 87%, followed by persons with IV drug use at 79%; persons on chronic hemodialysis had an HCV prevalence of around 10% [29]. Due to improvements in blood blank screening in 1990s, injection drug use now accounts for approximately 60% of the transmission of HCV infection [29].

Analysis of several NHANES cohorts demonstrated that persons born between 1945 and 1965 accounted for as high as 75% of individuals with HCV infection; the approximate prevalence of HCV in this birth cohort was 3.25%, three times that of the general population [30]. In order to improve yield of HCV screening, based upon the NHANES birth cohort and demographic findings, the Centers for Disease Control and Prevention (CDC) issued recommendations in 2012 to screen all individuals born in 1945 through 1965 for HCV infection [31].

Further risk factors identified by analysis of NHANES data included male gender and non-Hispanic black race/ethnicity (Fig. 6.3) [26]. The reason for the higher rate in blacks is unclear. Blacks have a twofold lower lifetime prevalence of injection drug use than whites (0.8% vs. 1.7%) but appear to clear the virus after an episode of acute hepatitis C less frequently [10]. Sequelae of chronic liver disease

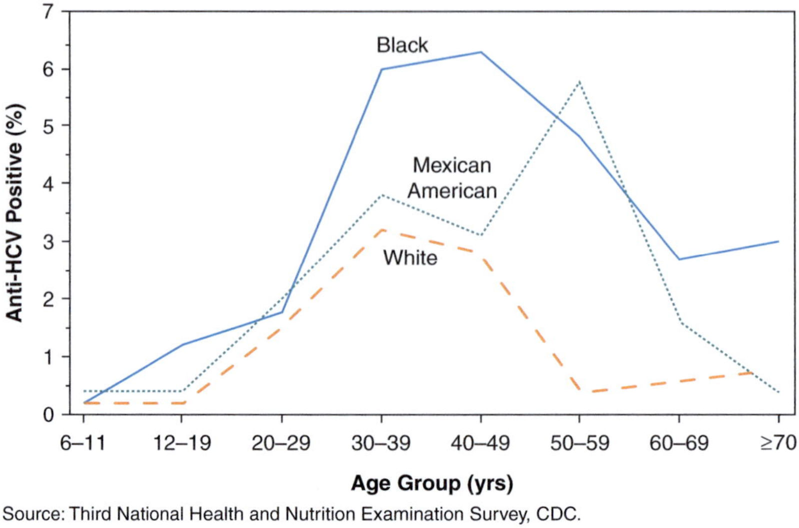

Fig. 6.3 Prevalence of hepatitis C virus (HCV) infection by age and race/ethnicity—United States, 1988–1994

Fig. 6.4 Cases of acute hepatitis C (2000–2013)

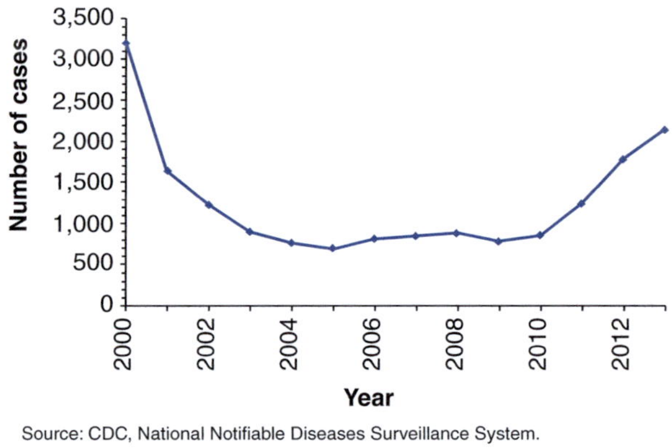

(e.g. cirrhosis) are more common in patients with chronic HCV who also ingest alcohol than in those with chronic HCV alone [2, 3].

Both outpatient and inpatient HCV diagnoses have greatly increased since hepatitis C received its own ICD code in the early 1990s. The number of hospitalizations prior to 1992 was too small to provide estimates. Much of the increase can be attributed to increasing recognition of the disease. There was also the introduction of antiviral therapy that required frequent patient monitoring.

Since most patients with acute hepatitis C are anicteric, the reported incidence rate underestimates the true burden of disease. The cases of acute hepatitis C declined until 2003, remained steady until 2010 and have increased through 2013 (Fig. 6.4). The incidence rate in 2013 was 0.7/100,000 with a death rate of 0.2% [32].

Utilizing Quest Diagnostics test results in individuals with HCV infection from 2010 through 2013, Klevens et al. estimated the proportion of patients that had advanced fibrosis or cirrhosis, defined as APRI score >1.5 or FIB-4 score >3.25 [33]. They estimated that among individuals with chronic infection, approximately 23% (27% in those born between 1945 and 1965) had advanced fibrosis at first diagnosis. Data from the United Network for Organ Sharing show that the proportion of liver transplants performed on patients with HCV-related end-stage liver disease increased from 12% in the 1990s to 35–40% in the last decade [34]. HCV is now the leading etiology for liver transplantation in the US [31].

In 2004, 85% of hepatitis-related deaths were from HCV. Hepatitis C was listed as a contributing cause of death more often than as the underlying cause. About two-thirds of deaths occurred between the ages of 45 and 64 years. Age-adjusted death rates among blacks were nearly twice those of whites, and males had more than double the death rate of females [7]. In 2013, the death rate for hepatitis C was 5.0/100,000 population compared with the death rate for hepatitis B (0.52/100,000) [32].

Further studies will need to be conducted to determine the impact of the new direct-acting anti-viral therapies on HCV prevalence and mortality.

6.5 Hepatitis B

Hepatitis B is a reportable infectious disease in the United States and the CDC conducts ongoing monitoring for its incidence [35]. Starting in 1982, the CDC began monitoring the incidence of acute viral hepatitis B in the Sentinel Counties Study of Viral Hepatitis. This survey incorporated four counties representative of the U.S. population, including Denver County, Colorado; Jefferson County, Alabama; Pierce County, Washington; and Pinellas County, Florida. Cases of HBV infection were reported to the health department by clinical providers and laboratories. Using data collected from this study, Goldstein et al. calculated incidence rates of acute hepatitis B using county-specific census data. They initially found an HBV incidence of 13.5/100,000 persons in 1982, with a decrease to 3.3/100,000 persons by 1998 and, and to 2.1/100,000 by 2004 [35, 36]. By 2013, the rate had dropped further, to 1.0/100,000. [31] Stratified by age group, individuals aged 10–19 years old had the greatest decline in incidence (72.5%), followed by individuals 20–29 years old (70.6%). In 2013, infections were most commonly recognized in those between ages 30 and 39 years (incidence of 2.4/100,000), and hospitalizations with the diagnosis occurred across the age range of adults. In 2013, the incidence was higher in men that women (1.21/100,000 vs. 0.73/100,000). Based on data from 2001 to 2005, approximately 79% of newly acquired cases of hepatitis B were associated with high-risk sexual exposure or injection drug use; other known exposures (occupational, household, travel, and health-care related) together accounted for 5% of new cases and 16% denied a specific risk factor for infection [37].

Fig. 6.5 Reportable cases of acute hepatitis B

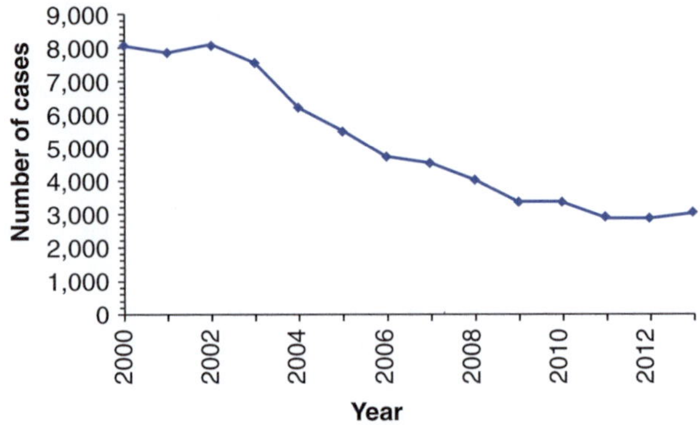

This reduction in HBV incidence in the United States (Fig. 6.5) may be attributed to several measures implemented since 1991. Elements of this strategy included (1) universal vaccination of infants beginning at birth, (2) prevention of perinatal HBV infection through routine screening of all pregnant women for hepatitis B surface antigen (HBsAg) and the provision of immunoprophylaxis to infants born to HBsAg-positive women, (3) routine vaccination of previously unvaccinated children and adolescents, and (4) vaccination of previously unvaccinated adults at increased risk for infection. The last group includes health care workers, dialysis patients, household contacts and sex partners of persons with chronic HBV infection, persons with a recent history of multiple sex partners or a sexually transmitted disease, men who have sex with men, and injection drug users [35]. While nationwide vaccination programs have decreased the incidence and prevalence of HBV in the young and adolescent population, the prevalence of chronic HBV infection has remained relatively unchanged, and is higher in non-Hispanic Asians and non-Hispanic black populations [38].

Utilizing similar strategies as described in the NHANES studies of chronic HCV above, NHANES demonstrated that prevalence of chronic HBV decreased after introduction of the vaccination program. In 6–19 year olds, prevalence of chronic HBV decreased from 0.24% in 1988–1994 to 0.05% in 1999–2006 [39]. However, the overall prevalence of chronic HBV infection was found to be fairly constant over the last two decades at approximately 0.3% [38]. This is thought to be due to the migration of foreign-born individuals with HBV infection into the United States who are thought to account for approximately 95% of new U.S. cases of chronic hepatitis B [40]. Notably, NHANES found that 3.1% of non-Hispanic Asians had chronic HBV infection, a prevalence tenfold higher than the general population; non-Hispanic black individuals had a prevalence two- to threefold higher than the general population [38].

NHANES data indicate that the prevalence of HBsAg-positive individuals is low (0.33% in 1976–1980 and 0.42% in 1988–1994). More recent unpublished data from 2005 to 2006 are similar (0.30%). The NHANES data did not include statistically valid samples from populations in which HBV is most common, such as Asians, Pacific Islander and Alaskan Natives, and also did not include institutionalized individuals, the homeless, and those in prison, all of whom would be expected to have a higher prevalence rate [35]. For instance, estimates of HBV prevalence in Asian and Pacific Island immigrants to the United States who reside in urban areas range from 10% to 15% [35]. Because of these limitations, the true prevalence of hepatitis B infection in the United States may be several times higher than estimated.

Through CDC's enhanced viral hepatitis surveillance which reported on chronic hepatitis B, 56% of reported cases were male and 43.4% were female; 35.4% were Asian or Pacific Islander; 65.4% of cases were among patients aged 25–54 [32]. Of those with country of birth recorded, 63.9% were born outside of the United States [32].

Rates of both ambulatory care visits and hospitalizations with hepatitis B were higher among blacks than whites and among males than females. Hepatitis B was rarely the first-listed hospital diagnosis. There has been a vaccine available for hepatitis B since the 1980s, but the rates of both ambulatory care and hospitalizations have increased markedly since 1999. This increase has also been attributed to increased rates of immigration of chronic carriers of hepatitis B virus.

A recent report on the burden of digestive diseases used the National Ambulatory Medical Care Survey and the National Hospital Ambulatory Medical Care Survey and estimated that outpatient visits for an HBV-related diagnosis in the United States occurred at a rate around 100 visits per 100,000 in 1992, which increased to roughly 250 visits per 100,000 by 2004 [41]. The National Hospital Discharge Survey data showed a similar increase in discharges with a HBV diagnosis: in 1992, the rate of hospitalization for a HBV-related illness was 5 per 100,000 in 1992, which increased to more than 20 per 100,000 in 2002. These data strongly suggest that the number of patients with HBV requiring in- and outpatient care increased substantially during the late 1990s and early 2000s [35, 41]. These increases were accompanied by increases in total charges. For hospitalizations, inflation-adjusted to 2006 US$, increased from $357 million in 1990 to $1.5 billion in 2003 [35].

The majority of deaths with HBV as either underlying or contributing cause occurred in middle age, between age 45 and 64 years. As with other forms of infections, HBV was more often listed as a contributing rather than as an underlying cause. In 2013, the hospitalization rate for reported cases of acute hepatitis B was 58.8% and the mortality rate was 0.9% For chronic HBV, the mortality rate was 0.5% between 2009 and 2013 [32].

6.6 Alcohol-Related Liver Disease

Several studies have previously identified a link between alcohol consumption and the development and mortality from alcohol-related liver disease (ALD).

In Europe, the Dionysos study was a cohort study conducted in two northern Italian communities of over 6000 participants aged 12–65 without viral liver disease. Using self-reported alcohol consumption levels, multivariate analysis showed that a threshold of ingesting greater than 30 g of alcohol daily was associated with an odds ratio of 7.5 for developing CLD, and 10.9 for developing

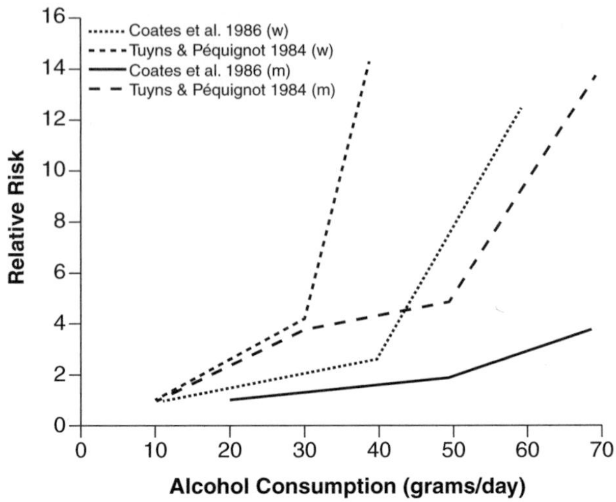

Fig. 6.6 Alcohol consumption and the Relative Risk of cirrhosis of the liver in men (m) and women (w). From Mann RE, Smart, RG, Govoni R. The Epidemiology of Alcoholic Liver Disease. Alcohol Research and Health. 2003;27(3):209–19

liver damage or cirrhosis [42]. The odds ratio of developing CLD or cirrhosis increased in a dose-dependent fashion (see Fig. 6.6) [43]. However, only a small proportion of individuals with high alcohol consumption developed ALD. For instance, in patients with >120 g/day of alcohol intake, approximately 14% developed chronic ALD.

A series of nationwide household surveys suggest that the proportion of incident cases of heavy drinkers in the United States between 1984 and 1992 was highest among Hispanics, followed by African Americans and then whites [44]. A subsequent analysis from 1984 to 1995 showed that nationwide declines in heavy alcohol consumption were different with respect to race. Whereas the prevalence of heavy alcohol drinking decreased among white men (20–12%) and women (5–2%) during the period, it remained unchanged for African American men (15%) and women (5%). Similarly, a reduction in heavy alcohol use was not observed in Hispanic men (17–18%) and women (2–3%) [45]. In contrast, data from the National Longitudinal Alcohol Epidemiologic Study suggest that heavy alcohol consumption (>5 drinks/day) did not vary significantly by race or ethnicity [46]. There is evidence to suggest that African Americans have a higher level of liver test elevation at all levels of alcohol consumption when compared with whites [10].

Accurate assessments in the literature of the use of alcohol and prevalence of ALD has faced several limitations, including the under-coding of alcohol use disorder in medical records, variable accuracy of self-reported alcohol consumption, and tendency of patients with excessive alcohol use to not seek medical care until a decompensation event has occurred.

Several studies assessing the etiologies of CLD have been based upon data from NHANES datasets (methodology as described above). Recently, Younossi et al. published a population-based study in 2011 utilizing NHANES data collected from 1998 through 2008. A diagnosis of alcohol-related liver disease was assumed if participants had self-reported excessive alcohol use, had an ALT >40 or AST >37 in men or either ALT or AST >31 in women, and no other identified etiology of liver disease. The study suggested a prevalence of ALD of 1.4% between 1988 and 1994, increasing to 2.2% between 1999 and 2004, and remaining stable at 2.0% between 2005 and 2008. Male gender, history of smoking, and hypertension were found to be associated with alcohol-related liver disease in multivariate analyses [6].

An outpatient population-based study by Bell et al. conducted from 1999 to 2001 identified patients in gastroenterology practices in three counties across the United States who had newly-diagnosed chronic liver disease as defined by elevated liver enzymes for six months or pathologic, clinical, or imaging findings consistent with CLD. Extrapolated to the U.S. population, the study suggested that approximately 150,000 individuals were newly diagnosed with CLD yearly between 1999 and 2001. Physician diagnoses and in-person interviews utilizing a self-reported lifetime alcohol consumption history revealed that approximately 8% of newly-diagnosed patients had ALD; approximately 22% had comorbid HCV and ALD [3]. These results suggest that in the United States, approximately 12,000 and 33,000 people were diagnosed with ALD alone, or alcohol- and HCV-related liver disease, respectively. Approximately 45% of patients with ALD had cirrhosis, whereas 20% of patients with HCV and ALD had cirrhosis at time of diagnosis. Patients with alcohol-related liver disease were mostly male (72%), white (84%), and without a college degree (90%). In a subgroup analysis of these data, we found that only 40.2% of patients who met criteria for alcohol-related liver disease attributed their liver disease to alcohol use [47]. Age-adjusted incidence rates of alcohol-related cirrhosis from 1970 through 1998 by gender and race are depicted in Fig. 6.7 [43].

Alcohol-related liver disease remains a main cause of CLD in the United States and is often associated with cirrhosis at the time of diagnosis.

6.7 Hepatocellular Carcinoma

In the United States, the annual incidence rate of hepatocellular carcinoma (HCC) was 1.5 cases per 100,000 in 1973 and rose to 6.2/100,000 in 2010, using Surveillance, Epidemiology, and End Results (SEER) data [48, 49]. The rate was threefold higher in men than in women (11.5 vs. 3.9 per 100,000 between 2008 and 2012). The highest age-adjusted incidence rates had been noted in Asian and Pacific Islanders. However, for the first time in 2011, Hispanics had the highest rate. The reasons for this recent trend are not clear but may be related to higher rates of HCV, alcoholic liver disease, NAFLD, and metabolic syndrome in Hispanics [50].

Although incidence rates had increased by approximately 3.1% per year, a slowing of the rate was noted beginning in 2006 [49, 51]. A significant survival improvement in HCC was also noted from 1973 to 2010, which seems to be driven by earlier detection of HCC at a curative stage (possibly driven by increased screening) and greater utilization of curative modalities (especially liver transplantation) [49].

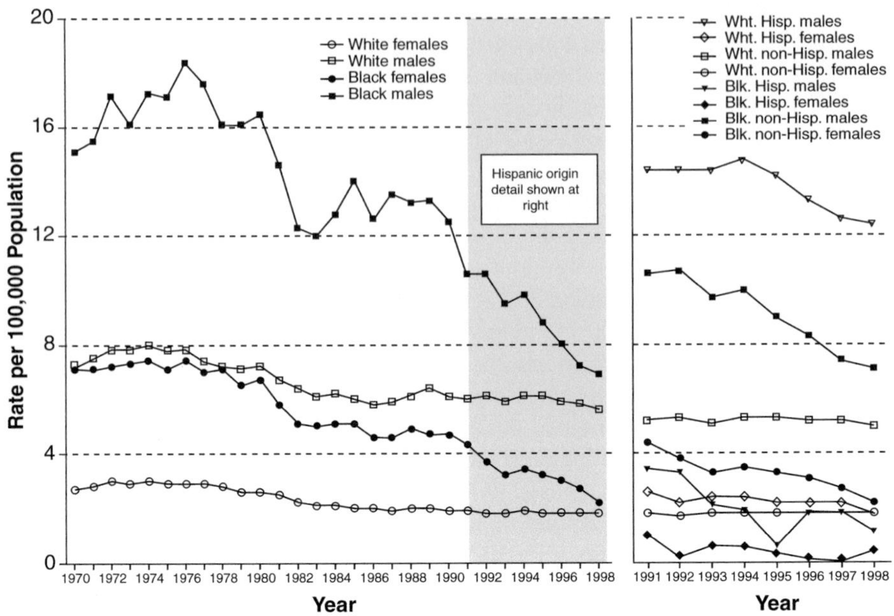

Fig. 6.7 Age-adjusted rates of alcohol related cirrhosis by gender and ethnic group in the United States, 1970–1998. From Mann RE, Smart, RGR, Govoni R. The Epidemiology of Alcoholic Liver Disease. Alcohol Research and Health. 2003;27(3):209–19

In the United States, the major risk factors for HCC include chronic infection with hepatitis B and hepatitis C viruses, excessive alcohol consumption, obesity, and type 2 diabetes mellitus [52]. In patients with pre-existing chronic liver disease, additional independent risk factors for hepatocellular carcinoma include age >40, male gender, presence of cirrhosis, lifetime smoking, and Asian ethnicity [53]. Among patients with HCC currently diagnosed in the US, 50–60% are infected with HCV, 10–15% are infected with HBV, and 20–25% have alcoholic liver disease. Approximately 20–30% of HCC cases do not have any of the previously mentioned factors but have some features of the metabolic syndrome [48]. Although most cases of HCC are seen in the setting of cirrhosis, HBV can lead to HCC in the absence of advanced fibrosis [48]. It is hoped that newer treatments for hepatitis C will change the trajectory of HCV-related HCC in the United States. However a lack of systematic screening and treatment of those infected with HCV may translate to a continued increase in HCC cases until after 2020, when it is hoped that incidence will decline [48].

Summary Table of Landmark Literature

Study title and authors	Study design	Summary results	Main limitations
Younossi, ZM, et al. Changes in the prevalence of the most common causes of chronic liver diseases in the United States from 1988 to 2008. Clinical Gastroenterology & Hepatology. 2011;9(6):524–30.	Repeated cross-sectional surveys using NHANES to determine trends in the etiologies of chronic liver disease in the United States from 1988 to 2008.	• Prevalence of HCV has remained stable • Prevalence of alcoholic liver disease has remained stable • NAFLD has increase in prevalence from 5.5% in 1988–1994 to 11.0% in 2005–2008	• NHANES only captures non-institutionalized adults • Immigrants, incarcerated persons, those in hospital or nursing homes, and the homeless are underrepresented
Bell BP, et al. The epidemiology of newly diagnosed chronic liver disease in gastroenterology practices in the United States: results from population-based surveillance. American Journal of Gastroenterology. 2008;103(11): 2727–36	Prospective study of patients newly diagnosed with chronic liver disease in specialty offices (gastroenterology and hepatology). Patients underwent a chart review, interview, and additional viral hepatitis testing	• Yearly incidence rate was 63.9/100,000 population between 1999 and 2001 • 42% were related to hepatitis C, 22% to hepatitis C and alcohol, 9% related to non-alcoholic liver disease, 8% from alcohol alone, and 3% to hepatitis B • 18% presented with cirrhosis	• Referral population • 49% of eligible patients participated • Three geographical areas in the United States were included • Patients with HIV infection were excluded
Lazo M, et al. Prevalence of nonalcoholic fatty liver disease in the United States: the Third National Health and Nutrition Examination Survey, 1988–1994. American Journal of Epidemiology. 2013;178(1):38–45.	Cross-sectional study using ultrasonography in the diagnosis of nonalcoholic fatty liver	• Prevalence of NAFLD was 19.0% • 28.8 million adults estimated to have NAFLD nationwide • More common in Mexican-Americans and in men compared with women • Independently associated with diabetes, insulin resistance dyslipidemia, and with obesity	• Cross-sectional so could not define causality • Unable to detect inflammation as used ultrasound alone • Data are 20 years old

Study title and authors	Study design	Summary results	Main limitations
Goldstein ST, Alter MJ, Williams IT, Moyer LA, Judson FN, Mottram K, et al. Incidence and risk factors for acute hepatitis B in the United States, 1982–1998: implications for vaccination programs. J Infect Dis. 2002;185(6):713–9.	Cross-sectional analysis of patient data from county-based health department reports of HBV infection in four U.S. counties from 1982 to 1998.	• Incidence of HBV decreased from 13.5/100,000 persons initially in 1982 to 3.3/100,000 by 1998 • Individuals aged 10–19 years old had the greatest decline in incidence (72.5%)	• Data are 20 years old
Roberts H, Kruszon-Moran D, Ly KN, Hughes E, Iqbal K, Jiles RB, et al. Prevalence of chronic hepatitis B virus (HBV) infection in U.S. households: National Health and Nutrition Examination Survey (NHANES), 1988–2012. Hepatology. 2016;63(2):388–97	Repeated cross-sectional surveys of NHANES data assessing the prevalence of hepatitis B in the United States from 1988 through 2012.	• Overall prevalence of chronic HBV infection was found to be fairly constant over the last two decades at approximately 0.3% • 3.1% of non-Hispanic Asians had chronic HBV infection, tenfold higher than the general population; non-Hispanic black individuals had a prevalence two- to threefold higher than the general population • In 6–19 year olds, prevalence of chronic HBV decreased from 0.24% in 1988–1994 to 0.05% in 1999–2006	• NHANES only captures non-institutionalized adults • Immigrants, incarcerated persons, those in hospital or nursing homes, and the homeless are underrepresented

Study title and authors	Study design	Summary results	Main limitations
Smith BD, Morgan RL, Beckett GA, Falck-Ytter Y, Holtzman D, Teo CG, et al. Recommendations for the identification of chronic hepatitis C virus infection among persons born during 1945–1965. MMWR Recommendations and reports: Morbidity and mortality weekly report Recommendations and reports. 2012;61(RR-4):1–32	Systematic Review. Guidelines based upon multiple population-based epidemiologic studies (mostly NHANES) on the prevalence of HCV by age corhort	• Individuals born between 1945 and 1965 have a threefold higher prevalence of HCV infection compared to the general population. Approximately 75% of individuals with chornic HCV infection were born during this time • CDC recommends one-time HCV screening of all individuals in this birth cohort	• NHANES only captures non-institutionalized adults • Immigrants, incarcerated persons, those in hospital or nursing homes, and the homeless are underrepresented
Denniston MM, Jiles RB, Drobeniuc J, Klevens RM, Ward JW, McQuillan GM et al. Chronic hepatitis C virus infection in the United States, National Health and Nutrition Examination Survey 2003 to 2010. Ann Intern Med. 2014;160(5): 293–300.	Repeated cross-sectional surveys using NHANES to determine trends in hepatitis C incidence and prevalence in the United States	• Chronic HCV infection affects approximately 1% of the U.S. population, or an estimated 2.7 million people • Individuals who use IV drugs, or who received blood transfusions prior 1992 were more likely to be infected than the general population	• NHANES only captures non-institutionalized adults • Immigrants, incarcerated persons, those in hospital or nursing homes, and the homeless are underrepresented

References

1. Kim WR, Brown RS Jr, Terrault NA, El-Serag H. Burden of liver disease in the United States: summary of a workshop. Hepatology. 2002;36(1):227–42.
2. Frieden TR, Ozick L, McCord C, Nainan OV, Workman S, Comer G, et al. Chronic liver disease in central Harlem: the role of alcohol and viral hepatitis. Hepatology. 1999;29(3):883–8.
3. Bell BP, Manos MM, Zaman A, Terrault N, Thomas A, Navarro VJ, et al. The epidemiology of newly diagnosed chronic liver disease in gastroenterology practices in the United States: results from population-based surveillance. Am J Gastroenterol. 2008;103(11):2727–36. quiz 37.
4. Navarro VJ, St Louis T, Bell BZ, Sofair AN. Chronic liver disease in the primary care practices of Waterbury, Connecticut. Hepatology. 2003;38(4):1062.
5. Lazo M, Hernaez R, Eberhardt MS, Bonekamp S, Kamel I, Guallar E, et al. Prevalence of nonalcoholic fatty liver disease in the United States: the Third National Health and Nutrition Examination Survey, 1988–1994. Am J Epidemiol. 2013;178(1):38–45.
6. Younossi ZM, Stepanova M, Afendy M, Fang Y, Younossi Y, Mir H, et al. Changes in the prevalence of the most common causes of chronic liver diseases in the United States from 1988 to 2008. Clin Gastroenterol Hepatol. 2011;9(6):524–30.e1. quiz e60.
7. Everhart JE, Ruhl CE. Burden of digestive diseases in the United States. Part 1: Overall and upper gastrointestinal diseases. Gastroenterology. 2009;136(2):376–86.
8. Vallin M, Guillaud O, Boillot O, Hervieu V, Scoazec JY, Dumortier J. Recurrent or de novo nonalcoholic fatty liver disease after liver transplantation: natural history based on liver biopsy analysis. Liver Transpl. 2014;20(9):1064–71.
9. Davis GL, Albright JE, Cook SF, Rosenberg DM. Projecting future complications of chronic hepatitis C in the United States. Liver Transpl. 2003;9(4):331–8.
10. Nguyen GC, Thuluvath PJ. Racial disparity in liver disease: biological, cultural, or socioeconomic factors. Hepatology. 2008;47(3):1058–66.
11. Chalasani N, Younossi Z, Lavine JE, Diehl AM, Brunt EM, Cusi K, et al. The diagnosis and management of non-alcoholic fatty liver disease: practice Guideline by the American Association for the Study of Liver Diseases, American College of Gastroenterology, and the American Gastroenterological Association. Hepatology. 2012;55(6):2005–23.
12. Carrion AF, Ghanta R, Carrasquillo O, Martin P. Chronic liver disease in the Hispanic population of the United States. Clin Gastroenterol Hepatol. 2011;9(10):834–41. quiz e109-10.
13. Beymer C, Kowdley KV, Larson A, Edmonson P, Dellinger EP, Flum DR. Prevalence and predictors of asymptomatic liver disease in patients undergoing gastric bypass surgery. Arch Surg. 2003;138(11):1240–4.
14. Machado M, Marques-Vidal P, Cortez-Pinto H. Hepatic histology in obese patients undergoing bariatric surgery. J Hepatol. 2006;45(4):600–6.
15. Boza C, Riquelme A, Ibanez L, Duarte I, Norero E, Viviani P, et al. Predictors of nonalcoholic steatohepatitis (NASH) in obese patients undergoing gastric bypass. Obes Surg. 2005;15(8):1148–53.
16. Kanwal F, Kramer JR, Duan Z, Yu X, White D, El-Serag HB. Trends in the burden of nonalcoholic fatty liver disease in a United States cohort of veterans. Clin Gastroenterol Hepatol. 2016;14(2):301–8.e1-2.
17. Williams CD, Stengel J, Asike MI, Torres DM, Shaw J, Contreras M, et al. Prevalence of nonalcoholic fatty liver disease and nonalcoholic steatohepatitis among a largely middle-aged population utilizing ultrasound and liver biopsy: a prospective study. Gastroenterology. 2011;140(1):124–31.
18. Adams LA, Lymp JF, St Sauver J, Sanderson SO, Lindor KD, Feldstein A, et al. The natural history of nonalcoholic fatty liver disease: a population-based cohort study. Gastroenterology. 2005;129(1):113–21.
19. Ekstedt M, Franzen LE, Mathiesen UL, Thorelius L, Holmqvist M, Bodemar G, et al. Long-term follow-up of patients with NAFLD and elevated liver enzymes. Hepatology. 2006;44(4):865–73.

20. Dam-Larsen S, Franzmann M, Andersen IB, Christoffersen P, Jensen LB, Sorensen TI, et al. Long term prognosis of fatty liver: risk of chronic liver disease and death. Gut. 2004;53(5):750–5.
21. Dam-Larsen S, Becker U, Franzmann MB, Larsen K, Christoffersen P, Bendtsen F. Final results of a long-term, clinical follow-up in fatty liver patients. Scand J Gastroenterol. 2009;44(10):1236–43.
22. Dunn W, Xu R, Wingard DL, Rogers C, Angulo P, Younossi ZM, et al. Suspected nonalcoholic fatty liver disease and mortality risk in a population-based cohort study. Am J Gastroenterol. 2008;103(9):2263–71.
23. Matteoni CA, Younossi ZM, Gramlich T, Boparai N, Liu YC, McCullough AJ. Nonalcoholic fatty liver disease: a spectrum of clinical and pathological severity. Gastroenterology. 1999;116(6):1413–9.
24. Rafiq N, Bai C, Fang Y, Srishord M, McCullough A, Gramlich T, et al. Long-term follow-up of patients with nonalcoholic fatty liver. Clin Gastroenterol Hepatol. 2009;7(2):234–8.
25. Stepanova M, Rafiq N, Younossi ZM. Components of metabolic syndrome are independent predictors of mortality in patients with chronic liver disease: a population-based study. Gut. 2010;59(10):1410–5.
26. Denniston MM, Jiles RB, Drobeniuc J, Klevens RM, Ward JW, McQuillan GM, et al. Chronic hepatitis C virus infection in the United States, National Health and Nutrition Examination Survey 2003 to 2010. Ann Intern Med. 2014;160(5):293–300.
27. Armstrong GL, Wasley A, Simard EP, McQuillan GM, Kuhnert WL, Alter MJ. The prevalence of hepatitis C virus infection in the United States, 1999 through 2002. Ann Intern Med. 2006;144(10):705–14.
28. Edlin BR, Eckhardt BJ, Shu MA, Holmberg SD, Swan T. Toward a more accurate estimate of the prevalence of hepatitis C in the United States. Hepatology. 2015;62(5):1353–63.
29. Centers for Disease Control and Prevention. Recommendations for prevention and control of hepatitis C virus (HCV) infection and HCV-related chronic disease. MMWR Recommendations and Reports: Morbidity and Mortality Weekly Report Recommendations and Reports. 1998;47(Rr-19):1–39.
30. Smith BD, Morgan RL, Beckett GA, Falck-Ytter Y, Holtzman D, Ward JW. Hepatitis C virus testing of persons born during 1945–1965: recommendations from the Centers for Disease Control and Prevention. Ann Intern Med. 2012;157(11):817–22.
31. Smith BD, Morgan RL, Beckett GA, Falck-Ytter Y, Holtzman D, Teo CG, et al. Recommendations for the identification of chronic hepatitis C virus infection among persons born during 1945–1965. MMWR Recommendations and Reports: Morbidity and Mortality Weekly Report Recommendations and Reports. 2012;61(Rr-4):1–32.
32. CDC. Surveillance for viral hepatitis—United States, 2013. Atlanta: CDC. https://www.cdc.gov/hepatitis/statistics/2013surveillance/index.htm#tabs-801937-5.
33. Klevens RM, Canary L, Huang X, Denniston MM, Yeo AE, Pesano RL, et al. The burden of hepatitis C infection-related liver fibrosis in the United States. Clin Infect Dis. 2016;63(8):1049–55.
34. Kim WR. The burden of hepatitis C in the United States. Hepatology. 2002;36(5 Suppl 1):S30–4.
35. Kim WR. Epidemiology of hepatitis B in the United States. Hepatology. 2009;49(5 Suppl):S28–34.
36. Goldstein ST, Alter MJ, Williams IT, Moyer LA, Judson FN, Mottram K, et al. Incidence and risk factors for acute hepatitis B in the United States, 1982–1998: implications for vaccination programs. J Infect Dis. 2002;185(6):713–9.
37. Mast EE, Weinbaum CM, Fiore AE, Alter MJ, Bell BP, Finelli L, et al. A comprehensive immunization strategy to eliminate transmission of hepatitis B virus infection in the United States: recommendations of the Advisory Committee on Immunization Practices (ACIP) Part II: immunization of adults. MMWR Recommendations and Reports: Morbidity and Mortality Weekly Report Recommendations and Reports. 2006;55(RR-16):1–33. quiz CE1-4.

38. Roberts H, Kruszon-Moran D, Ly KN, Hughes E, Iqbal K, Jiles RB, et al. Prevalence of chronic hepatitis B virus (HBV) infection in U.S. households: National Health and Nutrition Examination Survey (NHANES), 1988–2012. Hepatology. 2016;63(2):388–97.
39. Wasley A, Kruszon-Moran D, Kuhnert W, Simard EP, Finelli L, McQuillan G, et al. The prevalence of hepatitis B virus infection in the United States in the era of vaccination. J Infect Dis. 2010;202(2):192–201.
40. Mitchell T, Armstrong GL, Hu DJ, Wasley A, Painter JA. The increasing burden of imported chronic hepatitis B—United States, 1974–2008. PLoS One. 2011;6(12):e27717.
41. Everhart JE, editor. Liver disease (Chapter 21). In: The burden of digestive diseases in the United States. US Department of Health and Human Services, Public Health Service, National Institutes of Health, National Institute of Diabetes and Digestive and Kidney Diseases. Washington, DC: US Government Printing Office; 2008, NIH Publication No. 09-6443.
42. Bellentani S, Saccoccio G, Costa G, Tiribelli C, Manenti F, Sodde M, et al. Drinking habits as cofactors of risk for alcohol induced liver damage. The Dionysos Study Group. Gut. 1997;41(6):845–50.
43. Mann RE, Smart RG, Govoni R. The epidemiology of alcoholic liver disease. Alcohol Res Health. 2003;27(3):209–19.
44. Caetano R, Kaskutas LA. Changes in drinking patterns among whites, blacks and Hispanics, 1984-1992. J Stud Alcohol. 1995;56(5):558–65.
45. Galvan FH, Caetano R. Alcohol use and related problems among ethnic minorities in the United States. Alcohol Res Health. 2003;27(1):87–94.
46. Dawson DA, Grant BF, Chou SP, Pickering RP. Subgroup variation in U.S. drinking patterns: results of the 1992 national longitudinal alcohol epidemiologic study. J Subst Abuse. 1995;7(3):331–44.
47. Sofair AN, Barry V, Manos MM, Thomas A, Zaman A, Terrault NA, et al. The epidemiology and clinical characteristics of patients with newly diagnosed alcohol-related liver disease: results from population-based surveillance. J Clin Gastroenterol. 2010;44(4):301–7.
48. El-Serag HB, Kanwal F. Epidemiology of hepatocellular carcinoma in the United States: where are we? Where do we go? Hepatology (Baltimore, MD). 2014;60(5):1767–75.
49. Njei B, Rotman Y, Ditah I, Lim JK. Emerging trends in hepatocellular carcinoma incidence and mortality. Hepatology (Baltimore, MD). 2015;61(1):191–9.
50. White DL, Thrift AP, Kanwal F, Davila J, El-Serag HB. Incidence of hepatocellular carcinoma in all 50 United States, from 2000 through 2012. Gastroenterology. 2017;152(4):812–20. e5
51. Ryerson AB, Eheman CR, Altekruse SF, Ward JW, Jemal A, Sherman RL, et al. Annual report to the nation on the status of cancer, 1975–2012, featuring the increasing incidence of liver cancer. Cancer. 2016;122(9):1312–37.
52. Major JM, Sargent JD, Graubard BI, Carlos HA, Hollenbeck AR, Altekruse SF, et al. Local geographic variation in chronic liver disease and hepatocellular carcinoma: contributions of socioeconomic deprivation, alcohol retail outlets, and lifestyle. Ann Epidemiol. 2014;24(2):104–10.
53. Ha NB, Ha NB, Ahmed A, Ayoub W, Daugherty TJ, Chang ET, et al. Risk factors for hepatocellular carcinoma in patients with chronic liver disease: a case-control study. Cancer Causes Control. 2012;23(3):455–62.

Epidemiology of Alcoholic Liver Disease

7

C. Taylor Richardson and Ashwani K. Singal

Abstract

Alcohol abuse is recognized as a major determinant of public health outcomes. The use of alcohol accounted for 5.9% of all deaths worldwide in 2012. Only in the twentieth century has alcohol been found to be a direct hepatotoxin. A dose dependent relationship has been described in many studies across many countries between the consumption of alcohol and the development of alcoholic liver disease.

There is not a clear consumption threshold for development of liver disease, which spans a spectrum from steatosis to steatohepatitis to fibrosis to cirrhosis. Other factors for development of cirrhosis include type of alcohol, pattern of drinking, gender, age, ethnicity, obesity, viral hepatitis, genetics, smoking, coffee, and hepatic iron overload.

Worldwide data from 2010 indicate greater than 1 million deaths (2% of all deaths) and 31 million disability adjusted life years (DALYs) lost were related to liver cirrhosis and alcohol contributed to 493,300 of those deaths (47.9%). Often alcoholic liver disease affects a relatively more productive middle-aged cohort relative to other liver diseases and this effect poses unique societal and economic costs.

Regional variations in consumption and public policy have provided outcomes worthy of study and understanding the epidemiology of alcoholic liver disease is important to this end. In countries where the per capita consumption of alcohol decreases, there appears to be an associated drop in the burden of disease. Avoidance of alcohol remains the best treatment of alcoholic liver disease and the burden of this lethal disease is preventable.

C. Taylor Richardson · A. K. Singal (✉)
Division of Gastroenterology and Hepatology, Department of Medicine, University of Alabama at Birmingham, Birmingham, AL, USA
e-mail: asingal@uabmc.edu

R. J. Wong, R. G. Gish (eds.), *Clinical Epidemiology of Chronic Liver Diseases*,
https://doi.org/10.1007/978-3-319-94355-8_7

Keywords
Alcoholic cirrhosis · Alcoholic hepatitis · Liver cirrhosis · Liver cancer · Prevalence of disease · Burden of disease · Epidemiology

7.1 Introduction

The pathologic consumption of alcohol remains a major determinant of public health outcomes. Alcohol abuse is defined by a pattern of alcohol consumption that causes damage to physical and/or mental health. Alcohol dependence is defined as a syndrome that develops after repeated alcohol use which includes a strong desire to consume alcohol, difficulties in controlling its use, persistent use despite harmful consequences, increased tolerance, and sometimes a physiological withdrawal state. The *Diagnostic and Statistical Manual of Mental Disorders* (DSM) 5 combines alcohol use and dependence into a single entity called “alcohol use disorder”. In terms of specific amounts, heavy drinking is typically defined as three or more drinks per day in men and two or more drinks per day in women, where one drink equates to about 15 g of alcohol. Using this definition and given weight by volume percent alcohol content, one drink is contained in 12 ounces of beer (5% weight/volume or w/v), 6 ounces of wine (8% w/v), or 1.5 ounces of hard liquor (45% w/v) (Table 7.1) [1].

According to the World Health Organization (WHO), harmful use of alcohol is a factor in over 200 diseases and injuries, and one of the top five risk factors for disease. WHO data from 2012 show that alcohol accounted for 5.9% of all deaths and 5.1% of the global burden of disease measured in DALYs (disability-adjusted life years), with a total of 3.3 million deaths attributable to alcohol [2]. According to this data, alcohol has become the fifth leading cause of premature death and disability in 2010 (up from eighth place in 1990). Alcohol was outpaced only by hypertension, tobacco smoking, pollution, and diets low in fruit; while scoring higher than elevated body mass index, high fasting plasma glucose, and physical inactivity [3]. While this chapter will focus on alcoholic liver disease, it is important to remember the ill effects of pathologic alcohol consumption on multiple other organ systems (Table 7.2).

Table 7.1 National Institute on Alcohol Abuse and Alcoholism (NIAAA) definition of a standard drink

One drink of 1.5 oz. hard liquor	14 g alcohol
One glass or 5–6 oz. of wine	11 g alcohol
One 12 oz. can of beer	12.8 g alcohol

Table 7.2 Conditions associated with alcohol use

A.	Liver disease: fatty liver, steatohepatitis, alcoholic hepatitis, cirrhosis, and liver cancer
B.	Cardiovascular diseases: dilated cardiomyopathy, arrhythmias, hypertension
C.	Neurological diseases: stroke, neuropathy, myopathy, epilepsy, withdrawal
D.	Psychological diseases: depression, anxiety, psychosis
E.	Gastrointestinal diseases: pancreatitis, pancreatic cancer, malabsorption, alcoholic diarrhea
F.	Malignancy: oropharyngeal, esophagus, breast, liver, prostate, liver, pancreas
G.	Miscellaneous: psoriasis, sucicide, violence, abortion, fetal alcohol syndrome

7.2 Natural History of Alcoholic Liver Disease

The most common histologic abnormality in patients with harmful alcohol use is hepatic steatosis or alcoholic fatty liver. More than 90% of heavy drinkers develop macrovesicular or microvesicular steatosis without necrosis or inflammation [4]. These changes can occur within only two weeks of alcohol intake, but fortunately can resolve rapidly with complete alcohol cessation [5]. While the damage may be reversible, the presence of hepatic steatosis may not always be benign. One study showed that patients with hepatic steatosis alone have a 10% risk of progressing to cirrhosis and an 18% risk of progressing to fibrosis or cirrhosis over a median time period of 10.5 years. These risks were dramatically increased with heavier alcohol consumption [6].

Alcoholic hepatitis or steatohepatitis occurs less commonly than steatosis, and typically requires a heavier exposure to alcohol to develop. The true prevalence of this spectrum of disease is difficult to estimate, as many of these patients do not have any clinical symptoms with no epidemiologic reports available on patients with early alcoholic liver disease. In one study, histologic inflammation and necrosis consistent with alcoholic steatohepatitis was found in one-third of heavy drinkers [7]. Patients with alcoholic hepatitis will generally progress to cirrhosis at a rate of 10–20% a year and about 80–100% of patients with alcoholic hepatitis have or will eventually progress to cirrhosis [8, 9]. It is important to note that not all patients that progress from steatosis to cirrhosis will develop steatohepatitis.

Advanced fibrosis and cirrhosis is defined histologically by the presence of bridging fibrosis and the distortion of hepatic architecture with regeneration nodules. Alcohol remains the most common cause of cirrhosis and contributes to the highest proportion of cirrhosis mortality as compared to other liver diseases. According to 2009 data in the United States, 48% of all cirrhotic deaths were related to alcohol [10]. The five-year survival rate for compensated (no encephalopathy, variceal bleeding, or ascites) cirrhotics is 90% with alcohol cessation and 70% with persistent drinking. In decompensated cirrhotics, the five-year survival decreases to 60% with alcohol cessation and 30% with persistent drinking [1].

7.3 Historical Perspective of Alcohol Use

Alcohol has been present in human society for more than 10,000 years and initially served as a source of both water and calories at a time when available water sources were often contaminated and unreliable. Fermented alcoholic beverages were limited in their alcohol content by the ability of the yeasts to survive at higher alcoholic concentrations. This fact changes in the twelfth century in Europe when distillation was described allowing for the production of spirits [11].

Traditionally alcohol was produced and consumed on a same scale in the household where drinking occurred as communal activity. This pattern began to change with early industrialization in the European empires. With the development of distilled spirits and increased productive capacity, alcohol became more of a commodity. Effort was devoted to the promotion of alcohol and transportation improvements facilitated increased distribution and availability [12]. By the nineteenth century, many industrial leaders in modernizing countries viewed rampant alcohol abuse as an impediment to a sober and productive workforce.

As social leaders began to recognize the public health implications of changing alcohol consumption patterns, temperance movements gained some political traction in certain countries [2]. For example, the United States enacted a nation-wide ban on the production, importation, and sale of alcoholic beverages during the period of Prohibition from 1920 to 1933. Interestingly, the cirrhosis mortality rate in the United States, which had peaked in 1911, decreased significantly during Prohibition. After its ultimate repeal in 1933, both the per-capita consumption of alcohol and cirrhosis related mortality increased. A similar phenomenon occurred in Europe during the First and Second World Wars when rationing of alcohol was enforced [13].

At the turn of the twentieth century, the relationship between heavy drinking and increased mortality was beginning to be described. It was initially proposed that health outcomes were affected secondarily through poor nutrition in those who over indulged in alcohol. In the 1930s, lab rats were fed large amounts of alcohol and were discovered to subsequently develop liver disease [14]. The biochemical basis of alcohol as a primary hepatotoxin began to be established in the 1960s. It was understood that the oxidation of ethanol and profound metabolic effects on the liver contributed to development of liver disease as a result of harmful alcohol use [15]. These findings underscored the basis for further study of the misuse of alcohol at the population and global level.

7.4 Alcohol Consumption

Alcohol consumption is typically reported as per capita consumption, or the amount of alcohol consumed in liters per person. There are several limitations in the reporting of alcohol consumption. Individual studies often rely on self-reporting, which often are underestimates of true alcohol consumption. Global studies of disease burden often rely on ICD codes, which are not used consistently across the world.

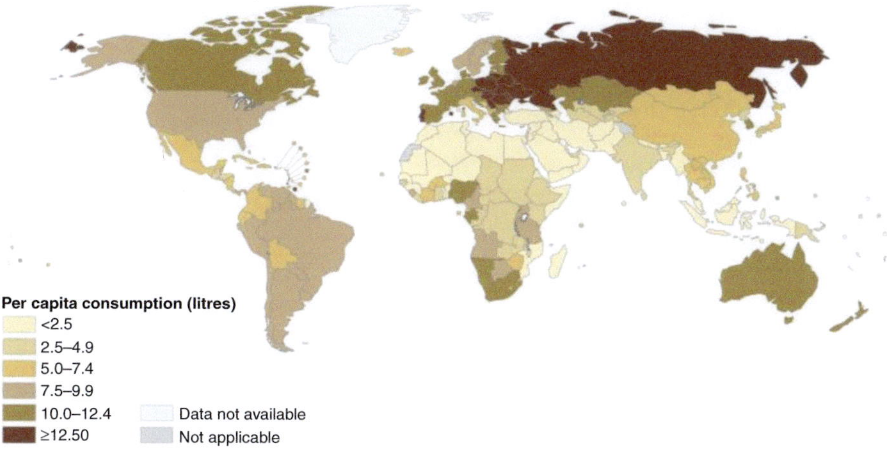

Fig. 7.1 Total alcohol consumed per capita consumption (L alcohol) in 15+ year/old in 2010. Reproduced with permission. World Health Organization. Global status report on alcohol and health. Geneva, Switzerland: World Health Organization; 2014

Review of ICD codes may also not capture individuals who do not seek medical care, of which alcohol abusers may be over represented. Lastly, reporting of national consumption figures rely on calculations of legal sales of alcohol, which do not account for alcohol that is illegally produced, smuggled, or home-brewed [1].

According to the most recent WHO data [2], about half of the world's population over 15 years old (48%) has never consumed alcohol, and 61.7% have not consumed alcohol in the past 12 months. Individuals drink on average 6.2 L of pure alcohol per year or 13.5 g of pure alcohol per day. Figure 7.1 shows the per capita consumption across WHO member states. The highest rates of drinking are in Eastern Europe and the former Soviet Union, while some of the lowest rates are seen in countries with significant Islamic populations (i.e. the Middle East and Southeast Asia). The type of alcohol consumed also has some geographic variation. Globally, 50.1% of total alcohol is spirits followed by beer (34.8%), wine (8%), and other (7.1%).

Countries with the highest consumption are not necessarily those where drinking rates are increasing (Fig. 7.2). Alcohol consumption in North America and Europe remains more or less stable over time. In the United States, 67.3% of the population over the age of 18 drinks alcohol each year and 7.4% of the U.S. population meets criteria for alcohol abuse or alcoholism [16]. Data from the U.S. National Institute on Alcohol Abuse and Alcoholism indicate a decrease in per capita consumption from the early 1980s to 1998 and then a slight uptrend since that time from 2.14 gallon/year to 2.18 gallon/year in 2001 [17]. In the countries that compose the European Union, one-fifth of the population over the age of 15 reported heavy episodic drinking (five or more drinks on an occasion or 60 g alcohol) at least once a week [2].

Perhaps more alarming, is that largely populated, developing countries like China and India are seeing significant growth in their per capita consumption of alcohol.

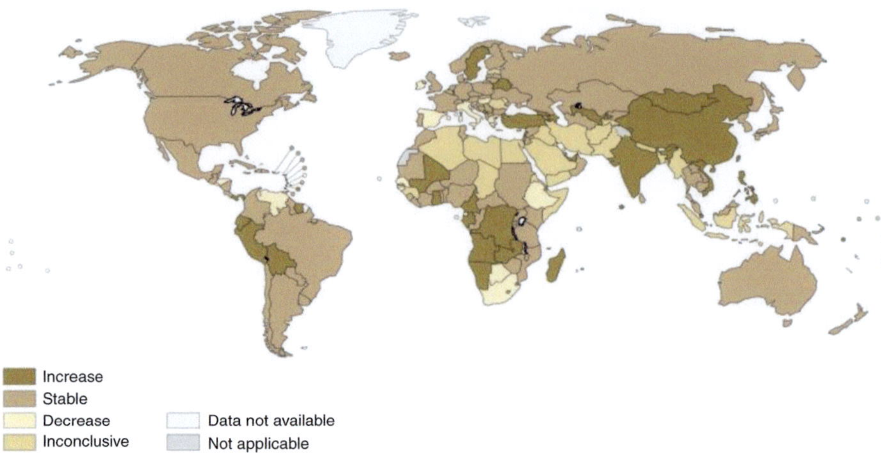

Fig. 7.2 Five-year change in recorded alcohol per capita (15+ years), 2006–2010. Reproduced with permission. World Health Organization. Global status report on alcohol and health. Geneva, Switzerland: World Health Organization; 2014

Drinking patterns in these countries reflect an increase in the use of spirits and episodic heavy drinking. In China, per capita consumption from 2003–2005 to 2008–2010 rose from 4.9 to 6.7 L of alcohol annually, with 69% of all alcohol consumed in the form of spirits. In India, per capita consumption from 2003–2005 to 2008–2010 rose from 3.6 to 4.3 L of alcohol annually, with 93% of all alcohol consumed in the form of spirits [2]. Projections by the WHO forecast that this trend will continue and suggest that increased marketing and disposable incomes may be factors in this change.

7.5 How Alcohol Causes Liver Disease?

Multiple studies have showed a dose dependent relationship between alcohol and the development of alcoholic liver disease. In 1974, Lelbach studied 319 alcoholics in Germany and discovered a relationship between the presence and severity of liver disease and the patient's mean daily alcohol intake and average duration of use. Patients with normal liver function had drank a mean 90 mg of alcohol per kg of body weight for an average duration of 7.7 years, and those with uncomplicated fatty liver had also drank a mean 109 mg of alcohol per kg of body weight for an average of 7.8 years. In contrast, individuals who developed liver cirrhosis consumed 147 mg of alcohol per kg of body weight for an average duration of 17.1 years [14]. More recently, the Dionysos study proposed that alcoholic liver disease does not develop below a lifetime alcohol ingestion of 100 kg, equivalent to an average daily alcohol intake of 30 g for 10 years. The Dionysos group selected two towns in Northern Italy (Compogaliano, Modena and Cormons, Gorizia) and studied 6917 of the 10,151 total inhabitants (70%) starting in 1991. Alcohol consumption was recorded on the basis of questionnaires and the subject's responses were validated by interviewing family members and the local alcohol sales during the time period of the study. The presence of liver disease was determined based on thorough history, physical exam, blood testing, and ultrasound of the liver if indicated. The study findings showed significant changes in the odds ratio for cirrhosis in persons who consumed greater than 30 g of alcohol daily, with dose dependent increase in the risk of liver disease. For consumption of 31–60 g/day and for >120 g/day the odds were 10.9 and 63.2, respectively [18].

Critiques of the Dionysos cohort have centered on whether the results of a Northern Italian cohort can be generalized to the rest of the world. A review of the mortality from cirrhosis in France between 1925 and 1964 showed that 14 per 100,000 persons who drank less than 80 g of alcohol daily died from cirrhosis as compared to 357 per 100,000 persons who drank more than 160 g of alcohol daily [19]. While an exact pathologic daily dose may be debated, there is sufficient evidence that above some amount of alcohol consumption, one has a progressive dose dependent risk for developing alcoholic liver disease and increased mortality in excess of any cardioprotective benefits of moderate alcohol use. The National Institute on Alcohol Abuse and Alcoholism, recommends no more than 28 g of alcohol daily for men (2 drinks) and 14 g of alcohol daily for women (1 drink). Many other factors outside of the volume and duration of alcohol consumed also appear to affect the development of liver disease given that only 8–20% of chronic alcoholics develop cirrhosis [20]. Factors including the amount of alcohol, pattern of alcohol, type of alcohol, host factors, and environmental factors may influence progression to advanced liver disease and cirrhosis.

7.6 Factors Associated with the Development of Alcoholic Liver Disease (Fig. 7.3)

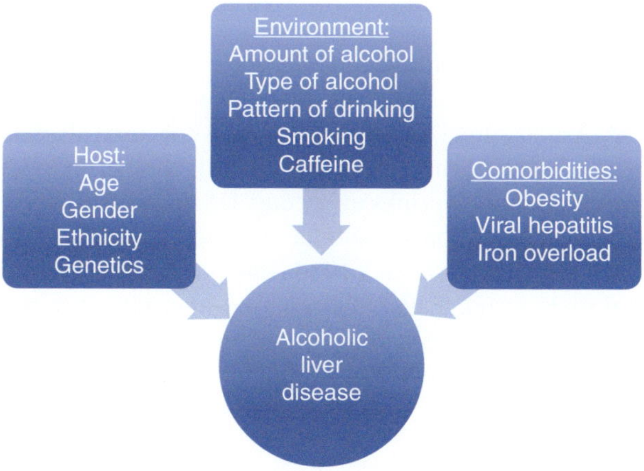

Fig. 7.3 Disease modifiers and co-actors associated with the development of alcoholic liver disease

7.6.1 Type of Alcohol

Many studies have examined association of the type of beverage consumed (i.e. beer, wine spirits) with the development of liver disease. In one study during the first half of the twentieth century in the United States, Canada, and the United Kingdom, an association was noted between mortality from liver cirrhosis and the variable consumption of wine and spirits [21]. However, the Dionysus study did not find a relationship between the choice of beer, wine, or spirits and the development of cirrhosis.

In a pooled data between 1953 and 1993 from Australia, Canada, New Zealand, United Kingdom, and United States, association between beverage specific alcohol consumption and cirrhosis mortality was analyzed. As expected, total alcohol consumption was significantly related to cirrhosis mortality rates. A 1 L increase in per capita alcohol consumption was associated with a 16% increase in cirrhosis mortality. Using attributable fraction analysis, total alcohol was found to account for 67% of cirrhosis deaths. When the analysis was stratified by beverage type, the beverage specific model coefficient was only statistically significant for spirits as opposed to beer and wine. Attributable fractions to cirrhosis mortality were 41% for spirits, 13% for wine, and 8% for beer [22]. Specifically in the United States, it has been noted that mortality from cirrhosis rose from 1950 to 1973 and then began to fall, but paradoxically per capita alcohol consumption continue to rise until 1980. While there are many explanations for this apparent discrepancy, closer analysis showed that per capita consumption of spirits followed the trend in cirrhosis mortality [23]. It is speculated that differences in behavioral patterns on drinking alcohol in spirit drinkers may explain the increased risk for liver disease. United States data suggest that consumers of spirits are older, less educated, and heavier drinkers, and that they more frequently engage in episodic heavy drinking and the use of alcohol without food [24–26]

7.6.2 Pattern of Drinking

Most population data is commonly reported in per capita amount or volume of alcohol consumed. However, given for equal amounts of alcohol consumed, drinking patterns may vary. For example, one individual may consume alcohol only 2 days a week but 7 drinks on each of these days. In contrast, another individual may drink all days of the week but only 2 drinks every day. Do these two individuals have different risk for liver disease in spite of similar amounts of total alcohol consumed? A study of over 5000 respondents from a 1984 National Alcohol Survey in the United States found that male respondents who reported intermittent heavy occasions of drinking (>8 drinks) or drinking to the point of intoxication were found to have a 70% increased risk of mortality while adjusting for age and ethnicity. The same pattern was present for females, but to a lesser degree [27]. It must be noted that all-cause mortality including mortality from accidents and injuries was reported in this study and not mortality specifically from liver disease.

The Dionysus group reported the effect of drinking pattern on the development of alcoholic liver disease in their Northern Italian cohort. On multivariate analysis, they showed that independent of the amount of alcohol consumed, those who drank multiple types of alcohol and alcohol outside of meal times had increased risk of liver disease. For those who drank multiple types of alcohol beverages, the odds ratio for cirrhosis was 23.2 compared to those who drank only one form of alcohol. For those who drank outside of meals, the odds ratio for non-cirrhotic liver disease was 5.0 and the odds ratio for cirrhosis was 3.4 [28]. A speculated mechanism for the differential risk of liver disease with pattern and type of alcohol use is that above particular blood alcohol content (BAC), the usual metabolic pathway for alcohol is overwhelmed with increased risk of alcohol related hepatotoxicity [29]. Thus, intuitively, it makes sense that binge drinking could be a factor in developing associated liver injury relative to other drinking patterns that do not achieve a similar BAC.

As epidemiologic studies suggest increased rates of cirrhosis in countries with a stronger tradition of binge drinking, there has also been research into cellular mechanisms for liver injury in binge drinking. Studies in rodents have shown decrease in hepatic glutathione after binging, which results in increased oxidative stress and damage to hepatic mitochondrial DNA. Recurrent hepatic mitochondrial degradation with repeated episodes of binging ultimately overwhelms the typical repair mechanisms. Other consequences of binge drinking include increased intestinal permeability, FAS-L expression leading to hepatic apoptosis, and sinusoidal endothelial cell dysfunction leading to ischemic injury [30].

7.6.3 Age

While not entirely understood, it is believed that children and the elderly are more susceptible to alcohol related harm from a given quantity of alcohol. A report in 2002 estimated that 19.7% of all alcohol was by underage drinkers [31]. Importantly from a public policy standpoint, it is known that those who consume alcohol earlier in life are at higher risk for engaging in heavy episodic drinking, and for developing problematic drinking habits later in life. WHO data shows that largest proportion of alcohol attributed deaths is in the age group from 40 to 49 years old. The age group at highest risk for hospitalization due to alcoholic liver disease is 45–64 years, with a prevalence of 94.8 per 10,000, while the prevalence among individuals aged 25–44 years is 60.4 per 10,000 [1]. Policy efforts in many countries aim to curtail the use of alcohol amongst youth by restricting access and marketing and setting a legal age limit for consumption. Additionally, there has been increased awareness for the existence of alcohol abuse among the elderly, and a need for screening in this population to prevent alcohol related harm.

7.6.4 Gender

In all parts of the world, men consume alcohol more frequently and are less likely to abstain as compared to women, with more frequent alcoholic liver disease and resultant mortality and morbidity among men. According to data from the WHO, trends on alcohol consumption show increasing alcohol use in women, likely due to

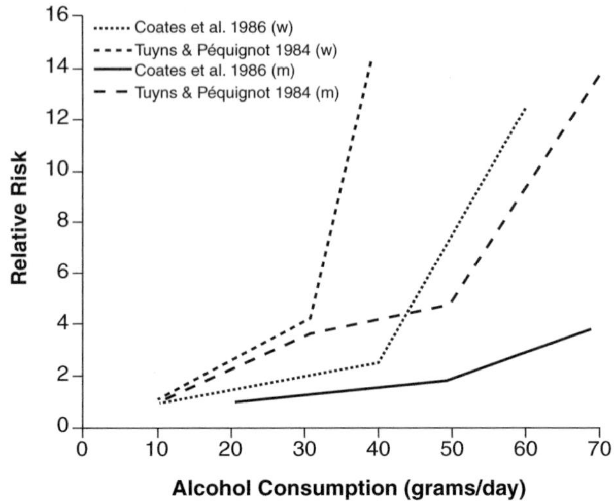

Fig. 7.4 Alcohol consumption and incidence of cirrhosis of liver in men (m) and women (w). Reproduced with permission. Mann et al. The epidemiology of alcoholic liver disease. Alcohol Research and Health. 2003; 27:212

redefinition of traditional gender roles [2]. Outside of gender based differences in drinking patterns and behaviors, women as compared to men are more susceptible to alcohol induced liver injury, with women developing advanced liver disease at a much lower amount of alcohol consumed compared to men (Fig. 7.4). In men, the risk of cirrhosis increases with daily alcohol intake greater than 40–80 g per day, but for women this figure is 20–60 g per day [1].

One explanation of this finding is that women achieve a higher BAC relative to men for a given amount of alcohol consumed and thus potentiates increased hepatotoxicity. It has been described that the gastric levels of alcohol dehydrogenase may be lower in females, resulting in decreased gastric oxidation of ethanol, decreased first pass metabolism, and increased systemic bioavailability [32]. Females also have a lower body size with increased percentage of body fat and decreased proportion of body water compared to men. Given that alcohol is water soluble, women will have higher blood levels for a given amount of alcohol consumed [33]. Estrogen is also thought to play a role. Alcohol is thought to make the gut leaky allowing for increased endotoxin levels in the portal blood flow that stimulate an inflammatory response in the liver resulting in hepatotoxicity. In rat models, estrogen has been shown to augment this inflammatory response. Rats who had been ovarectomized were relatively protected from histiologic liver injury after being fed ethanol and this effect was ultimately reversed with administration of exogenous estrogen hormone [34]. Other genetic factors may be involved in gender specific differences in alcohol metabolism and further research is ongoing.

7.6.5 Ethnicity

In the first part of the twentieth century, cirrhosis mortality rates were higher for whites than non-whites in the United States. This pattern reversed by the 1950s, with higher mortality rates from alcoholic cirrhosis among blacks and Hispanics as compared to whites. These findings were true for both men and women [35]. A longitudinal epidemiologic study of alcohol use in the United States in 1992 did not find significant differences in the prevalence of heavy drinking between whites, blacks, and Hispanics [36]. Demographic characteristics like income, education, employment, access to healthcare resources, and increased prevalence of chronic viral hepatitis have also been speculated to be possible explanations.

7.6.6 Obesity

The role of obesity in the development of alcoholic liver disease has been debated. Data from the Dionysus study from Northern Italy, with 25% prevalence of obesity in their cohort showed 2.8-fold risk for steatosis in non-obese heavy drinkers compared to non-obese non-drinker controls. The odds were 4.6-fold for obese, non-drinkers and 5.8 for obese heavy drinkers [18].

In a cohort of over 1600 French alcoholics with alcohol use of >50 g alcohol/day over the preceding year, being overweight (BMI >27 in males and >25 in females) was independently correlated with the presence of cirrhosis. Of 172 (10%) of overweight individuals, 60% had cirrhosis compared to 35% prevalence of cirrhosis among non-overweight patients ($P < 0.001$). On multivariate analysis, being overweight for >10 years was associated with 2.15-fold risk of cirrhosis relative to a non-overweight person, after adjusting for age, sex, amount and duration of alcohol consumption [37].

Obesity is known to be a predictor of fibrosis in non-alcoholic fatty liver disease and been shown to predict fibrosis in alcoholic liver disease as well. A group of 268 French alcoholics without chronic hepatitis underwent liver biopsy to assess for degree of fibrosis. After adjusting for daily alcohol use and duration of use, the authors found that BMI, fasting plasma glucose, and iron overload were all significantly associated with higher fibrosis scores [38]. This finding raises considerations for counseling and treatment especially in light of the growing, worldwide epidemic of obesity.

7.6.7 Viral Hepatitis

Concomitant hepatitis C virus (HCV) infection potentiates the development of alcoholic liver disease in heavy drinkers. The prevalence of HCV infection in alcoholics is high at 16–34%. Patients with HCV and alcohol abuse are more likely to develop more frequent and faster progression to advanced fibrosis or cirrhosis, complications of liver disease, and hepatocellular carcinoma. A study of patients with chronic HCV infection showed that severity of histologic injury was more likely to progress to worsening fibrosis or cirrhosis in patients with even moderate drinking. An alcohol use of 31–50 g per day in men and 21–50 g per day in women was independently associated with progression of liver injury [39]. A review of data from the Nationwide

Inpatient Sample dataset in the United States from 1998 to 2007 showed that in patients admitted with acute alcoholic hepatitis, infection with HCV was an independent predictor of mortality with and OR of 1.29 [40]. Additionally, in the era of interferon treatment, it was shown that alcohol use during therapy decreased response rates [41].

The interaction between HCV and alcohol in the development of cirrhosis has been shown to be multiplicative as opposed to additive, indicating synergy in creating pathology [42]. Patients with HCV infection should be counseled to completely abstain of alcohol, as even minimal or moderate alcohol use has been shown to be detrimental.

The effect of hepatitis B virus (HBV) on alcoholic liver disease is less well understood. Two small studies in the 1980s showed a higher prevalence of HBV infection [43, 44]. A larger case-control study from the same time period showed that alcohol use and unresolved HBV infection were independently associated with development of cirrhosis; however synergistic association could not be established as for HCV infection [45]. A more recent study from Portugal showed that alcohol use in patients with chronic HBV infection was associated with more severe liver disease [46]. In a case control study from Albania, that included about 300 patients, synergistic association was shown for patients with increased alcohol use (>67 g alcohol per day) and hepatitis B surface antigen positivity for the development of cirrhosis [47].

Based on pre-clinical data, alcohol use has been shown to augment signaling pathways resulting in higher replication of both HCV and HBV with more severe liver injury [48, 49]. Acetaldehyde derived from alcohol metabolism and micro-RNA upregulation by alcohol consumption both have been shown to inhibit the interferon-gamma pathway, a known mechanism for HCV clearance [50]. Further, damage associated molecular proteins released as a result of HCV related cell injury and oxidative stress mediated by both alcohol and HCV infection contribute to more severe liver injury with faster progression to fibrosis [51].

7.6.8 Genetic Factors

Genes involved in the metabolism of alcohol including genes encoding for alcohol dehydrogenase (ADH2, ADH3), aldehyde dehydrogenase (ALDH2), and microsomal ethanol oxidation system (cytochrome P4502E1 [CYP2E1]) have been examined for their association with development of alcoholic liver disease. In one study from Japan, a specific polymorphism of the ADH gene (ADH2*2) was associated with the development of alcoholism and alcoholic cirrhosis [52]. A meta-analysis of studies looking at possible effects of ADH2 and ADH3 genes on the risk of developing alcoholic liver disease showed an association with ADH2 allele type, especially in Asian subjects [53]. However, a subsequent Korean study did not show an association between ADH polymorphisms and the development of alcoholic cirrhosis [54].

There is a variant in the gene encoding aldehyde dehydrogenase, ALDH2*2, that has been found in Japanese, Taiwanese, and Han Chinese populations to result in severe reduction in its activity with increased levels of acetaldehyde after alcohol consumption. This allele appears to protect against alcohol dependence due to the aversive symptoms of acetaldehyde during drinking [29]. Rates of alcoholic cirrhosis are believed to be about 70% reduced in populations with ALDH2*2 [55].

In another study from China, allelic variants of the cytochrome P450 system were not associated with risk of alcoholic liver disease [56]. Data from the Dionysus cohort showed association of one allele C2 of CYP2E1 and homozygosity of ADH3*2 allele with risk of alcoholic liver disease [18]. In a study from Mexico, the C2 allele of CYP2E1 was associated with alcoholic cirrhosis relative to healthy control and also to the severity of liver damage suggesting possible prognostic value. The believed mechanism for injury stems from the propensity for alcohol induced oxidative stress and the resultant detrimental accumulation of acetaldehyde [57]. These studies are limited by small sample size and have yielded contradictory responses, underscoring need for further research.

Most recently, a systematic review and meta-analysis reviewed the relationship between a genetic polymorphism in the patatin-like phospholiapse domain protein 3 (PNPLA3) genes. An association between a specific mutation in PNPLA3 and increased hepatic fat content had been described. The pooled analysis of ten prior studies showed increased odds ratio for the presence of alcoholic liver injury, alcoholic cirrhosis, and hepatocellular carcinoma in patients with the studied polymorphism [58]. Further research into a genetic basis for alcoholic liver disease is ongoing and may have both screening and therapeutic implications.

7.6.9 Smoking

Smoking has been negatively associated with multiple medical conditions including development of liver disease. In a large Danish cohort of over 18,000 patients followed for over 20 years, smoking was associated with risk of liver disease from alcohol [59]. However, the relationship of smoking to liver disease is confounded due to the relationship of smoking to alcohol use. In this Danish study, smokers carried a higher risk of cirrhosis after adjusting for confounders including alcohol consumption [59]. In another case control study, smoking was associated with development of hepatocellular carcinoma, with risk increasing with degree of smoking. The impact of smoking and alcohol was multiplicative, suggesting a possible mechanism of carcinogenesis that is enhanced by the combination [60].

7.6.10 Coffee

Coffee is among the most consumed beverages in the world and has been recently shown to be protective from liver disease. A meta-analysis of nine studies found a relative risk of 0.56 for developing cirrhosis (of any type) in patients that consumed at least two cups of coffee a day [61]. These findings do not hold up in other caffeinated beverages and it is believed that the benefit is derived from coffee's antioxidant properties, which exerts an anti-fibrotic effect. In a recent study on a large population, consumption of more than 4 cups of coffee was associated 80% reduction in the development of alcoholic cirrhosis [62].

7.6.11 Iron

Iron overload negatively impacts the outcome of patients with alcoholic liver disease with more frequent progression to cirrhosis and development of hepatocellular carcinoma. In a French cohort, hepatic iron scores were associated with the development of hepatocellular carcinoma in alcoholic cirrhotics, and not in HCV related cirrhosis [63]. An exact mechanism of iron induced carcinogenesis is not understood, but it is hypothesized that iron results in oxidative stress and increased DNA mutations. Interestingly, the amount of alcohol consumed by the patient did not correlate with the burden of iron overload. Although, HFE gene mutations may play a role in mediating iron overload, the frequency of these mutations is not higher among alcoholics as compared to general population [63].

Hepcidin influences iron metabolism in that it blocks intestinal uptake of iron and release of iron by macrophages, effectively serving as a negative regulator. Hepcidin is produced in the liver and it is thought that oxidative stress and tissue hypoxia from chronic alcohol use suppresses its production. In a cohort of over 200 patients with alcoholic cirrhosis, lower hepcidin levels were associated with a statistically significant higher risk of hepatocellular carcinoma and death over the study period (hazard ratios 1.7 and 1.6, respectively). On multivariate analysis, lower hepcidin was independently associated with death in these patients [64].

7.7 Magnitude and Burden of Alcoholic Liver Disease

The prevalence of cirrhosis and the mortality from cirrhosis are associated with alcohol consumption throughout the world. Alcohol attributed costs (not isolated to solely liver disease) are tremendous with total costs estimated at 125 billion Euros in the European Union in 2003 and 233 billion dollars in the United States in 2006 [65, 66]. These figures have been noted to constitute 1.3–3.3% of gross domestic product [67].

While the costs of alcohol as a whole are staggering, the epidemiologic data pertaining to alcoholic liver disease and cirrhosis are equally troubling. In the United States in 2009, 48.2% of all cirrhosis deaths were alcohol related with most (70.6%) among individuals aged 35–44 [68]. Clearly, alcoholic liver disease disproportionately affects individuals in their most productive years of life, resulting in significant direct and indirect social costs. Centers for Disease Control (CDC) data from 2006 to 2010 attributed an average annual rate of 87,798 deaths and 2,560,290 years of potential life lost to excessive drinking. Tallying an economic cost of 223.5 billion dollars in 2006, this equated to a $1.90 cost per alcohol beverage consumed [69]. While the total cost to society is enormous, the direct healthcare costs are also concerning. An admission for acute alcoholic hepatitis, one of the more severe presentations of alcoholic liver disease, costs an average of $46,264 and resulted in a 6.1 day length of stay in 2010 in US hospitals [70].

The pattern in Europe is similar to the United States, with alcohol being the most common cause for advanced liver disease. In the United Kingdom, liver disease is the third leading cause of premature mortality and alcohol is responsible for three-quarters of the deaths from liver disease. It was calculated that the National Health Service (NHS) spends approximately £3.5 billion annually on complications related to alcoholic liver disease [71]. A report from Portugal in 2015 studied the admissions for cirrhosis to all state hospitals from 1993 to 2008 and found that 84% of the admissions were related to alcoholic liver disease. Over the time period studied, there was a disproportionate increase in admission for males aged 40–54 with alcoholic cirrhosis. These patients were found to have increased length of stay and mortality relative to the other patients identified [72]. These findings highlight not only the prevalence of alcoholic liver disease and the substantial resultant medical costs, but also the indirect opportunity cost given the relative incidence in middle aged patients who would otherwise be in their most productive years. As opposed to alcohol, non-alcoholic cirrhosis tends to most affect elderly patients.

Given its population, China has a large impact on the worldwide burden of liver disease and it is estimated that nearly 300 million Chinese people suffer from liver disease. Chronic viral hepatitis remains the largest cause of liver disease, but alcohol abuse is increasing and treatment and screening programs for viral hepatitis are being put in place. Nationwide epidemiologic data for alcoholic liver disease does not exist, but in specific, regional populations the prevalence has ranged from 2.3% to 6.1% of the total population. The annual incidence of alcoholic liver disease as a cause of hospitalization relative to other types of liver disease is steadily increasing and the number of patients undergoing liver transplantation for alcoholic liver disease is also growing [73].

In 2010 global data, it was found that greater than one million deaths (2% of all deaths) and 31 million disability adjusted life years (DALYs) lost were related to liver cirrhosis. Alcoholic cirrhosis accounted for 493,300 deaths or 47.9% of total cirrhosis related deaths. Alcoholic cirrhosis accounted for 1.2% of all male deaths and 0.7% of all female deaths overall. Central Europe had the highest proportion of alcohol related liver cirrhosis deaths and DALYs relative to total cirrhosis deaths and DALYs with 72.3% and 74.6%, respectively. At the other end of the spectrum, likely due to the influence of Islam, Northern Africa and the Middle East had the lowest proportion of liver cirrhosis deaths and DALYs due to alcohol with 14% and 15.9%, respectively. The incidence of death from alcoholic cirrhosis in 2010 was highest in Central Asia where 17.5 deaths per 100,000 persons occurred due to alcoholic liver disease and it was followed by Central Latin America with 15.8 deaths per 100,000 persons [74]. Epidemiologic studies aiming to understand how these figures have changed over time and the patterns that have emerged have important implications in driving public policy decisions to counteract the burden of alcoholic liver disease.

7.7.1 Worldwide Trends in Alcoholic Liver Disease

Any analysis of trends in the epidemiology of liver disease over the past several decades needs to account for the fact that viral hepatitis B and C were not recognized as distinct clinical entities prior to the 1980s. However, it is informative to look at different experiences around the world as pertains to alcoholic liver disease.

Natural experiments such as Prohibition in the United States or the relative scarcity of alcoholic beverages in Europe during the First World War suggest that a decrease in per capita consumption of alcoholic beverages results in a decrease in population mortality of alcoholic liver disease. An analysis of mortality data from 14 European Union countries from 1950 to 1995 show that, on average, a 1 L increase in per capita consumption was associated with a statistically significant increase in male cirrhosis of 12% and in female cirrhosis of 8%. When stratified by a regional gradient, these findings were more pronounced in Northern Europe and less so for Southern Europe, possibly reflecting a difference in pattern in drinking and/or differences in public policy and legislation at the governmental level. A similar analysis was conducted in Canada and revealed that an increase in 1 L of per capita alcohol consumption resulted in a 16% increase in male mortality and a 12% increase in female mortality [75]. Thus, when thinking about trends in the morbidity and mortality of alcoholic liver disease, it is paramount to consider trends in the consumption of alcohol.

In the United States, a study of alcohol consumption from 1949 to 1994 showed mortality from cirrhosis rose by 75% from 1950 to 1973 when it reached its peak and thereafter began to decline slowly. Per capita alcohol use also rose during this time but it reached its peak in 1980 with a decline thereafter. The authors explained these incongruent findings by showing that mortality more closely paralleled the consumption of spirits [23]. As discussed earlier, spirits may be more dangerous relative to other types of alcohol and may be associated with a more pathologic pattern of drinking. Another explanation offered by the authors was that there was an improvement in the treatment of alcoholism during this time that could account for a decrease in mortality a few years prior to the decrease in consumption [23]. While not discussed in the analysis, it is also worth remembering the possible effect of undiagnosed, chronic viral hepatitis.

United States data from 1970 to 2009 show a decrease in the death rate from cirrhosis from 17.8 to 9.4 deaths per 100,000 people (47.6% decrease). This finding was present across ethnicities and gender though to varying degrees. More specifically, the death rate from alcoholic cirrhosis decreased from 6.3 to 4.5 deaths per 100,000 people (28.6% decreases) [10]. Other than a decrease in alcohol consumption between 1980 and 1998, there was an increase in participation in Alcoholics Anonymous, an increase in the use of liver transplantation to treat alcoholic liver disease, and an increase in the diagnosis of hepatitis C after the introduction of testing in 1991 (patients' hepatitis C related liver disease may have been miscategorized as alcoholic liver disease) [76].

Recent trends in Australia are similar to the United States. From 1991 to 2005, mortality from alcoholic liver disease decreased by 21.7% for men and by 8.3% for women. During this same time period, it was observed that admissions for alcoholic liver disease increased by 20% suggesting either improved access to healthcare or improved healthcare outcomes [77]. According to government statistics, per capita alcohol consumption remained flat during this time period. Total alcohol consumption per capita trended from 10.6 to 10.5 L per year. Consumption of beer decreased, while that of wine and spirits increased.

In Japan, alcoholic liver disease was largely unheard of based on autopsy studies prior to 1955. Per capita annual alcohol consumption from 1955 to 1988 increased sixfold. By 1988, the annual per capita alcoholic consumption was 6.3 L, which is less than most European and North American countries. However, if you excluded persons with ALDH2 the figure approached the level seen in Western countries. Unsurprisingly, the estimated incidence of alcoholic liver disease rose from 5.1% of all liver disease to 14.1% during this time period. Additionally rates of cirrhosis mortality paralleled in the increase in consumption [78].

In Korea per capita alcohol consumption has increased from 1 L in 1960 to 7 L by 1980 with a male per capita consumption of 18.4 L and rate of frequent drinking of 34% among males. The pattern of drinking has also changed from the use of mildly fermented beverages to regular and heavier consumption of distilled spirits. The percent of patients with alcohol as the etiology of their chronic liver disease increased from 1.5% in 1980 to 24% by 1993 [79]. An analysis from 2000 to 2009 showed that the per capita alcohol consumption had increased by 2009 to 8.54 L and that mortality rate for alcoholic liver disease had increased from 2000 to 2009 from 2.98 per 100,000 persons to 7.29 per 100,000 persons. The mortality rate was higher for men and highest in the age range from 40 to 50 years old [80].

India serves as an important example due to the country's recent trends in pathologic alcohol use and its effect on the worldwide burden of disease given the large population. Per capita alcohol use in India by adults has increased 106.7% between the years of 1970–1972 and 1994–1996 [81]. Particularly in young adults, there is a growing culture of heavy and binge drinking. A large survey of cirrhosis admitted to a Northeast Indian hospital found that 72% of diagnosed cases of cirrhosis were related to alcohol. The patients with alcoholic cirrhosis tended to be younger, middle class, male, and non-Muslim relative to the non-alcoholic etiologies. Similar to other countries, this demographic is expected to be a more socially productive group and thus the negative health outcomes has a disproportionate effect on societal costs. They also found that relative to non-alcoholic cirrhosis, the alcoholics tended to have more episodes of hepatic encephalopathy, upper gastrointestinal bleeding, and ascites and secondarily worse overall mortality [82].

As shown above, changes in the incidence of alcoholic liver disease and mortality are affected by drinking patterns and consumption and these trends have geographic variations. There have likewise been changes in the medical treatment of alcohol abuse and liver disease that may have some impact. The identification of viral hepatitis and future treatment will also affect the morbidity and mortality of alcoholic liver disease. Another arena of intervention is that of public policy given the substantial social costs of alcoholic liver disease. Research highlighted by the WHO, found that the most "cost-effective" public policy intervention in terms of decreasing alcohol attributable deaths were taxation of alcoholic beverages, restricting the availability of alcoholic beverages and imposing bans or restrictions on alcohol advertising [2].

For instance, a dramatic increase in taxation of alcoholic products was imposed in 2002. The most common alcoholic beverage in Taiwan at the time was a domestic rice based spirit and in 2002 the rice alcohol tax was $0.73 per liter. The tax was increased to $6.16 per liter by 2003 meaning that retail prices increased sevenfold. There was a dramatic, immediate decrease in alcoholic consumption and analysis of hospital inpatient changes for alcohol attributable diseases showed a corresponding reduction that was sustained for several years despite a prior increasing rate of expenditures for alcoholic disease [83].

Other countries have employed multiple mechanisms for curbing alcohol consumption. There has been use of a legal drinking age, regulation in the density of alcohol selling outlets, and limitations on the days and hours when alcohol can be sold. Governments have also used monopoly and licensing power to control the supply of various alcoholic beverages. Laws against public consumption and drinking and driving further aim to limit the consumption of alcohol. In many countries, advertising in alcohol has been viewed as being causative in driving further consumption and an unhealthy pattern of drinking. Data from the WHO in 2012 from 166 different countries showed that 39.6% of those countries had no restrictions with regard to alcohol advertising while 10.1% imposed total bans with the majority somewhere in between with specific but not total regulation [2]. Enforced labeling of alcoholic beverages with a warning of possible medical risks is another avenue by which some countries warn prospective consumers. Many countries, particularly those with the highest and rising burdens of disease are utilizing the above interventions at population level.

Conclusion

Studying the changes in the epidemiology of alcoholic liver disease has led to many advances including the hypothesis that alcohol was a hepatotoxin in the first place. Understanding current trends is essential in recognizing the current burden of disease and in identifying strategies to combat alcoholic liver disease. Given current consumption patterns, alcohol is likely to remain a primary driver of liver disease for the decades to come. In contrast, hepatitis B now has effective therapies and ultimately there is a goal for universal vaccination against hepatitis B. Just recently, effective and safe therapies for hepatitis C are becoming more available and will likely further shift the epidemiology of liver disease. The connection between obesity and liver disease is now better understood and great deal of research has been performed for the purpose of finding therapies for non-alcoholic fatty liver disease. Projections in the United States suggest that alcohol consumption and the incidence of alcoholic cirrhosis will increase in the upcoming decades [84]. There remains a paucity of therapies directed at alcoholic liver disease.

Medically, the molecular mechanisms of alcoholic liver disease and alcoholic liver injury must be better understood in order to understand possible therapeutic interventions. The best current therapy remains complete abstinence of alcohol. The future of therapeutics for alcoholic liver disease depends on the availability and willingness to conduct clinical trials. It is hoped that with increased research efforts, there may be new drugs for managing this lethal disease. Socially, the opportunity exists for various societies to decide on public policy interventions that can affect the consumption of alcohol with direct health benefits and cost savings. The future of alcoholic liver disease worldwide will be determined by efforts in each of these realms.

Acknowledgments The work is supported by faculty development grant funding to AKS from the American College of Gastroenterology.

Summary Table of Landmark Literature

Study title and authors	Study design	Summary results	Main limitations
Bellentani S, et al. Journal of Hepatology. 1994; 20:1442–1449	Italian cohort study assessing the prevalence of liver disease and attributable risks	• Above the 30 g/day threshold, the incidence of alcoholic liver disease and of cirrhosis increases linearly with increasing alcohol intake	• Limited study population and unclear if results can be generalized to other populations
Corrao G, et al. Addiction Biology. 1998; 3:413–422	Descriptive study that assesses cirrhosis mortality trends in seven Eastern Europe countries relative to Europe as a whole	• In Europe the cirrhosis mortality rates were explained by their relationship with per capita alcohol consumption with a specific lag time	• Descriptive, epidemiologic study that does not address natural history of cirrhosis • Does not account for other factors like viral hepatitis?
Ramstedt M, et al. Addiction. 2001; 96:S19–34	Analysis of yearly changes in gender and age specific mortality rates from 1990 to 1995 in 14 European countries in relation to corresponding yearly changes in per capita alcohol consumption	• There exists a positive and statistically significant effect in changes of per capita consumption on changes in cirrhosis mortality, particularly in northern Europe	• Mortality data based on ICD codes • Per capita consumption data based on alcohol sales
Roizen R, et al. BMJ. 1999; 319:666–669	Trend analysis using data on US cirrhosis mortality and per capita alcohol consumption	• A relationship exists between per capita consumption of distilled spirits and mortality from cirrhosis in the United States	• Relationship between consumption and mortality does not establish a causal relationship

Study title and authors	Study design	Summary results	Main limitations
Kerr W, et al. Addiction. 2000; 95:339–346	Pooled cross-sectional time series analysis to compare beverage specific per capita consumption and cirrhosis mortality in multiple countries	• Associations between mortality and consumption were found for total alcohol and for distilled spirits specifically • Use of spirits may affect mortality more than wine and beer	• Multiple potential confounder factors exist (i.e. those who drink spirits may be more prone to binging, heavier drinking) • Does not establish a causal relationship
Rehm J, et al. Journal of Hepatology. 2013; 59:160–168	Review of global mortality and consumption data to calculate and report the global burden of alcoholic liver disease	• In 2010 alcohol attributable liver disease was responsible for 493,300 deaths and 14,544,000 DALYs	• Reliability of global data on consumption • The role of past consumption to the current burden of disease for a disease like cirrhosis
Naveau S, et al. Hepatology. 1997; 25:108–111	French cohort study to assess whether being overweight was a risk factor for the development of alcoholic liver disease	• In patients with alcohol abuse, being overweight for at least ten years was independently correlated with developing cirrhosis, acute alcoholic hepatitis, and steatosis	• Does not establish a causal relationship
Carrrao G, et al. Hepatology 1998; 27:914–919	Data used from two case control studies in Italy to assess the joint effect of alcohol and hepatitis C infection on the development of cirrhosis	• The interaction between lifetime daily alcohol intake and the presence of the hepatitis c virus was additive for low volume consumers, but multiplicative in high volume consumers suggesting a synergistic effect	• Small study size • Self-reported alcohol use. • Small presence of heavy drinkers who had hepatitis C in the control (non-cirrhosis) group
Singal AK. Eur J Gastroenterol Hepatol. 2012; 24:1178–1184	Data from the US Nationwide Inpatient Sample dataset (1998–2007) reviewed to identify patients with alcoholic hepatitis and factors associated with hepatitis C positivity and mortality	• Hepatitis C infection is an independent predictor of mortality in patients with alcoholic hepatitis	• Does not establish a mechanism for the impact of hepatitis C in patients with alcoholic hepatitis

References

1. Mandayam S, Jamal MM, Morgan TR. Epidemiology of alcoholic liver disease. Semin Liver Dis. 2004;24:217–32.
2. World Health Organization. Global status report on alcohol and health. Geneva, Switzerland: World Health Organization; 2014.
3. Lim SS, Vox T, Flaxman AD, et al. A comparative risk assessment of burden of disease and injury attributable to 67 risk factors and risk factor clusters in 21 regions, 1990–2010: a systematic assessment for the global burden of disease study 2010. Lancet. 2012;380:2224–60.
4. MacSween RN, Burt AD. Histological spectrum of alcoholic liver disease. Semin Liver Dis. 1986;6:221–32.
5. Lane BP, Lieber CS. Ultrastructural alterations in human hepatocytes following ingestion of ethanol with adequate diets. Am J Pathol. 1966;49:593–603.
6. Teli MR, Day CP, Burt AD, Bennett MK, James OF. Determinants of progression to cirrhosis or fibrosis in pure aloholic fatty liver. Lancet. 1995;346:987–90.
7. Barrio E, Tome S, Rodriguez I, et al. Liver disease in heavy drinkers with and without alcohol withdrawal syndrome. Alcohol Clin Exp Res. 2004;28:131–6.
8. Diehl AM. Alcoholic liver disease: natural history. Liver Transpl Surg. 1997;3:206–11.
9. Bird GL, Williams R. Factors determining cirrhosis in alcoholic liver disease. Mol Aspects Med. 1998;10:97–105.
10. Yoon YH. Survellaince report #75: liver cirrhosis mortality in the United States, 1970–2009. Bethesda, MD: National Institute of Alcohol Abuse and Alcoholism; 2009.
11. Schwartz JM, Reinus JF. Prevalence and natural history of alcoholic liver disease. Clin Liver Dis. 2012;16:659–66.
12. Jernigan D. Applying commodity chain analysis to changing modes of alcohol supply in a developing country. Addiction. 2000;95:465–75.
13. Saunders JB, Latt N. Epidemiology of alcoholic liver disease. Baillieres Clin Gastroenterol. 1993;7:555–79.
14. Lelbach WK. Organic pathology related to volume and patterns of alcohol use. In: Gibbins RS, Israel Y, Kalant H, et al., editors. Research advances in alcohol and drug problems, vol. 1. New York; London: Wiley; 1974. p. 93–198.
15. Lieber CS. Biochemical factors in alcoholic liver disease. Semin Liver Dis. 1993;13:136–53.
16. Kim WR, Brown RS Jr, Terrault NA. Burden of liver disease in the United States: summary of a workshop. Hepatology. 2002;36:227–42.
17. Nephew TM, Williams GD, Yi H, et al. Apparent per capita alcohol consumption: National, State, and Regional trends, 1977–2000. Bethesda, MD: National Institute on Alcohol Abuse and Alcoholism; 2003.
18. Bellentani S, Tiribelli C. The spectrum of liver disease in the general population: lesson from the Dionysos study. Hepatology. 2001;31:531–7.
19. Pequignot G. About the geographical aspects of cirrhosis. Stuttgart. Germany: Schattauer Verlag; 1971.
20. Lelbach WK. Epidemiology of alcoholic liver disease. In: Popper H, Schaffner F, editors. Progress in liver diseases. Philadelphia: Grune and Stratton; 1976. p. 434–515.
21. Terris M. Epidemiology of cirrhosis of the liver: national mortality data. Am J Public Health Nations Health. 1967;57:2076–88.
22. Kerr WC, Fillmore KM, Marvy P. Beverage-specific alcohol consumption and cirrhosis mortality in a group of English-speaking beer-drinking countries. Addiction. 2000;95:339–46.
23. Roizen R, Kerr WC, Fillmore KM. Cirrhosis mortality and per capita consumption of distilled spirits, United States, 1949–94: trend analysis. BMJ. 1999;319:666–70.
24. Hartford TC. Beverage specific drinking contexts. Int J Addict. 1979;14:197–205.
25. Klatsky AL, Armstrong MA, Kipp H. Correlates of alcoholic beverage preference: traits of persons who choose wine, liquor, or beer. Br J Addict. 1990;85:1279–89.

26. Wechsler H, McFadden M. Drinking among college students in New England: extent, social correlates and consequences of alcohol use. J Stud Alcohol. 1979;40:969–96.
27. Rehm J, Greenfield TK, Rogers JD. Average volume of alcohol consumption, pattern of drinking, and all cause mortality: results from the US national alcohol survey. Am J Epidemiol. 2001;153:64–71.
28. Bellentani A, Saccoccio G, Costa G, et al. Drinking habits as cofactors of risk for alcohol induced liver damage. Gut. 1997;41:845–50.
29. Zakhari S, Li TK. Determinants of alcohol use and abuse: impact of quantity and frequency patterns on liver disease. Hepatology. 2007;46:2032–9.
30. Mathurin P, Deltenre P. Effect of binge drinking on the liver: an alarming public health issue. Gut. 2009;58:613–7.
31. Pincock S. Binge drinking on rise in UK and elsewhere. Government report shows increases in alcohol consumption, cirrhosis, and premature deaths. Lancet. 2003;362:1126–7.
32. Frezza M, Di Padova C, Pozzato G, et al. High blood alcohol levels in women. The role of decreased gastric alcohol dehydrogenase activity and first pass metabolism. N Engl J Med. 1990;322:95–9.
33. Schenker S. Medical consequences of alcohol abuse: is gender a factor? Alcohol Clin Exp Res. 1997;21:179–81.
34. Sato N, Lindros KO, Baraona E, et al. Sex difference in alcohol related organ injury. Alcohol Clin Exp Res. 2001;25:40S–5S.
35. Stinson FS, Grant BF, Dufour MC. The critical dimension of ethnicity in liver cirrhosis mortality statistics. Alcohol Clin Exp Res. 2001;25:1181–7.
36. Caetano R, Kaskutas LA. Changes in drinking patterns among whites, blacks, and hispanics, 1984–1992. J Stud Alcohol. 1995;56:558–65.
37. Naveau S, Giraud V, Borotto E, et al. Excess weight risk factor for alcoholic liver disease. Hepatology. 1997;25:108–11.
38. Raynard B, Baian A, Fallik D, et al. Risk factors of fibrosis in alcohol-induced liver disease. Hepatology. 2002;35:635–8.
39. Hezode C, Lonjon I, Roudot-Thoraval F, et al. Impact of moderate alcohol consumption on histological activity and fibrosis in patients with chronic hepatitis C, and specific influence of steatosis: a prospective study. Aliment Pharmacol Therapeutics. 2003;17:1031–7.
40. Singal AK, Kuo YF, Anand BS. Hepatitis C virus infection in alcoholic hepatitis: prevalence patterns and impact on in-hospital mortality. Eur J Gastroenterol Hepatol. 2012;24:1178–84.
41. Bhattacharya R, Shuhart MC. Hepatitis C and alcohol: interactions, outcomes, and implications. J Clin Gastroenterol. 2003;36:242–52.
42. Carrao G, Arico A. Idependent and combined action of hepatitis C virus infection and alcohol consumption on the risk of symptomatic liver cirrhosis. Hepatology. 1998;27:914–9.
43. Calabrese E, Gonnelli E, Ambu S, et al. Role of hepatitis B infection in alcoholic patients. Ric Clin Lab. 1986;16:543–8.
44. Inoue K, Kojima T, Koyata H, et al. Hepatitis B virus antigen and antibodies in the alcoholics. Etiological role of HBV in liver diseases of alcoholic patients. Liver. 1985;5:247–52.
45. Chevillotte G, Durbec JP, Gerolami A, et al. Interaction between hepatitis B virus and alcohol consumption in liver cirrhosis. An epidemiologic study. Gastroenterology. 1983;85:141–5.
46. Mota A, Guedes F, Areias J, et al. Alcohol consumption among patients with hepatitis B infection in northern Portugal considering gender and hepatitis B virus genotype differences. Alcohol. 2010;44:149–56.
47. Kondili LA, Tosti ME, Szklo M, et al. The relationships of chronic hepatitis and cirrhosis to alcohol intake, hepatitis B and C, and delta virus infection: a case control study in Albania. Epidemiol Infect. 1998;121:391–5.
48. Gao B. Interaction of alcohol and hepatitis viral proteins: implication in synergistic effect of alcohol drinking and viral hepatitis on liver injury. Alcohol. 2002;27:69–72.
49. Larkin J, Clayton MM, Feitelson MA. Chronic ethanol consumption stimulates hepatitis B virus gene expression and replication in transgenic mice. Hepatology. 2001;34:792–7.

50. Szabo G, Aloman C, Polyak S, et al. Hepatitis C infection and alcohol use: a dangerous mix for the liver and antiviral immunity. Alcohol Clin Exp Res. 2006;30:709–19.
51. Singal A, Shah V. Therapeutic strategies for the treatment of alcoholic hepatitis. Semin Liver Dis. 2016;36:56–8.
52. Yamauchi M, Maezawa Y, Toda G, et al. Association of a restriction fragment length polymorphism in the alcohol dehydrogenase 2 gene with Japanese alcoholic liver cirrhosis. J Hepatol. 1995;23:519–23.
53. Whitfield JB. Meta-analysis of the effects of alcohol dehydrogenase genotype on alcohol dependence and alcoholic liver disease. Alcohol Alcohol. 1997;32:613–9.
54. Lee HC, Lee HS, Jung SH, et al. Association between polymorphisms of ethanol-metabolizing enzymes and susceptibility to alcoholic cirrhosis in a Korean male population. J Korean Med Sci. 2001;16:745–50.
55. Nagata N, Hiyoshi M, Shiozawa H, et al. Assessment of a difference in ALDH2 heterozygotes and alcoholic liver injury. Alcohol Clin Exp Res. 2002;26:11S–4S.
56. Chao YC, Young TH, Chang WK, et al. An investigation of whether polymorphisms of cytochrome P4502E1 are genetic markers of susceptibility to alcoholic end-stage organ damage in a Chinese population. Hepatology. 1995;22(5):1409–14.
57. Garcia-Baneulos J, Panduro A, Gordillo-Bastidas D, et al. Association of CYP2E1*c2/CYP2E1*5b allele with cirrhosis and liver function. Alcohol Clin Res Exp. 2012;36:425–31.
58. Salameh H, Raff E, Erwin A. PNPLA3 gene polymorphism is associated with predisposition to and severity of alcoholic liver disease. Am J Gastroenterol. 2015;110:846–56.
59. Dam M, Flensborg-Madsen T, Eliasen M. Smoking and risk of liver cirrhosis: a population based cohort study. Scand J Gastroenterol. 2013;48:585–91.
60. Kuper H, Tzonou A, Kaklamani E. Tobacco smoking, alcohol consumption and their interaction in the causation of hepatocellular carcinoma. Int J Cancer. 2000;85:498–502.
61. Kennedy O, Roderick P, Buchanan R. Systematic review with meta-analysis: coffee consumption and the risk of cirrhosis. Aliment Pharmacol Ther. 2016;43:562–74.
62. Klatsky A, Morton C, Udaltsova N. Coffee, cirrhosis, and transaminase enzymes. Arch Intern Med. 2006;166:110–1195.
63. Nahon P, Sutton A, Rufat P. Liver iron, HFE gene mutations, and hepatocellular carcinoma occurrence in patients with cirrhosis. Gastroenterology. 2008;134:102–10.
64. Nahon P, Nuraldeen R, Rufat P. In alcoholic cirrhosis, low-serum hepcidin levels associate with poor long term survival. Liver Int. 2016;36:185–8.
65. Anderson P, Baumberg B. Alcohol in Europe—a public health perspective. A report for the European Commission. England: Institute of Alcohol Studies; 2006.
66. Bouchery EE, Harwood HJ, Sacks JJ, et al. Economic costs of excessive alcohol consumption in the US. Am J Prev Med. 2006;41:516–24.
67. Rehm J, Mathers C, Popova S, et al. Global burden of disease and injury and economic cost attributable to alcohol use and alcohol use disorders. Lancet. 2009;373:2223–33.
68. Yoon YH, Yi H. Surveillance report #93: Liver cirrhosis mortality in the United States 1970–2009. Washington, DC: National Institute on Alcohol Abuse and Alcoholism; 2012.
69. Stahre M, Roeber J, Kanny D. Contribution of excessive alcohol consumption to deaths and years of potential life lost in the United States. Prev Chronic Dis. 2014;11:130293. https://doi.org/10.5888/pcd11.130293.
70. Jinjuvadia R, Liangpunsakul S. Trends in alcoholic hepatitis related hospitalizations, financial burden, and mortality in the United States. J Clin Gastroenterol. 2015;49(6):506–11.
71. Hazeldine S, Hydes T, Sheron N. Alcoholic liver disease—the extent of the problem and what you can do about it. Clin Med. 2015;15:179–85.
72. Marinho RT, Duarte H, Giria J, et al. The burden of alcoholism in fifteen years of cirrhosis hospital admissions in Portugal. Liver Int. 2014;35:746–55.
73. Wang FS, Fan JG, Zhang Z, et al. The global burden of liver disease: the major impact of China. Hepatology. 2014;60:2099–108.
74. Rehm J, Samokhvalov A, Shield K. Global burden of liver diseases. J Hepatol. 2013;59:160–8.

75. Norstrom T, Ramstedt M. Mortality and population drinking: a review of the literature. Drug Alcohol Rev. 2005;24:537–47.
76. Paula H, Asrani SK, Boetticher NC. Alcoholic liver disease-related mortality in the United States: 1980–2003. Am J Gastroenterol. 2010;105:1782–7.
77. Liang W, Chikritzhs T, Pascal R. Mortality rate of alcoholic liver disease and risk of hospitalization for alcoholic liver cirrhosis, alcoholic hepatitis, and alcoholic liver failure in Australia between 1993 and 2005. Intern Med J. 2011;41(1a):34–141.
78. Hasumura Y, Takeuchi J. Alcoholic liver disease in Japanese patients: a comparison with caucasians. J Gastroenterol Hepatol. 1991;6:520–7.
79. Park SC, Oh SI, Lee MS. Korean status of alcoholics and alcohol-related health problems. Alcohol Clin Exp Res. 1998;22:170S–2S.
80. Bang HA, Young-Hwan K, Lee MJ. Trends in the epidemiological aspects and mortality of alcoholic liver disease in Korea in the decade between 2000–2009. J Clin Med Res. 2015;7:91–6.
81. Das S, Balakrishnan V, Vasudevan D. Alcohol: its health and social impact in India. Natl Med J India. 2006;19:94–9.
82. Bhattacharyya M, Barman N, Goswami B. Survey of alcohol-related cirrhosis at a tertiary care center in northeast India. Indian J Gastroenterol. 2016;35:167–72.
83. Lin CM, Lian CM. Inpatient expenditures on alcohol-attributed disease and alcohol tax policy: a nationwide analysis in Taiwan from 1996 to 2010. Public Health. 2014;128:977–84.
84. Guirguis J, Chhatwal J, Dasarathy J, et al. Clinical impact of alcohol-related cirrhosis in the next decade: estimates based on current epidemiological trends in the United States. Alcohol Clin Exp Res. 2015;39:2085–94.

Hepatitis B Virus: Asian Perspective

8

Wai-Kay Seto and Man-Fung Yuen

Abstract

Chronic hepatitis B virus (HBV) infection is a major cause of liver cirrhosis and hepatocellular carcinoma in Asia. HBV is generally endemic in many parts of Asia. China has the largest number of chronic HBV patients worldwide (74.6 million), with hepatitis B surface antigen (HBsAg) seroprevalence in different regions of China ranging from 3.7% to 10.4%. Other Asian countries with a high HBsAg seroprevalence include Taiwan, Mongolia, Vietnam and Uzbekistan. Migratory and behavioral patterns influence HBsAg seroprevalence rates, and the impact of HBV vaccination is gradually emerging in the younger age groups. Seroprevalence of antibody to the hepatitis B core antigen (anti-HBc) is gaining epidemiological significance due to the risk of HBV reactivation during high-risk immunosuppressive therapy. HBV genotypes B and C are commonly found in East and South East Asia, while genotypes A and D are the common genotypes in South and Central Asia. Under-treatment of HBV might be common from a public health perspective, and there is currently a paucity of evidence on the epidemiological effect of nucleoside analogue therapy on HBV-related complications. Based on available prescription patterns, nucleoside analogue coverage could be improved among the elderly age groups.

Keywords

HBV · HBsAg · Anti-HBc · Epidemiology · Genotypes · Nucleoside analogues

W.-K. Seto · M.-F. Yuen (✉)
Department of Medicine, The University of Hong Kong, Pokfulam, Hong Kong
e-mail: wkseto@hku.hk; mfyuen@hku.hk; mfyuen@hkucc.hku.hk

R. J. Wong, R. G. Gish (eds.), *Clinical Epidemiology of Chronic Liver Diseases*,
https://doi.org/10.1007/978-3-319-94355-8_8

8.1 Introduction

Chronic hepatitis B virus (HBV) infection affects 248 million individuals worldwide, with a high prevalence found especially in Asia [1], and is a major cause of liver-related morbidity and mortality. Cirrhosis develops in untreated chronic HBV infection at an incidence rate of 838 per 100,000 person years [2], with 30% of cirrhosis worldwide attributed to HBV [3]. HBV is also a major determinant of hepatocellular carcinoma (HCC). Liver cancer is currently the fifth most common cancer in men and the seventh most common cancer in women worldwide [4], with 53% of HCCs globally attributed to HBV [3]. HBV-related HCC can also uniquely occur in non-cirrhotic individuals [5]. When compared to individuals without the infection, chronic HBV (CHB) patients have a 223-fold of increased risk of HCC [6].

While chronic HBV infection is generally endemic throughout many countries in Asia, regional and national variations do exist. The molecular epidemiology of different HBV genotypes also differs among ethnicities. Besides the seroprevalence of hepatitis B surface antigen (HBsAg), the seroprevalence of antibody to hepatitis B core antigen (anti-HBc) is also gaining clinical significance. The epidemiological impact of universal HBV vaccination is also gradually emerging. The following sections will describe the clinical epidemiology of CHB from an Asian perspective in detail.

8.2 Natural History

The natural history of chronic HBV infection is depicted in Fig. 8.1 [7]. In the first phase, the immune tolerant phase, patients are hepatitis B e antigen (HBeAg)-positive, with high serum HBV DNA levels, normal liver biochemistry and minimal

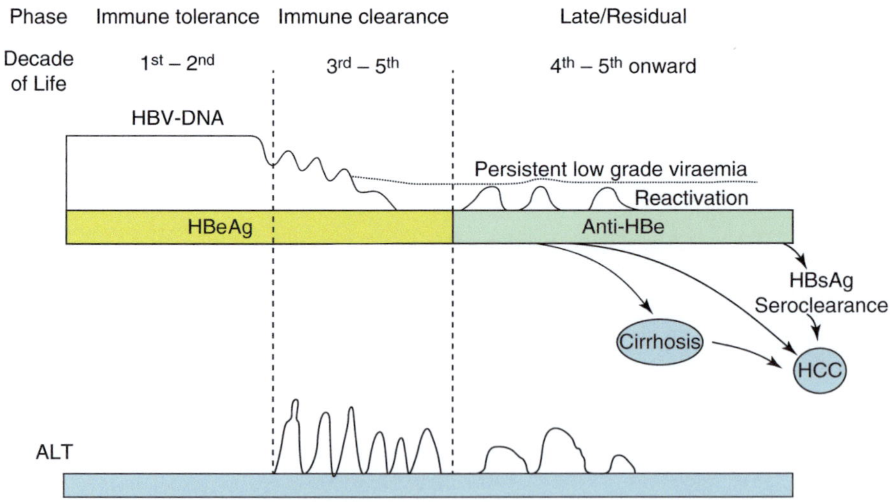

Fig. 8.1 The natural history of chronic hepatitis B infection with the depiction of different disease phases (adopted from Lai CL, Locarnini S 2008 with permission)

disease changes in liver histology [8]. The immune tolerant phase is markedly different between Asian HBV-infected patients and patients of European descent. Asian patients usually acquire the infection perinatally with the phase usually lasting for more than 20 years, unlike European patients who usually acquire the disease during adulthood and have a relatively shorter first phase [9]. The second disease phase, the immune clearance phase, is characterized by immune-mediated liver damage, with high serum alanine aminotransferase (ALT) and HBV DNA levels, and with active necroinflammatory changes in histology [10]. Patients then undergo HBeAg seroconversion, and in the subsequent late/residual HBeAg-negative phase, the disease could be quiescent, or could be characterized by intermittent virological or biochemical flares. Disease progression to cirrhosis or HCC is common during the HBeAg-negative phase [11].

A minority of patients will then proceed to the clearance of HBsAg from the sera. This HBsAg seroclearance occurs at a mean age of 50 years [12] and at a rate of 2.26% per year [13]. Intrahepatic HBV is still present at low transcriptional levels [12]. Nonetheless, serum HBV DNA is usually undetectable [14], with anti-HBc, an indication of past HBV exposure, being the only definite positive HBV serum marker. Therefore, for a newly-presenting HBsAg-negative, anti-HBc positive individual with no prior HBV-related assessment, it is extremely difficult to distinguish chronic HBV infection with past HBsAg seroclearance versus merely past exposure and without intrahepatic presence of HBV. The term "occult HBV infection" is used to define HBsAg-negative, anti-HBc positive individuals with underlying presence of intrahepatic HBV DNA [15]. These patients are at risk of HBV reactivation after high-risk immunosuppressive therapies including rituximab [16] and hematopoietic stem cell transplantation [17], rendering the seroprevalence of anti-HBc relevant from an epidemiological perspective to the disease burden of HBV.

8.3 Epidemiology: HBsAg Seroprevalence

The clinical epidemiology of chronic HBV infection is usually presented in terms of the seroprevalence of HBsAg. Other relevant HBV-related epidemiological parameters include the seroprevalence of anti-HBc, HBV genotype distribution and in the current era of long-term nucleoside analogue therapy, the coverage of nucleoside analogue treatment.

Many countries with a high HBsAg seroprevalence are found in Asia, as depicted in Fig. 8.2, of which selected countries will be described in the following sections.

8.3.1 Mainland China and Hong Kong

Historically China had a very high rate of HBsAg seroprevalence, quoted at 9.8% prior to the availability of HBV vaccination [18]. Nonetheless, it must be noted that China is a geographically and ethnically diverse country, with wide variations in HBsAg seroprevalences observed throughout different regions of China (Fig. 8.3).

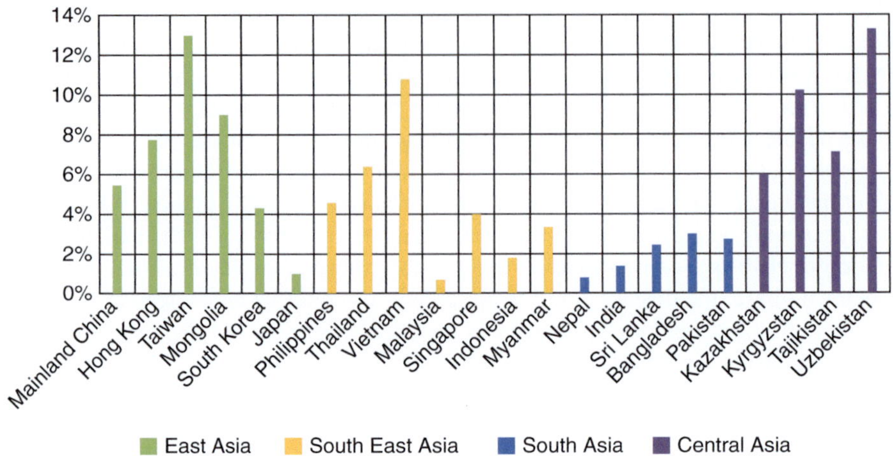

Seroprevalence data adopted from Hope et al. Epidemiol Infect 2014, Schweitzer et al. Lancet 2015, Chen et al. J Hepatol 2015 and Liu , et al. J Hepatol 2016 HBsAg, hepatitis B surface antigen

Fig. 8.2 Seroprevalence of HBsAg in Asia as categorized by different geographic regions

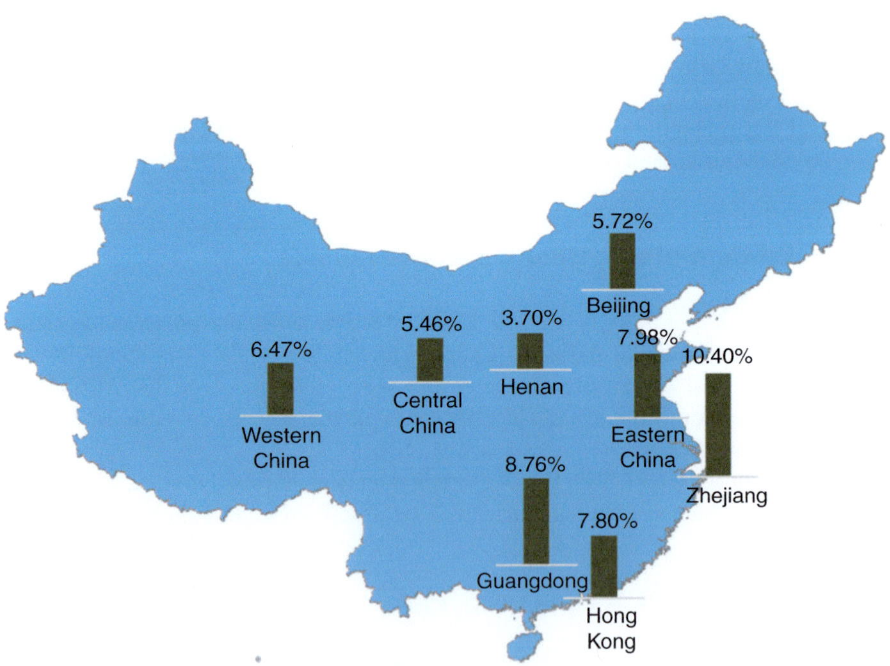

Seroprevalence data adopted from Chen et at. PLoS One 2013 Xu et al. PLoS One 2015 Zeng et at Sci Rep 2016 Liu et al. Lancet Infect Dis 2016 Yong Hao et al. J Med Virol 2017 Liu et al. J Hepatol 2016. HBsAg, hepatitis B surface antigen

Fig. 8.3 HBsAg seroprevalence in different geographical regions of China

China also has a huge burden of liver-related complications. HCC, of which 80% are HBV-related, is the second-leading cause of cancer mortality in China [19]. Currently, China accounts for 51% of deaths from liver cancer worldwide [20]. HBV is also responsible for 79% of liver cirrhosis in China [20].

A pooled analysis of published data estimated China to have the largest number of infected individuals worldwide (74.6 million) and a HBsAg seroprevalence of 5.49% (95% confidence interval (CI) 5.47–5.50%) [1]. A recent population-based study among Chinese men demonstrated the wide disparity in HBsAg seroprevalence still remaining present throughout different China regions. Eastern China had a higher HBsAg seroprevalence (7.98%) when compared to Central (5.46%) or Western China (6.47%) [21]. Local prevalence studies found HBsAg seroprevalence to be markedly higher in South and Southeast China, ranging from 8.76% in Guangdong [22] to 10.4% in Zhejiang [23]. Meanwhile, the HBsAg positivity rate in Beijing and Henan, Central China were only 5.72% [24] and 3.7% [25], respectively. As for Hong Kong, a population-based study of more than 10,000 participants found the HBsAg seroprevalence to be 7.8% [26]. HBsAg seroprevalence among high-risk groups were expectedly higher, with the prevalence among hemodialysis patients and HIV-positive patients being 11.9% and 12.49%, respectively [27].

HBsAg seroprevalence rates were consistent throughout different age groups born prior to the availability of neonatal HBV vaccination [21]. As for the younger age groups that benefited from neonatal HBV vaccination programs, HBsAg seroprevalence was much lower, ranging from 1% to 2.3% [18]. The coverage of HBV vaccination in Mainland China was variable, achieving up to 99% in major cities but only reaching 70% in more rural areas [18]. Hong Kong introduced universal neonatal HBV vaccination in 1988 and among individuals born in Hong Kong in or after 1988, HBsAg seroprevalence was greatly reduced to 1.8%. The actual HBsAg seroprevalence among the same age group, when including individuals born outside Hong Kong, was higher at 3.4% [26], an example of how migration can substantially impact HBV prevalence.

8.3.2 Taiwan

Similar to Mainland China, Taiwan historically also had very high rates of HBsAg seroprevalence, reported at 14.5% in the pre-HBV vaccination era [28]. Taiwan was also the first country to commence a nationwide HBV vaccination program since July 1984. Vaccination coverage rates were >95% [29]. By 1999, the impact of universal vaccination was evident, with HBsAg seroprevalence in children younger than 15 years of age dropping to only 0.7% [30]. The incidence of childhood HCC was also in decline [31].

A nationwide survey conducted in 2002–2007 involving 6602 participants found a HBsAg positivity rate of 13.7% (95% CI 12.5–14.5%) [32]. The results suggest, despite approximately 20 years since the commencement of nationwide HBV vaccination, chronic HBV infection would remain a substantial health care burden in Taiwan. In addition, among individuals born after the commencement of nationwide HBV vaccination,

HBsAg seroprevalence was 5.04% (95% CI 2.45–7.62%) [32]. The HBsAg seropositivity rate was significantly higher than the 1.2% found among 18,779 subjects born in or after 1984 in Taiwan and followed up from neonatal to adulthood [33]. A reason for this disparity could be due to the impact of migration, similar to the situation in Hong Kong. Another reason is the study by Ni et al. was confined to the capital city of Taipei, while Chen et al. included the rural areas of Taiwan as well as the Taiwanese aboriginal populations in which HBV vaccination coverage might had been incomplete.

8.3.3 Korea

Prior to the introduction of HBV vaccination programs in Korea in 1991, approximately 8% of the urban Korean population was HBsAg-positive [34]. The latest HBsAg seroprevalence estimate in South Korea based on pooled data is 4.36% (95% CI 4.36–4.37%) [1]. A population-based cross-sectional study conducted in 2007–2009 involving 18,091 individuals found the HBsAg positivity rate to be 6%. However, chronic HBV infection is no longer the most important cause of deranged liver biochemistry; 74.9% of elevated ALT cases were instead related to metabolic causes [35].

HBsAg seroprevalence is gradually decreasing in South Korea. A longitudinal study of 50,140 participants also showed a stepwise decrease in HBsAg seroprevalence, from 4.61% in 1998 to 2.98% in 2010. Significant decreases were only noted in the younger age groups of <50 years. Among participants age 50 years or above, HBsAg seroprevalence remained similar over time [36], implying HBV will remain an important health care issue in the middle-aged and elderly populations. Another large population study involving 11,513 subjects showed the seroprevalence of HBsAg decreasing from 5.5% in 1998–2001 to 4.2% in 2008–2011. Interestingly, females with the highest income and education levels exhibit the largest decreases, while no significant reduction was noted in males with a higher education level [37].

8.3.4 Japan

When comparing with nearby Asian countries, Japan has a relatively lower HBsAg seroprevalence. Currently the estimated HBsAg positivity rate is at 1.02% (95% CI 1.01–1.02) [1]. Prevalence studies among blood donors found the seroprevalence of HBsAg to be 0.71% [38]. Japan implemented a policy of selective HBV vaccination of infants born to HBsAg-positive mothers in 1986. A nationwide study conducted from 2005 to 2011 among children aged 4–15 years found the HBsAg positivity rate to be only 0.17% [39].

Adult-acquired HBV is emerging as an important route of transmission in Japan. In a study involving 212 patients acutely infected with HBV, 8 patients (4.2%) developed chronicity of infection with persistence of HBsAg for more than 12 months. The majority of patients developing chronic HBV infection were of genotype A, the predominant genotype of adult-acquired HBV in Western countries [40]. With horizontal transmission of HBV gaining importance in Japan, prevalence studies targeting high-risk groups will be required to accurately understand the future health care burden of HBV.

8.3.5 Mongolia

Mongolia has a high HBsAg seroprevalence of 9% [1]. In addition, co-infection with hepatitis C virus (HCV) and hepatitis delta virus (HDV) is common, reaching 7.7% and 26.6%, respectively among patients with known chronic liver disease. Mongolia is one of the few regions worldwide with patients possessing concomitant triple infections of HBV, HCV and HDV (30.0%) [41]. Mongolia has one of the highest incidences of HCC worldwide (78.1 per 100,000 persons) [42], of which many have underlying triple HBV/HCV/HDV infection [41].

8.3.6 South East Asia

Vietnam is the South East Asian country with the highest HBV burden, with HBsAg positivity estimated at 10.79% (95% CI 10.29–1.31%) [1]. HBsAg positive rates in the rural areas of Vietnam are even higher, reaching 19.0% [43]. Universal HBV vaccination only started in 2003 and its benefits are not expected to be reflected anytime soon. Based on the expected population growth in Vietnam, HBV-related mortality from 1990 to 2025 is expected to increase by more than threefold [44].

HBV is of intermediate endemicity in the remaining of South East Asia, with HBsAg seroprevalence ranging from 3.40% in Myanmar to 6.42% in Thailand. The exceptions are Malaysia and Indonesia, with low HBsAg positivity rates of 0.74% and 1.86%, respectively [1].

8.3.7 South Asia

India has the second-largest population of HBsAg-positive patients worldwide, with 37.6 million infected individuals, and an HBsAg seroprevalence rate estimated at 1.46% (95% CI 1.44–1.47%) [1]. This is however likely an underestimation, since majority of Indian prevalence studies are based on blood donors, and with professional blood donors constituting 40% of the blood donor population, bias from a large healthy donor pool would be anticipated [45].

HBsAg seroprevalence estimates in other South Asian countries ranges from 0.82% in Nepal to 3.10% in Bangladesh [1]. A weighted average of HBsAg seroprevalence in Pakistan was 2.4%, and with coverage of HBV vaccination suboptimal, HBV-related disease will still be present in the foreseeable future [46].

8.3.8 Central Asia

HBV is prevalent in Central Asian countries, with HBsAg seroprevalence estimates ranging from 6.05% in Kazakhstan [1] to 13.3% in Uzbekistan [47]. Unlike other parts of Asia, the predominant method of transmission is horizontal [48]. A similarly high HBsAg seroprevalence was noted among high-risk groups for horizontal transmission, including people who inject drugs and men who have sex with men [47]. While currently most Central Asian countries have universal HBV vaccination programs for newborn infants, vaccination coverage remains variable. Extension of HBV vaccination to high-risk groups remains a challenge [48].

8.4 Epidemiology: Anti-HBc Seroprevalence

Without antiviral prophylaxis, HBV reactivation rates in Asian HBsAg-negative, anti-HBc positive individuals after high-risk immunosuppressive therapy exceeds 40% [16, 17]. At the same time, accessibility to high-risk immunosuppressive therapy in Asia is improving. Asia is facing an aging population, and increasing numbers of elderly individuals are being treated with rituximab or other B-cell depleting agents [49]. The percentage of hematopoietic stem cell transplants being performed in the Asia-Pacific region also increased from 5.6% in 1985 to 17.5% in 2012 [50]. All these signify that the clinical significance of anti-HBc positivity, the marker of past HBV exposure, in Asia will continue to rise.

The available data on anti-HBc seroprevalence in Asia is depicted in Fig. 8.4 [26, 32, 43, 51–58]. Generally speaking, for regions with HBsAg seroprevalence exceeding 10%, (e.g. Taiwan and Vietnam), anti-HBc seroprevalence would be >60% [32, 43]. Regions with HBsAg seroprevalence between 5% and 8% (e.g. China) would demonstrate an anti-HBc seroprevalence of >35%. In India,

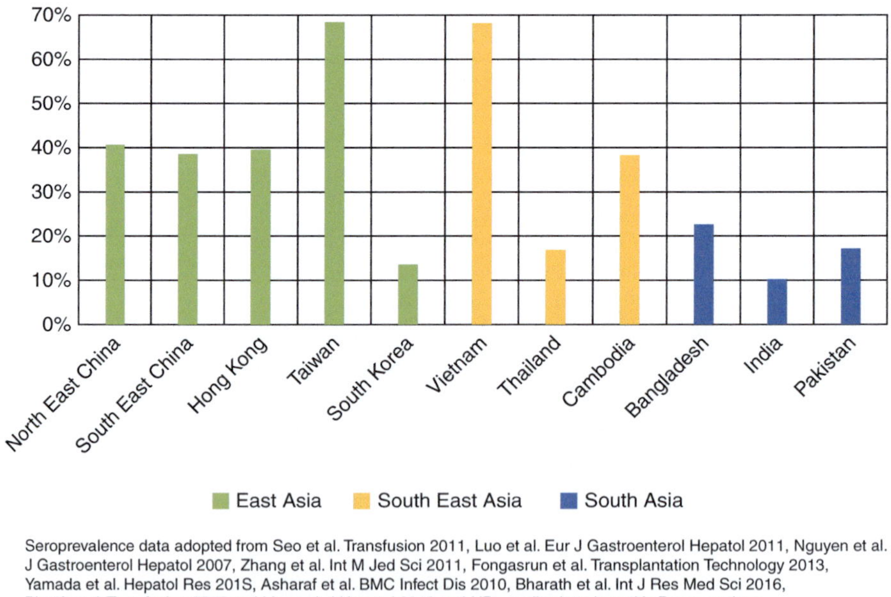

Fig. 8.4 Seroprevalence of anti-HBc in Asia as categorized by different geographic regions

where HBsAg seroprevalence is below 2%, different sources of anti-HBc seroprevalences consistently exceeded 10% [58, 59]. All recorded anti-HBc positivity levels are substantially higher than the 4.6–7.3% seropositive rates of Western countries [60, 61].

Population-based data is still lacking from many regions of Asia, including the whole of Central Asia. Nonetheless, since Kazakhstan has one of Asia's highest anti-HBc positivity rates among intravenous drug users (79.5%) [62], the general anti-HBc seroprevalence in Central Asia should expectedly be high. An important determinant of anti-HBc positivity is age. While the reported prevalence of anti-HBc in Hong Kong is reported to be 37.3%, positivity rates increases significantly with age, reaching 44.7%, 57.8% and 74.0% among individuals aged 55–65 years, 66–75 years and >75 years, respectively [26].

8.5 Molecular Epidemiology

HBV is a molecularly diverse virus, with HBV genotypes defined as a viral genomic sequence divergence greater than 8% of the entire HBV genome, and subgenotypes defined genomic sequence divergence between 4% and 8% [63]. Currently there are eight well-defined HBV genotypes (A to H), with a ninth (I) and tenth (J) recently described in Vietnam and the Ryukyu Islands, Japan, respectively [64]. The distinct geographic distribution of HBV genotypes in Asia is depicted in Fig. 8.5. Genotypes B and C are found in East Asia and South East Asia, with genotype C being the more common genotype, with the exception of Taiwan and Indonesia where genotype B is more common. South Asia and Central Asia mainly consists of genotypes A and D, with genotype D being the more common genotype [64]. There are Asian countries with exclusively one HBV genotype: Korea only has genotype C, while Mongolia only has genotype D [65].

HBV genotypes are clinically important as they influence the disease progression, and to a certain extent, the treatment response of chronic HBV. When comparing genotypes B and C, hepatitis B e antigen (HBeAg) seroconversion occurs much earlier in genotype B [66]. Genotype C is associated with a higher risk of HCC development [67], although the apparently higher risk of HCC is due to the close association of the core promoter mutation [68]. As for genotypes A and D, genotype A is associated with a more quiescent disease after HBeAg seroconversion [69], while a study from the Indian subcontinent showed genotype D to have more severe liver disease and an increased probability of developing HCC [70]. In terms of treatment response, HBV genotype A has a higher chance of response during pegylated interferon therapy when compared to genotypes B to D [71]; as for nucleoside analogue therapy, the predominant treatment of choice nowadays, HBV genotypes are not an important determinant to successful treatment [72].

Behavioral and migratory patterns are continuously influencing the geographical distribution of HBV genotypes. An example is Japan where genotype A is gaining

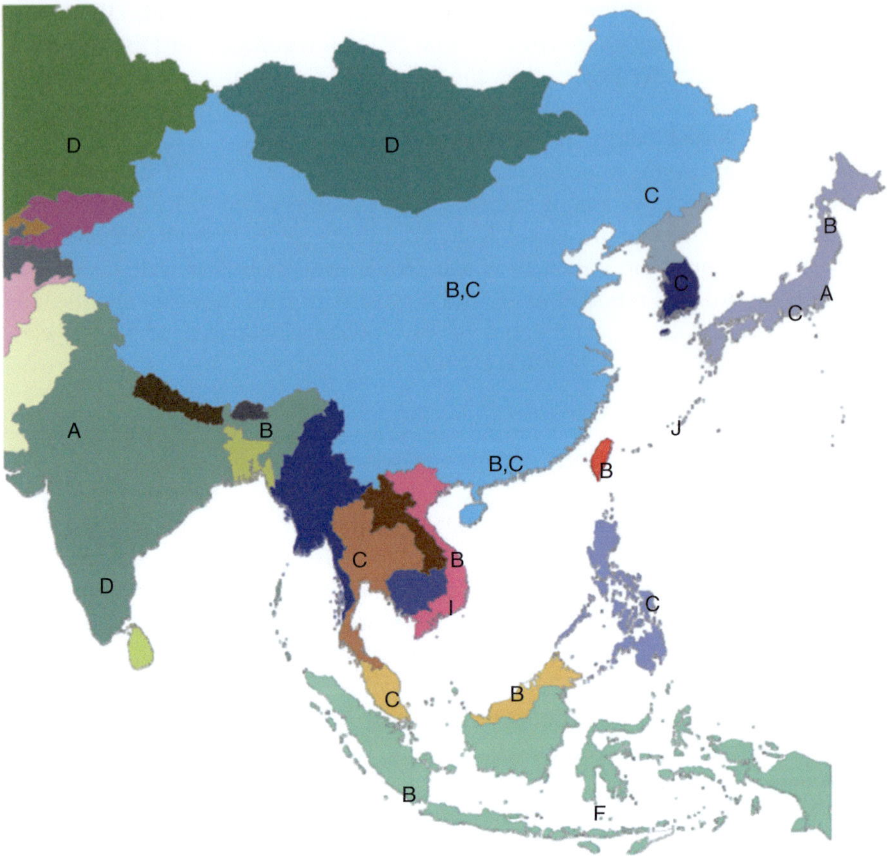

Fig. 8.5 Geographical distribution of HBV genotypes in Asia. Genotypes B and C are the most common in East Asia and South East Asia, while genotypes D and A and predominant in South Asia and Central Asia. Genotype A is currently increasing in Japan. Newly-described genotypes include genotype I from Vietnam and genotype J from Ryukyu Islands, Japan

prominence as a result of increased adult-acquired infection via horizontal transmission [40]. Bangladesh now has all four common HBV genotypes A to D, possibly due to its close geographical proximity with South East Asia [73].

8.6 Nucleoside Analogue Prescription Coverage

Besides the serological prevalence of HBV, the health care burden of HBV is also reflected through the morbidity and mortality of liver-related complications (acute decompensation, cirrhosis, HCC). Long-term nucleoside analogue therapy for chronic HBV infection is effective in achieving virological suppression, reduce liver-related complications and reverse liver fibrosis [74, 75]. However, the impact of nucleoside analogue therapy in Asia at an epidemiological level has not been well-reported.

Based on treatment recommendations from international guidelines, up to 59% of chronic HBV patients followed up in specialist clinics could be eligible for therapy [76]. Yet under-treatment of HBV is common worldwide [77], with only 27% of chronic HBV patients in the United States being treated with nucleoside analogues [78]. From Taiwan's national health insurance database, 41% of chronic HBV patients were nucleoside analogue-experienced, but the mean treatment duration was only 1.44 years [79]. Data on HBV nationwide treatment coverage in other Asian countries is otherwise lacking, but is essential from a public health perspective in order to determine the epidemiological efficacy of nucleoside analogue therapy in reducing HBV-related liver complications.

A recent study analyzed nucleoside analogue prescription patterns from 1999 to 2012 within the public hospital network of Hong Kong, which covers 90% of health care in the territory. While nucleoside analogue prescription patient headcount increased at 2006 patients per year to 26,411 patients in 2012, prescription volume mainly concentrated in the 55–64 years and 45–54 years age groups (Fig. 8.6). The age group of ≥65 years only took up 18.8% of prescription volume, but had the highest liver cancer burden with 52% of newly diagnosed liver cancers in the territory. Nucleoside analogue prescription was ecologically associated with a decreased incidence in liver cancer overall, although this association was not present among patients ≥65 years [80]. The results imply HBV treatment coverage not only needs to be enhanced, but also should be expanded especially in the elderly chronic HBV population in order to maximize the oncoprotective effects of nucleoside analogue therapy against HCC.

8.7 Concluding Remarks

HBV endemicity is steadily on the decline in Asia, largely due to the impact of HBV vaccination programs. However, due to differences in public health policy and vaccine the efficacy of vaccination differs from country to country. Other factors, including migration and behavioral patterns, can influence HBV prevalence. Given the effectiveness of long-term nucleoside analogue therapy, data on HBV treatment coverage among different Asian populations will be valuable in understanding whether current treatment regimens can effectively reduce liver-related morbidity and mortality at a public health level and decrease the global burden of HBV.

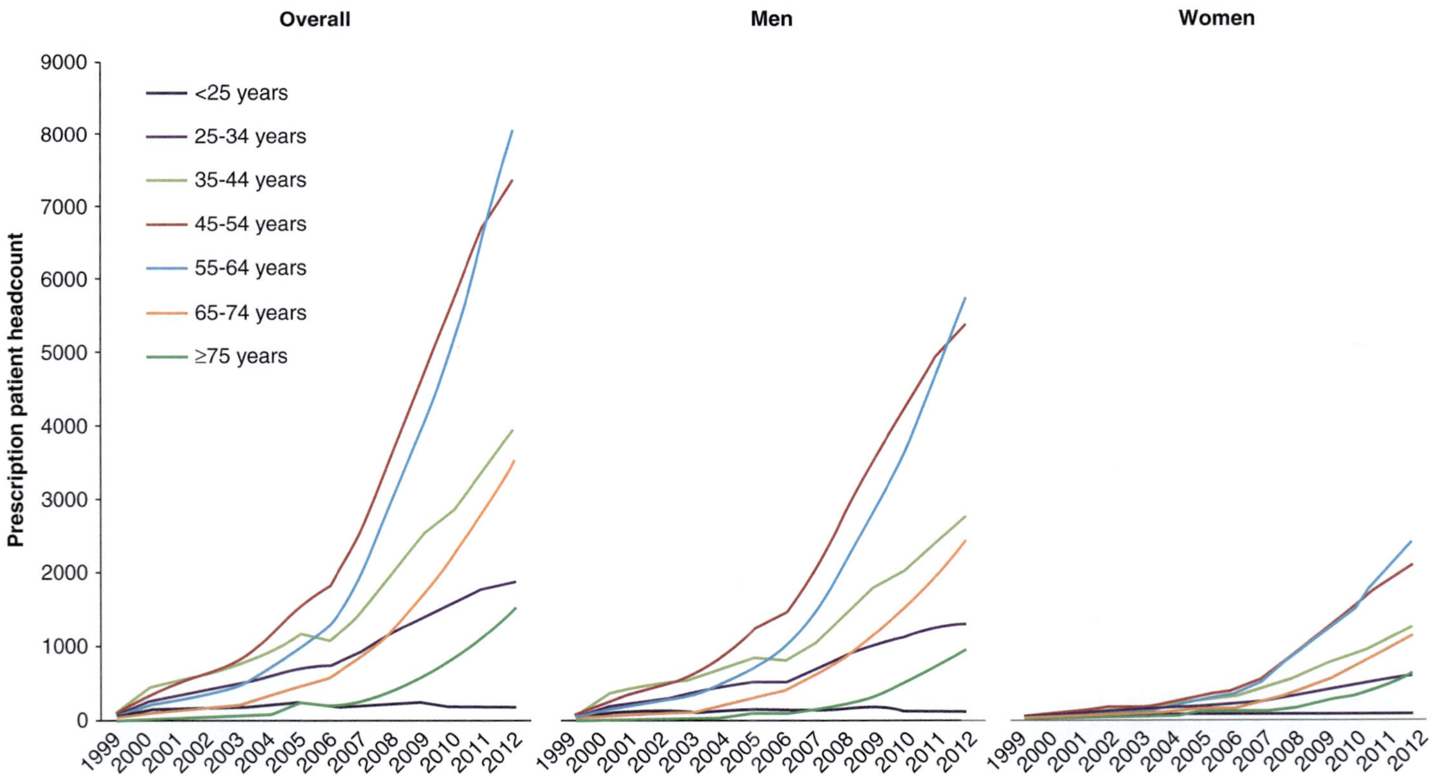

Fig. 8.6 Nucleoside analogue prescription in the Hospital Authority, Hong Kong from 1999 to 2012. 58.2% of prescriptions were among the age groups of 45–64 years. Liver cancer was most frequent in the ≥65 years age group, which only took up 18.8% of prescriptions (adopted from Seto WK et al. 2017 with permission)

Summary Table of Landmark Literature

Study title and authors	Study design	Summary results	Main limitations
Schweitzer A et al. Lancet 2015;386(10003):1546–1555	Systematic review and pooled analysis of worldwide chronic HBV prevalence published between 1965 and 2013	• Asia-Pacific regions had highest rates of HBsAg seroprevalence (5.26%, 95% CI 5.26–5.26) • Asian countries with high HBV endemicity include China, Vietnam, Mongolia, Kyrgyzstan and Uzbekistan	• Paucity of prevalence data might affect extrapolated prevalence estimates in some regions
Liu J et al. Lancet Infect Dis 2016;16(1):80–86	Population-based prevalence study of HBV prevalence among Chinese men from different regions of China	• HBsAg seroprevalence overall was 6% • HBV markers were more prevalence in the eastern regions of China when compared to the central or western regions	• Only married men aged 21–49 enrolling into family planning programs were included
Ito K et al. Hepatology 2014;59(1):89–97	Nationwide cohort study on the clinical course of acute hepatitis B in Japan	• >50% of acute hepatitis B infections were of HBV genotype A • Time to disappearance of HBsAg and progression to chronicity was higher in genotype A when compared to other genotypes	• Clinical outcomes were mainly retrospective and descriptive in nature
Chen CL et al. J Hepatol 2015;63(2):354-363	Nationwide survey on the prevalence of HBV markers in both vaccinated and unvaccinated populations in Taiwan	• Overall HBsAg seroprevalence was high, at 13.7% • HBsAg seroprevalence among vaccinated individuals was 5.04%, significantly lower, but still a substantial rate	• Vaccination history among certain cohorts might not be accurate

Study title and authors	Study design	Summary results	Main limitations
Seto WK et al. Aliment Pharmacol Ther 2017;45(4):501–509	Ecological study evaluating the territory-wide association of nucleoside analogue prescription for chronic hepatitis B with liver cancer incidence in Hong Kong	• Nucleoside analogue prescription was overall associated with reduced liver cancer incidence • No association was noted in elderly age groups, which had the highest liver cancer burden	• Ecological study design, which might affect the control of confounding factors

References

1. Schweitzer A, Horn J, Mikolajczyk RT, Krause G, Ott JJ. Estimations of worldwide prevalence of chronic hepatitis B virus infection: a systematic review of data published between 1965 and 2013. Lancet. 2015;386(10003):1546–55.
2. Lee MH, Yang HI, Liu J, Batrla-Utermann R, Jen CL, Iloeje UH, et al. Prediction models of long-term cirrhosis and hepatocellular carcinoma risk in chronic hepatitis B patients: risk scores integrating host and virus profiles. Hepatology. 2013;58(2):546–54.
3. Perz JF, Armstrong GL, Farrington LA, Hutin YJ, Bell BP. The contributions of hepatitis B virus and hepatitis C virus infections to cirrhosis and primary liver cancer worldwide. J Hepatol. 2006;45(4):529–38.
4. El-Serag HB. Epidemiology of viral hepatitis and hepatocellular carcinoma. Gastroenterology. 2012;142(6):1264–73. e1
5. Do AL, Wong CR, Nguyen LH, Nguyen VG, Trinh H, Nguyen MH. Hepatocellular carcinoma incidence in noncirrhotic patients with chronic hepatitis B and patients with cirrhosis of all etiologies. J Clin Gastroenterol. 2014;48(7):644–9.
6. Beasley RP, Hwang LY, Lin CC, Chien CS. Hepatocellular carcinoma and hepatitis B virus. A prospective study of 22 707 men in Taiwan. Lancet. 1981;2(8256):1129–33.
7. Lai CL, Yuen M-F. Chapter 12: The natural history of chronic hepatitis B. In: Lai CL, Locarnini S, editors. Hepatitis B virus. Second ed. London, Atlanta: International Medical Press; 2008.
8. Andreani T, Serfaty L, Mohand D, Dernaika S, Wendum D, Chazouilleres O, et al. Chronic hepatitis B virus carriers in the immunotolerant phase of infection: histologic findings and outcome. Clin Gastroenterol Hepatol. 2007;5(5):636–41.
9. Lai CL, Ratziu V, Yuen MF, Poynard T. Viral hepatitis B. Lancet. 2003;362(9401): 2089–94.
10. Seto WK, Lai CL, Ip PP, Fung J, Wong DK, Yuen JC, et al. A large population histology study showing the lack of association between ALT elevation and significant fibrosis in chronic hepatitis B. PLoS One. 2012;7(2):e32622.
11. Yuen MF, Yuan HJ, Wong DK, Yuen JC, Wong WM, Chan AO, et al. Prognostic determinants for chronic hepatitis B in Asians: therapeutic implications. Gut. 2005;54(11):1610–4.
12. Yuen MF, Wong DK, Fung J, Ip P, But D, Hung I, et al. HBsAg Seroclearance in chronic hepatitis B in Asian patients: replicative level and risk of hepatocellular carcinoma. Gastroenterology. 2008;135(4):1192–9.
13. Liu J, Yang HI, Lee MH, Lu SN, Jen CL, Wang LY, et al. Incidence and determinants of spontaneous hepatitis B surface antigen seroclearance: a community-based follow-up study. Gastroenterology. 2010;139(2):474–82.

14. Seto WK, Wong DK, Fung J, Hung IF, Fong DY, Yuen JC, et al. A large case-control study on the predictability of hepatitis B surface antigen levels three years before hepatitis B surface antigen seroclearance. Hepatology. 2012;56(3):812–9.
15. Raimondo G, Pollicino T, Cacciola I, Squadrito G. Occult hepatitis B virus infection. J Hepatol. 2007;46(1):160–70.
16. Seto WK, Chan TS, Hwang YY, Wong DK, Fung J, Liu KS, et al. Hepatitis B reactivation in patients with previous hepatitis B virus exposure undergoing rituximab-containing chemotherapy for lymphoma: a prospective study. J Clin Oncol. 2014;32(33):3736–43.
17. Seto WK, Chan TS, Hwang YY, Wong DK, Fung J, Liu KS, et al. Hepatitis B reactivation in occult viral carriers undergoing hematopoietic stem cell transplantation: a prospective study. Hepatology. 2017;65:1451–61.
18. Luo Z, Li L, Ruan B. Impact of the implementation of a vaccination strategy on hepatitis B virus infections in China over a 20-year period. Int J Infect Dis. 2012;16(2):e82–8.
19. Chen W, Zheng R, Zeng H, Zhang S. The incidence and mortality of major cancers in China, 2012. Chin J Cancer. 2016;35(1):73.
20. Wang FS, Fan JG, Zhang Z, Gao B, Wang HY. The global burden of liver disease: the major impact of China. Hepatology. 2014;60(6):2099–108.
21. Liu J, Zhang S, Wang Q, Shen H, Zhang M, Zhang Y, et al. Seroepidemiology of hepatitis B virus infection in 2 million men aged 21–49 years in rural China: a population-based, cross-sectional study. Lancet Infect Dis. 2016;16(1):80–6.
22. Zeng F, Guo P, Huang Y, Xin W, Du Z, Zhu S, et al. Epidemiology of hepatitis B virus infection: results from a community-based study of 0.15 million residents in South China. Sci Rep. 2016;6:36,186.
23. Chen P, Yu C, Ruan B, Yang S, Ren J, Xu W, et al. Prevalence of hepatitis B in insular regions of southeast China: a community-based study. PLoS One. 2013;8(2):e56444.
24. Xu S, Wang Q, Zhang W, Qiu Z, Cui J, Yan W, et al. Seroprevalence of the hepatitis B, hepatitis C, and human immunodeficiency viruses and treponema pallidum at the Beijing General Hospital from 2010 to 2014: a cross-sectional study. PLoS One. 2015;10(10):e0140854.
25. Yong Hao G, Da Xing F, Jin X, Xiu Hong F, Pu Mei D, Jun L, et al. The prevalence of hepatitis B infection in central China: an adult population-based serological survey of a large sample size. J Med Virol. 2017;89:450–7.
26. Liu KS, Seto WK, Wong DK, Yuen JC, Lam YF, Cheung KS, et al. A territory-wide study on the seroprevalence of hepatitis B virus in the general population after universal hepatitis B immunization era in Hong Kong, China (abstract). J Hepatol. 2016;64((2):S378.
27. Cui Y, Jia J. Update on epidemiology of hepatitis B and C in China. J Gastroenterol Hepatol. 2013;28(Suppl 1):7–10.
28. Sung JL. Hepatitis B virus infection and its sequelae in Taiwan. Gastroenterol Jpn. 1984;19(4):363–6.
29. Chien YC, Jan CF, Kuo HS, Chen CJ. Nationwide hepatitis B vaccination program in Taiwan: effectiveness in the 20 years after it was launched. Epidemiol Rev. 2006;28:126–35.
30. Hsu HM, Lu CF, Lee SC, Lin SR, Chen DS. Seroepidemiologic survey for hepatitis B virus infection in Taiwan: the effect of hepatitis B mass immunization. J Infect Dis. 1999;179(2):367–70.
31. Chang MH, Shau WY, Chen CJ, Wu TC, Kong MS, Liang DC, et al. Hepatitis B vaccination and hepatocellular carcinoma rates in boys and girls. JAMA. 2000;284(23):3040–2.
32. Chen CL, Yang JY, Lin SF, Sun CA, Bai CH, You SL, et al. Slow decline of hepatitis B burden in general population: results from a population-based survey and longitudinal follow-up study in Taiwan. J Hepatol. 2015;63(2):354–63.
33. Ni YH, Huang LM, Chang MH, Yen CJ, Lu CY, You SL, et al. Two decades of universal hepatitis B vaccination in taiwan: impact and implication for future strategies. Gastroenterology. 2007;132(4):1287–93.
34. Kang JK, Jang KM, Woo SH, Yun DH, Lee KR, Kwon YO, et al. Seroepidemiologic survey on type B viral hepatitis in inchon area, Department of Internal Medicine, Inchon Christian Hospital. Korean J Med. 1983;26:1331–6.

35. Hyun HJ, Shim JJ, Kim JW, Lee JS, Lee CK, Jang JY, et al. The prevalence of elevated alanine transaminase and its possible causes in the general Korean population. J Clin Gastroenterol. 2014;48(6):534–9.
36. Kim H, Shin AR, Chung HH, Kim MK, Lee JS, Shim JJ, et al. Recent trends in hepatitis B virus infection in the general Korean population. Korean J Intern Med. 2013;28(4):413–9.
37. Park B, Jung KW, Oh CM, Choi KS, Suh M, Jun JK. Ten-year changes in the hepatitis B prevalence in the birth cohorts in Korea: results from nationally representative cross-sectional surveys. Medicine (Baltimore). 2015;94(41):e1469.
38. Tanaka J, Koyama T, Mizui M, Uchida S, Katayama K, Matsuo J, et al. Total numbers of undiagnosed carriers of hepatitis C and B viruses in Japan estimated by age- and area-specific prevalence on the national scale. Intervirology. 2011;54(4):185–95.
39. Kiyohara T, Ishii K, Mizokami M, Sugiyama M, Wakita T. Seroepidemiological study of hepatitis B virus markers in Japan. Vaccine. 2015;33(45):6037–42.
40. Ito K, Yotsuyanagi H, Yatsuhashi H, Karino Y, Takikawa Y, Saito T, et al. Risk factors for long-term persistence of serum hepatitis B surface antigen following acute hepatitis B virus infection in Japanese adults. Hepatology. 2014;59(1):89–97.
41. Tsatsralt-Od B, Takahashi M, Nishizawa T, Endo K, Inoue J, Okamoto H. High prevalence of dual or triple infection of hepatitis B, C, and delta viruses among patients with chronic liver disease in Mongolia. J Med Virol. 2005;77(4):491–9.
42. Kim YA, Estevez J, Le A, Israelski D, Baatarkhuu O, Sarantuya T, et al. Screening and management of viral hepatitis and hepatocellular carcinoma in Mongolia: results from a survey of Mongolian physicians from all major provinces of Mongolia. BMJ Open Gastroenterol. 2016;3(1):e000119.
43. Nguyen VT, McLaws ML, Dore GJ. Highly endemic hepatitis B infection in rural Vietnam. J Gastroenterol Hepatol. 2007;22(12):2093–100.
44. Nguyen VT, Law MG, Dore GJ. An enormous hepatitis B virus-related liver disease burden projected in Vietnam by 2025. Liver Int. 2008;28(4):525–31.
45. Tandon BN, Acharya SK, Tandon A. Epidemiology of hepatitis B virus infection in India. Gut. 1996;38(Suppl 2):S56–9.
46. Ali SA, Donahue RM, Qureshi H, Vermund SH. Hepatitis B and hepatitis C in Pakistan: prevalence and risk factors. Int J Infect Dis. 2009;13(1):9–19.
47. Hope VD, Eramova I, Capurro D, Donoghoe MC. Prevalence and estimation of hepatitis B and C infections in the WHO European Region: a review of data focusing on the countries outside the European Union and the European Free Trade Association. Epidemiol Infect. 2014;142(2):270–86.
48. Avazova D, Kurbanov F, Tanaka Y, Sugiyama M, Radchenko I, Ruziev D, et al. Hepatitis B virus transmission pattern and vaccination efficiency in Uzbekistan. J Med Virol. 2008;80(2):217–24.
49. Jones B. Haematological cancer: rituximab maintenance improves the outcome of elderly patients with FL. Nat Rev Clin Oncol. 2013;10(11):607.
50. Gratwohl A, Pasquini MC, Aljurf M, Atsuta Y, Baldomero H, Foeken L, et al. One million haemopoietic stem-cell transplants: a retrospective observational study. Lancet Haematol. 2015;2(3):e91–e100.
51. Seo DH, Whang DH, Song EY, Kim HS, Park Q. Prevalence of antibodies to hepatitis B core antigen and occult hepatitis B virus infections in Korean blood donors. Transfusion. 2011;51(8):1840–6.
52. Luo Z, Xie Y, Deng M, Zhou X, Ruan B. Prevalence of hepatitis B in the southeast of China: a population-based study with a large sample size. Eur J Gastroenterol Hepatol. 2011;23(8):695–700.
53. Zhang H, Li Q, Sun J, Wang C, Gu Q, Feng X, et al. Seroprevalence and risk factors for hepatitis B infection in an adult population in Northeast China. Int J Med Sci. 2011;8(4):321–31.
54. Fongsarun J, Ekkapongpisit M, Paisan M, Chanthachorn S, Papadopoulos KI. Prevalence of transmissible viral disease in maternal blood samples of autologous umbilical cord blood in a private cord blood bank. Transplant Technol. 2013;1:1.

55. Yamada H, Fujimoto M, Svay S, Lim O, Hok S, Goto N, et al. Seroprevalence, genotypic distribution and potential risk factors of hepatitis B and C virus infections among adults in Siem Reap, Cambodia. Hepatol Res. 2015;45(4):480–7.
56. Ashraf H, Alam NH, Rothermundt C, Brooks A, Bardhan P, Hossain L, et al. Prevalence and risk factors of hepatitis B and C virus infections in an impoverished urban community in Dhaka, Bangladesh. BMC Infect Dis. 2010;10(1):208.
57. Bhatti FA, Ullah Z, Salamat N, Ayub M, Ghani E. Anti-hepatits B core antigen testing, viral markers, and occult hepatitis B virus infection in Pakistani blood donors: implications for transfusion practice. Transfusion. 2007;47(1):74–9.
58. Bharath RR, Krishnan V. A study in the seroprevalence of hepatitis B core antibody and other transfusion transmitted infections in blood donors. Int J Res Med Sci. 2016;4(6):2337–40.
59. Lavanya V, Viswanathan T, Malar SAS, Malarvizhi A, Moorthy K. Prevalence of hepatitis B virus infection among blood donors with antibodies to hepatitis B core antigen. Int J Med Med Sci. 2012;4(6):128–37.
60. Meffre C, Le Strat Y, Delarocque-Astagneau E, Dubois F, Antona D, Lemasson JM, et al. Prevalence of hepatitis B and hepatitis C virus infections in France in 2004: social factors are important predictors after adjusting for known risk factors. J Med Virol. 2010;82(4): 546–55.
61. Ioannou GN. Hepatitis B virus in the United States: infection, exposure, and immunity rates in a nationally representative survey. Ann Intern Med. 2011;154(5):319–28.
62. Nelson PK, Mathers BM, Cowie B, Hagan H, Des Jarlais D, Horyniak D, et al. Global epidemiology of hepatitis B and hepatitis C in people who inject drugs: results of systematic reviews. Lancet. 2011;378(9791):571–83.
63. Glebe D. Hepatitis B virus taxonomy and hepatitis B virus genotypes. World J Gastroentrol. 2007;13(1):14–21.
64. Kim BK, Revill PA, Ahn SH. HBV genotypes: relevance to natural history, pathogenesis and treatment of chronic hepatitis B. Antivir Ther. 2011;16(8):1169–86.
65. Miyakawa Y, Mizokami M. Classifying hepatitis B virus genotypes. Intervirology. 2003;46(6):329–38.
66. Yuen MF, Sablon E, Yuan HJ, Wong DK, Hui CK, Wong BC, et al. Significance of hepatitis B genotype in acute exacerbation, HBeAg seroconversion, cirrhosis-related complications, and hepatocellular carcinoma. Hepatology. 2003;37(3):562–7.
67. Yuen MF, Tanaka Y, Shinkai N, Poon RT, But DY, Fong DY, et al. Risk for hepatocellular carcinoma with respect to hepatitis B virus genotypes B/C, specific mutations of enhancer II/core promoter/precore regions and HBV DNA levels. Gut. 2008;57(1):98–102.
68. Yuen MF, Tanaka Y, Mizokami M, Yuen JC, Wong DK, Yuan HJ, et al. Role of hepatitis B virus genotypes Ba and C, core promoter and precore mutations on hepatocellular carcinoma: a case control study. Carcinogenesis. 2004;25(9):1593–8.
69. Sanchez-Tapias JM, Costa J, Mas A, Bruguera M, Rodes J. Influence of hepatitis B virus genotype on the long-term outcome of chronic hepatitis B in western patients. Gastroenterology. 2002;123(6):1848–56.
70. Thakur V, Guptan RC, Kazim SN, Malhotra V, Sarin SK. Profile, spectrum and significance of HBV genotypes in chronic liver disease patients in the Indian subcontinent. J Gastroenterol Hepatol. 2002;17(2):165–70.
71. Buster EH, Hansen BE, Lau GK, Piratvisuth T, Zeuzem S, Steyerberg EW, et al. Factors that predict response of patients with hepatitis B e antigen-positive chronic hepatitis B to peginterferon-alfa. Gastroenterology. 2009;137(6):2002–9.
72. Lu T, Seto WK, Zhu RX, Lai CL, Yuen MF. Prevention of hepatocellular carcinoma in chronic viral hepatitis B and C infection. World J Gastroenterol. 2013;19(47):8887–94.
73. Jazayeri SM, Carman WF. Evolution of hepatitis B genotype D in the Middle east and South Asia. Hepat Mon. 2009;9(1):9–11.
74. Yuen MF, Seto WK, Chow DH, Tsui K, Wong DK, Ngai VW, et al. Long-term lamivudine therapy reduces the risk of long-term complications of chronic hepatitis B infection even in patients without advanced disease. Antivir Ther. 2007;12(8):1295–303.

75. Marcellin P, Gane E, Buti M, Afdhal N, Sievert W, Jacobson IM, et al. Regression of cirrhosis during treatment with tenofovir disoproxil fumarate for chronic hepatitis B: a 5-year open-label follow-up study. Lancet. 2013;381(9865):468–75.
76. Fung J, Seto WK, Lai CL, Yuen J, Wong DK, Yuen MF. Profiles of HBV DNA in a large population of Chinese patients with chronic hepatitis B: implications for antiviral therapy. J Hepatol. 2011;54(2):195–200.
77. Cohen C, Holmberg SD, McMahon BJ, Block JM, Brosgart CL, Gish RG, et al. Is chronic hepatitis B being undertreated in the United States? J Viral Hepat. 2011;18(6):377–83.
78. Spradling PR, Xing J, Rupp LB, Moorman AC, Gordon SC, Teshale ET, et al. Distribution of disease phase, treatment prescription and severe liver disease among 1598 patients with chronic hepatitis B in the Chronic Hepatitis Cohort Study, 2006–2013. Aliment Pharmacol Ther. 2016;44(10):1080–9.
79. Wu CY, Lin JT, Ho HJ, Su CW, Lee TY, SY W, et al. Association of nucleos(t)ide analogue therapy with reduced risk of hepatocellular carcinoma in patients with chronic hepatitis B: a nationwide cohort study. Gastroenterology. 2014;147(1):143–51.e5.
80. Seto WK, Lau EH, Wu JT, Hung IF, Leung WK, Cheung KS, et al. Effects of nucleoside analogue prescription for hepatitis B on the incidence of liver cancer in Hong Kong: a territory-wide ecological study. Aliment Pharmacol Ther. 2017;45(4):501–9.

9 Viral Hepatitis: The African Experience

Ramou Njie

9.1 Introduction

It is estimated that chronic viral hepatitis affects nearly 550 million people worldwide. While previous studies report approximately 350 million individuals are infected with hepatitis B virus (HBV), 185 million with hepatitis C virus (HCV) and 15 million with hepatitis delta virus [1, 2], recent updates from the World Health Organization (WHO) have revised estimates placing worldwide burden of chronic HBV at 257 million individuals. Viral hepatitis causes substantial mortality, globally accounting for more than 1 million deaths each year. Chronic viral infection is the primary cause of hepatocellular carcinoma (HCC), which is one of the most common cancers in developing countries and the second cause of cancer-related mortality worldwide [3].

The vast majority of individuals infected with viral hepatitis live in Africa and Asia, where screening and access to care and treatment are not readily available. In Africa, about 100 million individuals are estimated to be infected with HBV or HCV compared to 23 million HBV or HCV-infected individuals in more developed regions of the world [4]. In The Gambia, West Africa, the prevalence of chronic HBV infection in adults exceeds 8% [5] and HCC is the most frequent type of malignancy. There is strong epidemiological evidence that nearly 70% of HCC in sub-Saharan Africa is due to chronic infection with HBV, with fewer cases due to HCV [6].

R. Njie
Gambia Hepatitis Intervention Study (GHIS), International Agency for Research in Cancer, Lyon, France

C/O MRC Unit, The Gambia, Serrekunda, Gambia
e-mail: NjieR@iarc.fr; ranjie@mrc.gm

R. J. Wong, R. G. Gish (eds.), *Clinical Epidemiology of Chronic Liver Diseases*,
https://doi.org/10.1007/978-3-319-94355-8_9

9.2 The Devastating Burden of Viral Hepatitis in Africa

In Africa, HBV and HCV infections are highly endemic and responsible for 80% of cirrhosis and HCC cases, with HBV being the main cause of end-stage liver disease [2, 6, 7]. HCC has been reported as the most common cancer in males, the second most common in females and affects young individuals often below 40 years of age with a rapid and fatal outcome. HCV is steadily becoming an important cause of HCC; chronic viral hepatitis leading to HCC is enhanced by widespread exposure to aflatoxin, a carcinogenic mycotoxin that contaminates staple crops in many African countries [8]. There is lack of accurate data in Africa on the exact burden of cirrhosis and end-stage liver disease due to viral hepatitis because of a lack of infrastructure and skilled personnel, inadequate disease surveillance, and poor resources for proper data collection and management. Recent estimates show that, with 1.4 million attributed deaths in 2010, viral hepatitis poses a greater mortality threat than tuberculosis or malaria worldwide; most of these deaths occur in Africa [7].

The WHO estimates that HBV infection affects more than 5% of the local population in Sub-Saharan Africa and more than 8% in West Africa, reaching up to 15% in some areas [1, 7]. The transmission of the virus occurs early in life and is associated with a low rate of spontaneous viral clearance and a high risk of chronic liver disease. It is estimated that 25% of young adults, infected during childhood, will die prematurely from HBV-related cirrhosis or HCC [9]. The prevalence of HCV infection varies geographically with estimates between 3% and 5.3% [10]. Egypt bears the highest prevalence worldwide with a recent estimation of 14.7% in subjects aged 15–59 years [11]. This epidemic was the result of nosocomial transmission following mass treatment of schistosomiasis with the injectable drug antimony potassium tartrate during the 1960s. East and Central African countries, such as Burundi, Cameroon and Gabon, are also highly endemic for HCV with a prevalence in some areas reaching 11%, 13%, and 5% in the three respective countries [10]. In HIV infected individuals or other specific populations, such as drug users, sex workers, men who have sex with men, prisoners or patients with multiple transfusions secondary to sickle cell disease, estimates can even reach up to 50% [7, 12, 13]. The distribution of HCV genotypes in Africa also varies by sub-regions and is characterized by a considerable HCV subtype diversity. In West Africa, genotypes 1, 2, and 3 are predominant, whereas in Central Africa genotype 4 is more frequent. Genotype 5 is more frequently observed in Southern Africa [13].

9.3 Preventative Strategies

9.3.1 Vaccination

Major progress in the global response to viral hepatitis has been achieved through the expansion of routine hepatitis B vaccination, which was facilitated by the introduction of new combination vaccines. In 2015, global coverage with three doses of hepatitis B vaccine during infancy reached 84%. Between the date of introduction of the vaccine, (ranging from the 1980s in The Gambia, West Africa to the early 2000s in different countries) and 2015, the proportion of children <5 years of age who became chronically infected fell from 4.7% to 1.3 % [14]. However, in those African countries where high hepatitis B vaccination coverage has not been achieved, children continue to have intermediate or high hepatitis B surface antigen (HBsAg) prevalence. A substantial burden of chronic HBV infection persists because the global coverage with the birth vaccine dose is still low, estimated globally at 39% in 2015 [14]; in The Gambia, one of the first countries to introduce mass infant HBV vaccination, less than 3% of children received the birth dose within 24 h of birth [15]. In the absence of the universal birth dose or other effective interventions, the transmission of HBV infection from mother to child remains a major source of chronic liver disease when infected children become adults [14].

9.3.2 Prevention of Transmission

Nosocomial transmission at medical and dental facilities is an important route of viral hepatitis transmission in Africa. The World Health Organisation estimates that 24% of blood donations in low-income countries are not systematically screened for HBV or HCV and 2 million new HCV infections worldwide result from unsafe injections each year. In 2000, about 20% of medical injections were estimated to be administrated under unsafe conditions. Transmission of HCV through medical or dental procedures has also been documented in many African countries. A tragic illustration of such transmission is Egypt where the national campaign to eradicate schistosomiasis using reusable syringes led to the rapid spread of HCV. Similar health campaigns have led to iatrogenic spread of HCV in Cameroon and Gabon [7, 16]. Intravenous drug use, though not a major mode of transmission in Africa, has nevertheless been observed in some major cities. More research is needed to map out in more detail the HCV transmission routes in Africa. In the meantime, adopting universal infection control measures in all health facilities, blood donor screening, safe injection practices, routine antenatal screening as well as screening of high risk groups will be critical to prevent further transmission in the community.

9.3.3 Screening

Halting the transmission of HBV and HCV in Africa will require, in addition to the measures outlined above, screening and treatment of infected persons. WHO published recommendations on viral hepatitis testing in February 2017, in which it stated that testing and diagnosis of HBV and HCV infection is the gateway for access to both prevention and treatment services, and is a crucial component of an effective response to the viral hepatitis epidemic. Early identification of persons with chronic HBV or HCV infection enables them to receive the necessary care and treatment to prevent or delay progression of liver disease. Testing also provides an opportunity to link people to interventions to reduce transmission, through counselling on risk behaviours and provision of prevention commodities (such as sterile needles and syringes) and HBV vaccination. Overall, the guidelines recommend the use of a single quality-assured serological in vitro diagnostic test (i.e. either a laboratory-based immunoassay [enzyme immunoassay or chemiluminiscence immunoassay] or rapid diagnostic test [RDT]) to detect HBsAg and HCV antibody. RDTs used should meet minimum performance standards, and be delivered at the point of care to improve access and linkage to care and treatment. Access to affordable hepatitis testing is limited in Africa. There are very few comprehensive screening programmes that offer screening and treatment, in part because the assays, and effective treatments, are quite expensive and not accessible to those who need them the most. This is further compounded by lack of skilled manpower to undertake clinical liver assessment. There is thus a paucity of data from Africa on screening and treatment of viral hepatitis. In The Gambia, a small country in West Africa, two population-based, HBV preventative programs were set up to address this issue, and will be briefly described below.

9.4 Population-Based Approaches: The Gambian Experience

The Gambia is the smallest country in the African continent with a population of 1.8 million people. Two population-based intervention studies to control HBV infection, namely, the Gambia Hepatitis Intervention Study (GHIS) and Prevention of Liver Fibrosis and Cancer in Africa (PROLIFICA) have been undertaken [17] to generate data that will hopefully guide policy in the fight against viral hepatitis in Africa.

The GHIS started in 1986 as a nation-wide trial of the HBV vaccine to evaluate the effectiveness of infant HBV vaccination in preventing infection and chronic HBsAg carriage in childhood, and in preventing HCC in adulthood. The vaccination phase began in August 1986. Over the subsequent four years the vaccination was gradually introduced to each immunization team on a team by team basis in a cluster-randomized, "step-wedge" design. This resulted in half the children born over these four years receiving HBV vaccination (approximately 60,000) and the other half only receiving the other routine WHO expanded program on immunization (EPI) vaccinations. A second phase of assessment of the effect of vaccination on rates of infection with HBV began in 1986 with a cohort of 1000 vaccinated children who were followed until they were 9 years old. They were compared to cross sectional samples of unvaccinated children at the ages of 5 and 9 years. These studies showed a high effectiveness of the vaccine against acute infection (90%) and in particular against chronic infection (95%). Two further cross sectional surveys of both vaccinated and unvaccinated individuals have been made at the age of 15 years and at the age of 20 years. These studies have shown that although the surface antibody induced by vaccination is no longer detectable in more than half of the individuals, they continue to have 70% protection against infection and 95% protection against chronic infection. No case of acute HBV has been seen in any vaccinated individual—all infections have been sub-clinical and only detected on serology

[18]. The third phase of the study consists of the identification of cases of HCC and chronic liver disease in the study groups and linkage to their vaccination status. A national cancer registry has been running in The Gambia since 1986 to track outcomes of this study. To improve the quality of diagnosis of HCC cases and provide an outcome to the study this author was recruited as a hepatologist to lead the GHIS program, among other things, to improve the diagnostic capacity, provide training to local staff, improve the care and management of patients with liver disease (including palliative care for HCC) and enhance registration over the next 5–10 years; the study participants are now in their mid- to late twenties. It is estimated that a clear quantitative estimate of the protective efficacy of vaccination against cancer will be possible in this time. There is only one other study globally addressing this question in China and uses a similar cluster randomized design but on the background of a very different epidemiology of HBV infection.

Despite the introduction of mass immunization for HBV since 1990, HBV-related morbidity and mortality remains high in The Gambia. The number cases of HCC and end-stage liver disease have not declined as individuals chronically infected with HBV prior to the immunization program continue to present with advanced disease. The PROLIFICA project was set up in 2011 in The Gambia and Senegal initially for 5 years with the primary objective of assessing whether antiviral therapy using oral Tenofovir would reduce the incidence of HCC in West Africa. An additional objective was to determine the applicability and effectiveness of a population-based screening, clinical assessment and treatment in West Africa. Between Dec 7, 2011, and Jan 24, 2014, individuals living in randomly selected communities in western Gambia were offered hepatitis B surface antigen (HBsAg) screening via a point-of-care test. The test was also offered to potential blood donors attending the central hospital in the capital, Banjul. HBsAg-positive individuals were invited for a comprehensive liver assessment and were offered treatment according to the European Association for the Study of the Liver (EASL) 2012 guidelines. Linkage to care was defined as visiting the liver clinic at least once. Of the over 11,500 individuals screened (5980 from the community and 6832 blood donors) HBsAg was detected in 9% of individuals from the communities and 13.0% of blood donors, who were all almost exclusively male. Overall prevalence was higher in men (10.5%) versus women (7.6%). Linkage to care was high in the communities, with 81.3% of HBsAg-positive individuals attending the liver clinic but only 41.6% of HBsAg-positive people (mainly men) screened at the blood bank, linked into care. Overall less than 10% of all those who tested positive for HBsAg met the EASL criteria for treatment. Male sex was strongly associated with treatment eligibility. The PROLIFICA project confirmed that an HBV screen-and-treat programme targeting the general population is a feasible and realistic public health intervention in The Gambia. Such an intervention deserves to be assessed on a larger scale in sub-Saharan Africa and in other resource-limited countries, with eventual integration into international and national guidelines to fight against the burden of HBV infection in endemic areas [5]. The PROLIFICA programme in The Gambia and Senegal is one of very few addressing the issue of HBV testing, combined with assessment of the severity of chronic HBV and the screening of liver cancer. It also aims at demonstrating the efficacy of tenofovir-based antiviral therapy for preventing cirrhosis and HCC in West Africa; the on-going clinical follow-up of the treatment and observation cohorts is expected to yield valuable data on treatment outcomes in an African setting and contribute towards the further development of guidelines in this part of the world.

9.5 Future Strategies

The Gambia, like much of Africa, carries a disproportionate burden of viral hepatitis, with high mortality and morbidity from liver cancer and end-stage liver disease. However, it has very limited access to innovative new diagnostic tools and highly effective antiviral drugs that other regions of the world take for granted. This needs urgent attention from local governments, but the scale of the problem is such that the assistance of the global community will be crucial if any meaningful progress is to be made. Future strategies to improve prevention, screening, care and treatment can be achieved through existing health care infrastructure. Operational programs and clinical trials should be conducted in countries in Africa with the support of local governments and the international health community. WHO's elimination strategy by 2030 aims to reduce mortality from chronic infection with HBV and HCV by 65%. To achieve this goal, it is essential to scale up antiviral treatment programmes in low-income and middle-income countries, where most deaths due to viral hepatitis occur. These programmes must identify, engage, and retain infected populations. The recent call for action by WHO, through the Global Hepatitis Programme and Global Partners needs indeed to be translated into concrete action.

Summary Table of Landmark Literature

Study title and authors	Study design	Summary results	Main limitations
Lemoine M, et al. Lancet Glob Health. 2016;4(8):e559–67	Population-based prospective study from December 7, 2011 to January 24, 2014 evaluating the effectiveness of point of care HBsAg testing among individuals in randomly selected communites in western Gambia and potential blood donors in the central hospital of Banjul.	• Among the community-based cohort that underwent testing, HBsAg prevalence was 8.8%. • Among the cohort of potential blood donors, HBsAg prevalence was 13.0%. • HBsAg prevalence was significantly higher in men compared to women (10.5% vs. 7.6%, $p = 0.004$)	• Single country study among select populations may not be generalizable to populations in other African countries. • Overall test acceptance rates were 68.9% among the community-based cohort and 81.4% among the blood donor-based cohort

Study title and authors	Study design	Summary results	Main limitations
Kirk GD, et al. Hepatology 2004;39:211–9	The Gambia Liver Cancer Study (GLCS) was conducted in conjunction with The Gambia Hepatitis Intervention Study, an international collaborative project designed to evaluate the efficacy of phased introduction of hepatitis B vaccine into The Gambia's national immunization program in preventing chronic HBV infection, chronic liver disease, and HCC from September 1997 through January 2001	• 216 incidence cases of HCC and 408 controls were recruited into the study. • HBsAg prevalence was 61% among incidence HCC patients and 165 among non-HCC controls. • Overall, 57% of HCC cases were attributed to chronic HBV infection	• Single country study among select populations may not be generalizable to populations in other African countries • Relatively small sample size and may not reflect larger population-based HBV prevalence
Lemoine M, et al. J Hepatol 2015;62:469–76	Review paper highlighting the burden of viral hepatitis in Africa and discussion on potential strategies to achieve eradication among this high prevalence region	• According to WHO, HBV infection affects more than 5% of the local population in Sub-Saharan Africa and more than 8% in West Africa, reaching up to 15% in some areas • WHO estimates that very few countries have implemented an HBV birth dose vaccine strategy and that only 23% of children born in the African continent benefit from the early birth dose • Nosocomial transmission is another major route of viral hepatitis transmission in Africa. WHO estimates that 24% of blood donations in low-income countries are not systematically screened for HBV	• Review paper is limited by the lack of epidemiological data in many parts of the African continent. • Lack of epidemiological studies prevents an accurate assessment of HBV prevalence in many regions of Africa.

References

1. Ott JJ, Stevens GA, Groeger J, Wiersma ST. Global epidemiology of hepatitis B virus infection: new estimates of age-specific HBsAg seroprevalence and endemicity. Vaccine. 2012;30:2212–9.
2. Mohd Hanafiah K, Groeger J, Flaxman AD, Wiersma ST. Global epidemiology of hepatitis C virus infection: new estimates of age-specific antibody to HCV seroprevalence. Hepatology. 2013;57:1333–42.
3. Jemal A, Bray F, Forman D, O'Brien M, Ferlay J, Center M, et al. Cancer burden in Africa and opportunities for prevention. Cancer. 2012;118(18):4372–84.
4. Blachier M, Leleu H, Peck-Radosavljevic M, Valla DC, Roudot-Thoraval F. The burden of liver disease in Europe: a review of available epidemiological data. J Hepatol. 2013;58:593–608.
5. Lemoine M, et al. Acceptability and feasibility of a screen-and-treat programme for hepatitis B virus infection in The Gambia: the Prevention of Liver Fibrosis and Cancer in Africa (PROLIFICA) study. Lancet Glob Health. 2016;4(8):e559–67. https://doi.org/10.1016/S2214-109X(16)30130-9.
6. Kirk GD, Lesi OA, Mendy M, Akano AO, Sam O, Goedert JJ, et al. The Gambia Liver Cancer Study: Infection with hepatitis B and C and the risk of hepatocellular carcinoma in West Africa. Hepatology. 2004;39:211–9.
7. Lemoine M, Eholié S, Lacombe K. Reducing the neglected burden of viral hepatitis in Africa: strategies for a global approach. J Hepatol. 2015;62(2):469–76. https://doi.org/10.1016/j.jhep.2014.10.008.
8. Hainaut P, Boyle P. Curbing the liver cancer epidemic in Africa. Lancet. 2008;371:367–8.
9. Kane M. Global programme for control of hepatitis B infection. Vaccine. 1995;13:S47–9.
10. Madhava V, Burgess C, Drucker E. Epidemiology of chronic hepatitis C virus infection in sub-Saharan Africa. Lancet Infect Dis. 2002;2:293–302.
11. Guerra J, Garenne M, Mohamed MK, Fontanet A. HCV burden of infection in Egypt: results from a nationwide survey. J Viral Hepat. 2012;19:560–7.
12. Nelson PK, Mathers BM, Cowie B, Hagan H, Des Jarlais D, Horyniak D, et al. Global epidemiology of hepatitis B and hepatitis C in people who inject drugs: results of systematic reviews. Lancet. 2011;378:571–83.
13. Barth RE, Huijgen Q, Taljaard J, Hoepelman AI. Hepatitis B/C and HIV in sub-Saharan Africa: an association between highly prevalent infectious diseases. A systematic review and meta-analysis. Int J Infect Dis. 2010;14:e1024–31.
14. Global Hepatitis Report, World Health Organization, Geneva. 2017. http://apps.who.int/iris/bitstream/10665/255016/1/9789241565455-eng.
15. Miyahara R, Jasseh M, Gomez P, Shimakawa Y, Greenwood B, Keita K, Ceesay S, D'Alessandro U, Roca A. Barriers to timely administration of birth dose vaccines in The Gambia, West Africa. Vaccine. 2016;34(29):3335–41. https://doi.org/10.1016/j.vaccine.2016.
16. Njouom R, Caron M, Besson G, Ndong-Atome GR, Makuwa M, Pouillot R, et al. Phylogeography, risk factors and genetic history of hepatitis C virus in Gabon, central Africa. PLoS One. 2012;7:e42002.
17. Shimakawa Y, Lemoine M, Mendy M, Njai HF, D'Alessandro U, Hall A, Thursz M, Njie R. Population-based interventions to reduce the public health burden related with hepatitis B virus infection in the Gambia, west Africa. Trop Med Health. 2014;42(2 Suppl):59–64. https://doi.org/10.2149/tmh.2014-S08.
18. Peto TJ, Mendy ME, Lowe Y, Webb EL, Whittle HC, Hall AJ. Efficacy and effectiveness of infant vaccination against chronic hepatitis B in the Gambia Hepatitis Intervention Study (1986–90) and in the nationwide immunisation program. BMC Infect Dis. 2014;14:7.

10 Hepatitis B: The Western Perspective

Elana Rosenthal and Rachel Baden

Abstract

Chronic infection with hepatitis B virus (HBV) is present in approximately 257 million individuals worldwide and is a major cause of liver disease, liver cancer, and liver-related mortality. The prevalence of chronic hepatitis B (CHB) varies by region, and is often difficult to define due to limited surveillance. In highly endemic regions in Europe and the Americas, which have immigrants from endemic regions, a predominant cause of transmission remains perinatal infection. In low prevalence regions, sexual transmission has historically been a major source of HBV acquisition. More recently, implementation of widespread vaccination campaigns in some regions has dramatically reduced HBV prevalence and rates of acute HBV in children and young adults. However, due to high-risk behaviors and limited access to health services, marginalized populations—such as injection drug users (IDUs) and incarcerated individuals—continue to suffer from disproportionate rates of infection relative to the general population, with new outbreaks of HBV in IDUs in the United States becoming a health care crisis.

Keywords

Chronic HBV · Acute HBV · Perinatal transmission · HBV vaccination · PWID · Incarcerated individuals

E. Rosenthal
Division of Clinical Care and Research, Institute of Human Virology, University of Maryland School of Medicine, Baltimore, MD, USA

R. Baden (✉)
Department of Medicine, Highland Hospital, Alameda Health System, Oakland, CA, USA
e-mail: rbaden@alamedahealthsystem.org

R. J. Wong, R. G. Gish (eds.), *Clinical Epidemiology of Chronic Liver Diseases*,
https://doi.org/10.1007/978-3-319-94355-8_10

10.1 Introduction

Chronic infection with hepatitis B virus (HBV) is present in approximately 257 million individuals worldwide and caused 887,000 deaths in 2015 [1]. There are over 2 billion people who have been exposed to HBV, as indicated by antibody to the hepatitis B core antigen (anti-HBc), and are at risk for HBV reactivation with changes in their immune system. Overall burden in the Western hemisphere is difficult to fully quantify due to lack of surveillance and screening programs in certain regions and in various populations. However, understanding the epidemiology of chronic hepatitis B (CHB) allows for better screening and early intervention so appropriate monitoring and treatment can be implemented to avoid complications from this disease.

10.2 Prevalence: The Americas

Overall, most countries in the Americas, including the United States (U.S.), have a low prevalence of CHB as defined by HBsAg seroprevalence of less than 2%. However, certain regions such as Belize, Colombia, the Dominican Republic, Ecuador, and Peru have a low-intermediate prevalence of 2–4.99%. Importantly, Haiti is the one outlier across the Americas with recent data revealing a prevalence as high as 13.55% [2]. The most recent (2007–2012) U.S. National Health and Nutrition Examination Survey (NHANES) data shows that 3.9% of noninstitutionalized U.S. residents had anti-HBc, indicating approximately 10.8 million who have ever been infected; prevalence of CHB has remained constant since 1999 with an estimated prevalence in 2012 of 0.3% (847,000 residents) [3]. However, population-based surveys such as NHANES likely underestimate the burden of disease from CHB as they do not account for individuals who are institutionalized, incarcerated or not currently housed. The highest reported prevalence in the United States is in non-Hispanic Asians who have a tenfold higher rate of chronic infection than the general population. Non-Hispanic Asians accounted for 50% of cases in the U.S. from 2011 to 2012. Among the non-Hispanic Asians with CHB in the United States identified during 2011–2012, 93.1% were foreign-born. Higher rates of chronic infection are also reported in non-Hispanic blacks in the U.S., with a two to threefold greater prevalence than the general population. Among the non-Hispanic blacks in the U.S. with CHB, prevalence was 2.5% among those who were foreign-born compared to only 0.4% among the U.S.-born [3]. CHB disproportionately affects the immigrant population in the U.S. Over 90% of all new cases are in individuals born outside the country [4]. Importantly, attempts at accurately accounting for individuals with CHB who have migrated to the U.S. over the last several decades reveal that the prevalence may be much higher than previously reported. Taking into account these important populations, it is estimated that currently there are 2.2 million individuals living in the U.S. with chronic hepatitis B [5, 6].

10.3 Prevalence: Europe

Across Europe, there is geographic variation in the incidence and prevalence of CHB. Some of this variation is due to differences in surveillance and reporting. Additionally, the epidemiology of this disease is changing in this region. Much of Europe has a low HBsAg seroprevalence of 2% or less. However, some countries such as Azerbaijan, Belarus, Bulgaria, Cyprus, Georgia, Italy, Kosovo, Russia, and Turkey have a reported low-intermediate prevalence of 2–4.99%. Albania, Kazakhstan, Moldova, Romania, Tajikistan and Uzbekistan have a high-intermediate seroprevalence of 5–7.99%. Kyrgyzstan has the highest rate of CHB in the region with an estimated prevalence of 10.32% [2]. In 2013, 28 EU/EEA member states reported 19,101 cases of hepatitis B, approximately 3000 of which were acute [7]. Overall, the rate of acute cases declined from 2006 when it was 1.3/100,000 to 2013 when the reported rate was 0.7/100,000. However, the reported rate of chronic infections increased from 5.7/100,000 in 2006 to 7.4/100,000 in 2013. This increase in reported chronic infections is thought to be in part from increased surveillance. Additionally, as in the U.S., many European countries have seen an influx of CHB from migration of individuals from more highly endemic countries. In the six European countries studied by Chu and colleagues (Denmark, Finland, Germany, the Netherlands, Sweden, and the United Kingdom of Great Britain and Northern Ireland), incident infection was decreasing overall. However, migration into these regions has had a major impact on HBV prevalence. In the UK, for instance, it was estimated that 96% of newly identified chronic HBV infections were in individuals who had immigrated from more highly endemic regions. Similarly, in the other five countries studied a majority of individuals with CHB were born abroad [8].

10.4 Vaccination and Pregnancy

In the U.S., rates of acute hepatitis B have decreased significantly since the early 1980s when the first hepatitis B vaccine was introduced and have continued to decline since 1991 when the recommendation to vaccinate all infants born in the U.S. was first implemented [9]. Since 1995, guideline recommendations in the U.S. have expanded to include vaccination of all adolescents and to give stronger recommendations for all high-risk adult populations, including adults with diabetes in 2011 [10]. However, HBV vaccination coverage for higher risk adults remains low in the U.S. In adults with up to 3–4 risk factors for HBV, only 54.5% are vaccinated [11]. Strikingly, only 63.8% of health care workers have completed the full HBV vaccine series [12]. While the incidence of acute infection in the U.S. is the lowest it has been in decades, it is estimated that in 2014 there were still approximately 19,000 new cases of HBV, with 1200 cases of HBV from maternal fetal transmission (CDC 2017) [9]. Hepatitis B immunoglobulin and an initial dose of hepatitis B vaccine within 12 h of delivery should be given to infants who are born to mothers with CHB. This combination of hepatitis B immunoglobulin and vaccination at birth has decreased the rate of perinatal transmission from over 90% to less than 10% [13]. Other countries in the Americas have also gradually introduced hepatitis B vaccine into their childhood immunization schedules since 1991 with the last being Bonaire, Haiti, and Saba in 2012. However, as of 2016, only 69% of countries in the Americas include the birth dose vaccine in the schedule. Six countries have employed catch-up vaccination and, like the U.S., expanded vaccination to include older age groups. Moreover, Argentina, Cuba and Brazil have expanded their HBV vaccination recommendations to include the entire population, regardless of risk or age. For the period of 2010–2015, vaccine coverage rate in the Americas for infants and children ranged from as low as 36% in Haiti (likely owing to the fact that the national vaccination efforts for this age group were just introduced in 2012) to 99% in countries like Nicaragua, Anguilla and St. Lucia. Of the countries which had policies in place for vaccination for that entire time period, 74% reported a vaccination rate in children over 90% [14]. Of 29 European Union countries including Iceland and Norway reporting in 2010, all had implemented childhood HBV vaccination programs. However, seven countries in the EU report only risk-based vaccination programs, namely the United Kingdom, Sweden, Norway, The Netherlands, Iceland, Denmark, and Finland. All others either mandate or recommend universal HBV vaccination in childhood [15]. Data suggest that infants who still acquire hepatitis B despite immunoglobulin and vaccination at birth are more likely to be born to a mother with a high HBV viral load. To further combat perinatal transmission, current guidelines in Europe and the U.S. now also support the use of antivirals in pregnancy in women with baseline viral loads greater than 200,000 IU/mL [13, 16, 17].

10.5 Transmission

The largest burden of hepatitis B lies in the population of individuals living with chronic infection as 15–25% of these individuals are at risk for premature death from complications from their CHB including end-stage liver disease and hepatocellular carcinoma. Worldwide, hepatitis B accounts for 47% of viral hepatitis-associated mortality [18]. The risk of developing chronic infection depends on the age of infection. Up to 90% of perinatal infections become chronic while only 5–10% of adults and older children will develop chronic infection [19]. Risk factors for infection vary by region and by demographics. In highly endemic regions, for instance, vertical transmission is the most common cause of infection. For acute cases identified in Europe in 2013, heterosexual transmission, nosocomial transmission, injection drug use and transmission among men who have sex with men were reported as common causes of infection. However, likely reflecting that many individuals in the EU region with CHB were born in more highly endemic regions, vertical transmission was the most common etiology of infection, accounting for 43.5% of infections in individuals with CHB [7]. For the acute cases of HBV identified in the U.S. in 2014, sexual transmission and especially injection drug use were among the most common risk factors that could be identified [9].

10.6 Special Populations at Risk: Injection Drug Users

HBV is found in the highest concentrations in the blood and can be viable and infectious in the environment for as long as a week. Therefore, injection drug users (IDUs) are at particular risk of HBV transmission due to microtransfusions that occur when sharing injection equipment such as needles and syringes. In addition, transmission can occur from backloading, sharing cookers, cottons, and injecting water, even after several days without use. Up to 80% of IDUs who have injected for five or more years have evidence of exposure to HBV [20]. Prevalence of HBV in IDUs increases with duration of drug use, injection frequency, and prior history of sharing drug preparation equipment [20].

Worldwide there are 13 million IDUs, of whom 1.2 million are estimated to be chronically infected with hepatitis B [21]. In Europe, the estimated HBsAg prevalence in IDUs has been shown to be as high as 34% in some studies, with estimates nine times that of the general population [22, 23]. In the EU/EFTA region, 3.7% are estimated to have HBsAg, while outside the EU/EFTA that prevalence is believed to be 21% [23]. Higher prevalence among IDUs in these regions may reflect higher prevalence in the general population, as well as decreased access to vaccination and harm reduction strategies for IDUs. In the U.S., the prevalence of CHB in IDUs is estimated as 2.7–11%; IDUs with HIV have estimated prevalence of 7.1% [24]. Among all U.S. citizens known to have CHB, 4–12% report a history of injection drug use [24].

While injection drug use historically accounted for 15–20% of reported cases of acute HBV in the U.S., from the 1980–1990s, the predominant risk factors were high risk heterosexual sex, and sex between men who have sex with men [20, 25]. However, as overall incidence of HBV in the U.S. declined from the 1980s through the 2010s, the proportion of incidence attributable to drug use has increased. In a CDC study of seven surveillance sites in the U.S. between 2006 and 2011, the predominant risk factor for transmission was drug use, with the majority of cases in men who were aged 30–49, of white non-Hispanic race, and born in the U.S. [25].

Of note, declining HBV incidence has not been consistent across the US. In fact, between 2009 and 2013, HBV incidence increased 114% in three states: Kentucky, Tennessee, and West Virginia. In a review of these cases, the proportion of white individuals, aged 30–39, from non-urban counties increased. Further, the proportion of injection drug use as the predominant risk factor increased from 53% to 75%. This rise in incidence paralleled an increase in HCV infection in the Appalachian region, and an HIV outbreak in Indiana, all believed to be associated with the rising opioid epidemic currently impacting the US. Both opioid use disorders and viral hepatitis are particularly marked in regions with limited access to opioid use disorder treatment and harm reduction strategies such as needle and syringe programs [26].

IDUs with HBV infection are more likely to be coinfected with hepatitis delta than the general population, with HDV often identified during incident infection with HBV. Prior to widespread HBV vaccination, hepatitis delta coinfection in IDUs with CHB was found to be as high as 64% in Italy, 44% in Denmark, 33% in

Switzerland, and 31% in Ireland [27]. In an HBV outbreak in Washington state in the U.S., 34.5% of all IDUs identified as having acute HBV had evidence of HDV coinfection [20]. These individuals were more likely to inject more than four time per day, share cookers with more than two people in an average week, and have more than one sex partner in the previous 6 months [20]. However, more recent data from Spain indicate that HDV infection has dramatically declined amongst IDUs, largely the result of universal HBV vaccination and introduction of needle and syringe programs [28]. Measures have been taken to address HBV in IDUs, but prevention and harm reduction strategies remain suboptimal. While a history of injecting drug use is an indication for HBV immunization, immunization rates remain low among IDUs, even among the young [29, 30]. Further, the value of needle and syringe programs is incompletely understood. A study in the 1990s of needle and syringe programs in Seattle failed to demonstrate an impact of program enrollment on HBV acquisition [31]. Despite this, anti-HBc prevalence in IDUs in Seattle declined from 43% to 15% from 1994 to 2004 [29]. This decline was correlated with increases in self-reported needle exchange use, condom use, and HBV vaccination, without change in sharing of injecting equipment [29]. A comparison of IDUs in Newark, where syringe distribution was illegal, and NYC, where syringe distribution was legal, found higher prevalence of anti-HBc in IDUs in Newark [32]. Taken together, these data indicate that comprehensive programs to immunize and reduce harm in IDUs may contribute to a declining prevalence of CHB in this population. However, while these benefits have been seen in urban opioid epidemics in the U.S., HBV continues to spread in IDUs in non-urban regions and European regions with limited access to vaccines and needle and syringe programs.

10.7 Special Populations at Risk: Incarcerated Individuals

Due to a combination of factors including criminalization of drug use, criminalization of sex work, and disproportionate incarceration of marginalized populations people who are incarcerated have a higher prevalence of HBV infection than the general population [33]. As such, of the 10.2 million people worldwide estimated to be incarcerated on any given day, 491,500 (4.8%) have CHB [34]. In the U.S., HBsAg prevalence is 2% among jail and prison inmates, compared to 0.5% in the non-inmate population [24, 35]. Anti-HBc prevalence among adult inmates ranges from 13% to 47% [35]. Further, 12–39% of all individuals with CHB or chronic hepatitis C in the US were released during the previous year [35]. Outbreaks of acute HBV have been identified in prisons, with associated risk behaviors including tattooing, sharing a razor, condom-less sex, and injection drug use [34, 36]. HBV incidence in U.S. correctional settings ranges from 0.82% to 3.8% per year, with the highest risk of transmission attributable to sex with another inmate [35].

While immunization of inmates is recommended, immunization programs are not found in all correctional settings, and programs that exist vary in size and scope

[35]. However, when implemented, these programs have found relative success. In states offering universal vaccine coverage, 60–80% of inmates accept vaccination [35]. Further, studies of accelerated vaccination schedules in the Los Angeles county jail and in Denmark both demonstrated improved completion rates compared to the standard schedule [37]. In Scottish prisons, universal HBV vaccination of inmates was introduced and resulted in a complete elimination of acute HBV outbreaks among IDUs over 5 years [38]. Overall, incarcerated individuals remain a high risk population for HBV infection, in whom universal vaccination has the potential to dramatically limit HBV transmission both during incarceration and upon return to the community.

Summary Table of Landmark Literature

Study title and authors	Study design	Summary results	Main limitations
Schweitzer A, et al. Lancet. 2015;386(10003): 1546–55	Systematic review and pooled analysis of HBV prevalence in 1965 and in 2013 in 161 countries	Comprehensive evaluation of country-specific HBV prevalence data	Lack of data for some regions and much of the available data did not likely represent the population on a national level as certain groups were not included in analysis
Mitchell T, et al. PLoS One. 2011;6(12):e27717	Country specific prevalence was multiplied by yearly number of immigrants from each country between 1974 and 2008 to estimate the number of imported cased of HBV	Imported cased of HBV make up approximately 95% of new cases in the US Important to account for burden of disease in foreign-born Americans	Epidemiologic data from many countries still limited and may not necessarily represent the prevalence in the immigrant population from that region
Chu JJ, et al. Eur J Public Health. 2013;23(4):642–7	Literature review and statistical analysis on migration and HBV infection in six European countries	Incidence of HBV decreasing Similar prevalence in three largest migrant groups in all six countries of about 4% Immigrants from countries with high/intermediate endemicity makes up a substantial portion of all chronic cases of HBV	Overall prevalence of HBV is likely underestimated due to under-reporting Great heterogeneity in reporting across the six countries studied

Study title and authors	Study design	Summary results	Main limitations
Ropero Alvarez AM, et al. BMC Public Health. 2017;17(1):325	Data and survey collection regarding HBV vaccination schedules and strategies in 51 countries in the Americas	All countries and territories in the Americas have HBV vaccination in the immunization schedules Significant opportunities still exist ahead in birth dose vaccination and vaccination of high risk adults	
Harris AM, et al. MMWR Morb Mortal Wkly Rep. 2016;65(3):47–50	Analysis of data available on cases of acute HBV infection reported to CDC from Kentucky, Tennessee, and West Virginia during 2006–2013	Three states in the Appalachian region reported an increase in cases of acute HBV infection, among non-Hispanic whites, persons aged 30–39 years, and injection drug users. A significant increase in the proportion of cases from injection drug use was reported during 2010–2013	Not all cases are reported and asymptomatic cases excluded May underrepresent most vulnerable populations who may note present for care or have cases reported
Dolan K, et al. Lancet. 2016;388(10049):1089–102	Meta-analysis of studies identifying infections in incarcerated individuals	Prevalence of HBV, is higher in prison populations than in the general population and is estimated to be 4.8% Higher prevalence of infection in incarcerated individuals likely from the criminalization of drug use and the detention of people who inject drugs	Heterogeneity of reporting and lack of data in some regions

References

1. Global Hepatitis Report. World Health Organization. 2017. http://apps.who.int/iris/bitstream/10665/255016/1/9789241565455-eng.pdf?ua=1.
2. Schweitzer A, Horn J, Mikolajczyk RT, Krause G, Ott JJ. Estimations of worldwide prevalence of chronic hepatitis B virus infection: a systematic review of data published between 1965 and 2013. Lancet. 2015;386(10003):1546–55.
3. Roberts H, Kruszon-Moran D, Ly KN, Hughes E, Iqbal K, Jiles RB, et al. Prevalence of chronic hepatitis B virus (HBV) infection in U.S. households: National Health and Nutrition Examination Survey (NHANES), 1988–2012. Hepatology. 2016;63(2):388–97.
4. Mitchell T, Armstrong GL, Hu DJ, Wasley A, Painter JA. The increasing burden of imported chronic hepatitis B—United States, 1974–2008. PLoS One. 2011;6(12):e27717.

5. Kowdley KV, Wang CC, Welch S, Roberts H, Brosgart CL. Prevalence of chronic hepatitis B among foreign-born persons living in the United States by country of origin. Hepatology. 2012;56(2):422–33.
6. Gish RG, Cohen CA, Block JM, Brosgart CL, Block TM, Clary R, Le LT, Ninburg MH, Sandt L, Kowdley KY. Data supporting updating estimates of the prevalence of chronic hepatitis B and C in the United States. Hepatology 2015;62:1339–1341. https://doi.org/10.1002/hep.28026.
7. European Centre for Disease Prevention and Control. Hepatitis B surveillance in Europe—2013. Stockholm: ECDC; 2015.
8. Chu JJ, Wormann T, Popp J, Patzelt G, Akmatov MK, Kramer A, et al. Changing epidemiology of hepatitis B and migration—a comparison of six Northern and North-Western European countries. Eur J Pub Health. 2013;23(4):642–7.
9. Surveillance Data, CDC. https://www.cdc.gov/hepatitis/statistics/2014surveillance/commentary.htm#hepatitisB.
10. Centers for Disease Control and Prevention (CDC). Use of hepatitis B vaccination for adults with diabetes mellitus: recommendations of the Advisory Committee on Immunization Practices (ACIP). MMWR Morb Mortal Wkly Rep. 2011;60(50):1709–11.
11. Annunziata K, Rak A, Del Buono H, DiBonaventura M, Krishnarajah G. Vaccination rates among the general adult population and high-risk groups in the United States. PLoS One. 2012;7(11):e50553.
12. Buckley GJ, Stron BL. Eliminating the public health problem of hepatitis B and C in the United States: phase one report. Washington, DC: National Academies Press (US); 2016.
13. Terrault NA, Bzowej NH, Chang KM, Hwang JP, Jonas MM, Murad MH; American Association for the Study of Liver Diseases. AASLD guidelines for treatment of chronic hepatitis B. Hepatology. 2016;63(1):261–83. https://doi.org/10.1002/hep.28156.
14. Ropero Alvarez AM, Perez-Vilar S, Pacis-Tirso C, Contreras M, El Omeiri N, Ruiz-Matus C, et al. Progress in vaccination towards hepatitis B control and elimination in the Region of the Americas. BMC Public Health. 2017;17(1):325.
15. Haverkate M, D'Ancona F, Giambi C, Johansen K, Lopalco PL, Cozza V, et al. Mandatory and recommended vaccination in the EU, Iceland and Norway: results of the VENICE 2010 survey on the ways of implementing national vaccination programmes. Euro Surveill. 2012;17(22):1–6.
16. Brown RS Jr, McMahon BJ, Lok AS, Wong JB, Ahmed AT, Mouchli MA, Wang Z, Prokop LJ, Murad MH, Mohammed K. Antiviral therapy in chronic hepatitis B viral infection during pregnancy: a systematic review and meta-analysis. Hepatology. 2016;63(1):319–33. https://doi.org/10.1002/hep.28302.
17. European Association for the Study of the Liver. EASL 2017 Clinical Practice Guidelines on the management of hepatitis B virus infection. J Hepatol. 2017;67(2):370–98. https://doi.org/10.1016/j.jhep.2017.03.021.
18. Stanaway JD, Flaxman AD, Naghavi M, Fitzmaurice C, Vos T, Abubakar I, et al. The global burden of viral hepatitis from 1990 to 2013: findings from the Global Burden of Disease Study 2013. Lancet. 2016;388(10049):1081–8.
19. Nelson NP, Easterbrook PJ, McMahon BJ. Epidemiology of hepatitis B virus infection and impact of vaccination on disease. Clin Liver Dis. 2016;20(4):607–28.
20. Bialek SR, Bower WA, Mottram K, Purchase D, Nakano T, Nainan O, et al. Risk factors for hepatitis B in an outbreak of hepatitis B and D among injection drug users. J Urban Health. 2005;82(3):468–78.
21. Nelson PK, Mathers BM, Cowie B, Hagan H, Des Jarlais D, Horyniak D, et al. Global epidemiology of hepatitis B and hepatitis C in people who inject drugs: results of systematic reviews. Lancet. 2011;378(9791):571–83.
22. Hahne SJ, Veldhuijzen IK, Wiessing L, Lim TA, Salminen M, Laar M. Infection with hepatitis B and C virus in Europe: a systematic review of prevalence and cost-effectiveness of screening. BMC Infect Dis. 2013;13:181.
23. Hope VD, Eramova I, Capurro D, Donoghoe MC. Prevalence and estimation of hepatitis B and C infections in the WHO European Region: a review of data focusing on the countries

outside the European Union and the European Free Trade Association. Epidemiol Infect. 2014;142(2):270–86.
24. Weinbaum CM, Williams I, Mast EE, Wang SA, Finelli L, Wasley A, et al. Recommendations for identification and public health management of persons with chronic hepatitis B virus infection. MMWR Recomm Rep. 2008;57(RR-8):1–20.
25. Iqbal K, Klevens RM, Kainer MA, Baumgartner J, Gerard K, Poissant T, et al. Epidemiology of acute hepatitis B in the United States from population-based surveillance, 2006–2011. Clin Infect Dis. 2015;61(4):584–92.
26. Harris AM, Iqbal K, Schillie S, Britton J, Kainer MA, Tressler S, et al. Increases in acute hepatitis B virus infections—Kentucky, Tennessee, and West Virginia, 2006–2013. MMWR Morb Mortal Wkly Rep. 2016;65(3):47–50.
27. Zeldis JB, Jain S, Kuramoto IK, Richards C, Sazama K, Samuels S, et al. Seroepidemiology of viral infections among intravenous drug users in northern California. West J Med. 1992;156(1):30–5.
28. Aguilera A, Trastoy R, Barreiro P, Costa JJ, de Mendoza C, Pena JM, et al. Decline and changing profile of hepatitis delta among injection drug users in Spain. Antivir Ther. 2018;23(1):87–90.
29. Burt RD, Hagan H, Garfein RS, Sabin K, Weinbaum C, Thiede H. Trends in hepatitis B virus, hepatitis C virus, and human immunodeficiency virus prevalence, risk behaviors, and preventive measures among Seattle injection drug users aged 18–30 years, 1994–2004. J Urban Health. 2007;84(3):436–54.
30. Lum PJ, Hahn JA, Shafer KP, Evans JL, Davidson PJ, Stein E, et al. Hepatitis B virus infection and immunization status in a new generation of injection drug users in San Francisco. J Viral Hepat. 2008;15(3):229–36.
31. Hagan H, McGough JP, Thiede H, Weiss NS, Hopkins S, Alexander ER. Syringe exchange and risk of infection with hepatitis B and C viruses. Am J Epidemiol. 1999;149(3):203–13.
32. Neaigus A, Zhao M, Gyarmathy VA, Cisek L, Friedman SR, Baxter RC. Greater drug injecting risk for HIV, HBV, and HCV infection in a city where syringe exchange and pharmacy syringe distribution are illegal. J Urban Health. 2008;85(3):309–22.
33. Rich JD, Beckwith CG, Macmadu A, Marshall BD, Brinkley-Rubinstein L, Amon JJ, et al. Clinical care of incarcerated people with HIV, viral hepatitis, or tuberculosis. Lancet. 2016;388(10049):1103–14.
34. Dolan K, Wirtz AL, Moazen B, Ndeffo-Mbah M, Galvani A, Kinner SA, et al. Global burden of HIV, viral hepatitis, and tuberculosis in prisoners and detainees. Lancet. 2016;388(10049):1089–102.
35. Weinbaum C, Lyerla R, Margolis HS, Centers for Disease Control and Prevention. Prevention and control of infections with hepatitis viruses in correctional settings. Centers for Disease Control and Prevention. MMWR Recomm Rep. 2003;52(RR-1):1–36; quiz CE1–4.
36. Hutchinson SJ, Wadd S, Taylor A, Bird SM, Mitchell A, Morrison DS, et al. Sudden rise in uptake of hepatitis B vaccination among injecting drug users associated with a universal vaccine programme in prisons. Vaccine. 2004;23(2):210–4.
37. Costumbrado J, Stirland A, Cox G, El-Amin AN, Miranda A, Carter A, et al. Implementation of a hepatitis A/B vaccination program using an accelerated schedule among high-risk inmates, Los Angeles County Jail, 2007–2010. Vaccine. 2012;30(48):6878–82.
38. Beck CR, Cloke R, O'Moore E, Puleston R. Hepatitis B vaccination coverage and uptake in prisons across England and Wales 2003–2010: a retrospective ecological study. Vaccine. 2012;30(11):1965–71.

11 Hepatitis D Virus

Mario Rizzetto

Abstract

Hepatitis D is caused by the hepatitis D virus (HDV), a ubiquitous RNA agent which depends upon the envelope proteins of the hepatitis B virus (HBV) for assembly of progeny virus. The infection is transmitted parenterally as well as sexually. Intravenous drug users are at the highest risk of infection. HBV infected patients who become superinfected with HDV are the major reservoir of the virus due to the high rate of chronicity. With the advent of universal HBV vaccination, the incidence of hepatitis D has declined in developed and developing countries. Residual disease persists in the aging domestic population of Southern Europe and in injection drug users and immigrants throughout Europe and the United States, with high concentrations in Mongolia and northwestern Amazonia as well as pockets of high-risk people in other countries. The prevalence of hepatitis D remains high and has a major medical impact in many areas of the developing world where HBV remains endemic and not controlled.

Keywords

Hepatitis D virus · Hepatitis delta virus · Hepatitis D epidemiology · HBsAg

11.1 Introduction

The discovery of the hepatitis D virus (HDV, also known as hepatitis Delta virus) dates back to the mid-1970s [1]. It was characterized as a defective viroid like-agent relying on a concomitant infection with the hepatitis B virus (HBV) to become pathogenic [2]. Assays for the antibody to HDV (anti-HD), the serological signature

M. Rizzetto
Division of Gastroenterology, University of Torino, Torino, Italy

R. J. Wong, R. G. Gish (eds.), *Clinical Epidemiology of Chronic Liver Diseases*,
https://doi.org/10.1007/978-3-319-94355-8_11

of its infection, became available commercially in 1984 [3], expediting epidemiological surveys. HDV was endemic throughout the Mediterranean basin and in the Middle East, Turkey, Central Africa, the Amazon Basin and Taiwan. Worldwide, no less than 5% of chronic hepatitis B patients (defined as HBsAg-positive) were estimated to be HDV-infected, corresponding to approximately 15,000,000 individuals. Prevalence was highest in injection drug users (IDUs) sharing needles. HDV seroprevalence rates among HBsAg-positive IDUs reached 90% in Taiwan and Thailand. The burden was also high in IDUs in the United States where 42–67% of chronic hepatitis B (CHB) patients had anti-HD (total antibody to HDV) in studies from 1972 to 1988. Outbreaks of fulminant hepatitis D in drug-using communities were reported in the United States, the United Kingdom, Sweden, Ireland, and Italy.

Clinical scrutiny showed that chronic hepatitis D ran a severe course progressive to cirrhosis in most patients [4]. This ominous feature was confirmed in virtually all subsequent studies [5] and the finding of anti-HD has become synonymous with a virulent type of liver disease [6]. However, almost 40 years later, the prevalence and medical impact of hepatitis D has been determined only in the developed world. Both remain largely unknown in many parts of the developing world, although fragmentary evidence indicates that these areas, including Mongolia, bear the highest brunt of hepatitis D.

11.2 The Unique Biology of HDV

HDV is the smallest virus in human virology. It has a circular RNA genome of about 1700 nucleotides [7]. The diminutive HDV has no replicative machinery of its own. Its genome is copied by host DNA-dependent RNA polymerases deceived to reproduce the viral RNA as if it were a cellular DNA [8]. It does not require HBV viremia. From the partner HBV all that is required is a supply of HBsAg for virion formation. As a rule, HDV inhibits HBV-DNA production while maintaining the synthesis of HBsAg. The affinity of HDV for the surface antigen is very high. HBsAg acts as a magnet that traps HDV RNA with only infinitesimal amounts of HDV present. For example, HDV has been shown to be transmitted to chimpanzees carrying HBsAg by a 10^{-11} dilution of infectious serum [9], representing the highest infectivity titer recorded in human disease.

11.3 The Complex Epidemiology of HDV

Since hepatitis D disease results from the double infection of HDV with HBV, the epidemiological and clinical approach must take into account the variables related to either infection and to the interplay of this dual viral infection. The critical variable determining the epidemiologic pattern of hepatitis D is the prevalence of chronic HBV infections in a given population [2]; the tighter the mesh of HBsAg carriers with concomitant blood exposure in a given population, the more rapid, extensive and virulent is the spread of HDV. However, despite the extreme infectivity of HDV in the HBsAg-positive setting, the epidemiology of HDV is not simply a replica of the epidemiology of HBV. Prevalence rates overlap but do not coincide. Early surveys showed that the prevalence of HDV was high in areas of Africa and of the Amazon basin where the prevalence of HBV was also high, but was low throughout Southeast Asia where HBV was endemic, with genotypes B and C and vertical transmission dominant [3]. In follow-up studies in Japan [10] and Korea [11], HDV did not spread to these countries as expected from modern migratory exchanges in spite of a consistent number of CHB patients. Therefore, genuine differences appear to exist in the capacity of HDV to infect HBV populations. Whether these are related to variable virulence of HDV, different genetic susceptibility of the HBsAg carrier, HBV genotypes, or local socio-cultural constraints remains unknown.

Eight genotypes of HDV have been identified [12] with 81–89% homology in nucleotide sequences within the same genotype and as much as 35% divergence between different genotypes. Genotype 1 is widely distributed and predominates in Europe, North America, the Mediterranean basin, Iran and Nigeria. Genotype 2 is found mainly in East and Northern Asia. Genotype 3 has been found only in the Amazon basin. Genotype 4 is present in Taiwan and Okinawa. Genotypes 5–8 have been isolated in West and Central Africa; genotype 8 was also isolated in two Brazilian patients who presumably arrived in Brazil through the slave migration from Africa [13]. The different genotypes are credited with differing pathogenic potential. Genotype 3 appears to be the most virulent and has been associated with outbreaks of fulminant hepatitis in South America [14]. Genotype 1 has variable pathogenicity; in Taiwan, patients with genotype 1 had a more adverse outcome than those infected with genotype 2 [15].

11.4 Problems in the Clinical–Epidemiological Analysis

Major problems with clinical-epidemiological analyses are how to interpret the different serological patterns resulting from the interactions of HDV with HBV, and determining the correlations between serological profiles and clinical outcomes [16]. Diagnosis relies only on serology; no clinical, histological or biochemical feature distinguishes HDV from HBV. Although HDV patients may display the whole spectrum of HBV markers, the prototype patient at risk of HDV exhibits anti-HBe in serum and has no or low levels of circulating HBV-DNA. The lack of replicative markers of HBV may provide a clue to the differential diagnosis from hepatitis B.

Diagnosis is made by the finding of total or IgG anti-HD but this assay is not robust enough for screening for overall exposure [17]. Testing for HDV in acute HBsAg-positive hepatitis D (i.e., acute hepatitis D acquired by coinfection) is unreliable. In this setting, the expression of HDV markers (IgM, IgG and total anti-HD) is weak and transitory and does not persist after the clearance of HBsAg. It is common practice to test for all hepatitis markers at onset of the acute disease, including IgM anti-HD and total anti-HD; for patients who present with chronic disease, remote from their acute or high-risk exposure, total anti-HD. Clearly, due to under-testing and missed diagnoses that are due to incorrect use of HDV testing for acute disease, incidence figures from early samples of acute HBV underestimate the impact of HDV coinfection. HDV superinfection of HBsAg carriers is accompanied by a brisk total and IgM anti-HD response; the IgG persists over time and can be measured in random samples of the patient; therefore, chronic HBsAg carriers are the most reliable source of information on the prevalence of HDV. However, not all HBV carriers are suitable for testing. HDV is directly pathogenic and upon superinfection patients usually develop a chronic hepatitis with progressive liver disease [18]. Therefore, surveys for the prevalence of HDV should be oriented to HBsAg-positive carriers with liver disease. Studies of the prevalence of anti-HD in HBsAg carriers without liver disease, such as the blood donors who often represent the reference population for serologic surveys, are unrewarding because HDV superinfection results in a chronic hepatitis and an illness pattern that would preclude blood donation. Finally, while in most cases total anti-HD reflects an underlying HDV infection, in some carriers the antibody may represent a serological marker of past infection with no clinical significance. Thus, the presence or absence of HDV RNA determined by PCR is the ultimately confirmatory test.

Several in-house and commercial assays have been developed to detect viremia [19] but testing for HDV RNA is still not generally available. Though improvements in the reverse transcription polymerase chain reaction has increased sensitivity, allowing detection of serum HDV-RNA in up to 100% of patients with chronic HDV infection who are truly viremic, the generalized use of qualitative and quantitative HDV RNA tests is limited by lack of standardization, restricted genotype coverage with primers or probe mismatches related to the high genetic variability of HDV, and lack of internal controls. In 2013, the first WHO International Standard of HDV RNA for nucleic acid amplification technique (NAT)-based assays has been developed [20]. Taking advantage of this standard, the first international external quality control for HDV quantification was recently performed [21]. Panels of HDV-RNA samples were sent to 28 laboratories in 17 countries worldwide. The comprehensive analysis revealed a very high heterogeneity of assay characteristics and results, including variable technical steps and inconsistent technologies. Thirteen labs (46.3%) properly quantified all 18 positive samples; 16 (57.1%) failed to detect at least one positive specimen. In some cases up to 10 samples were deemed negative, and several laboratories underestimated by >3 log IU/mL HDV of African genotypes [1, 5–8].

11.5 The Clinical–Epidemiological Scenarios

With the background of an epidemic of HDV infection among IDUs worldwide, three epidemiologic scenarios were recognized in the 1980s based on the prevalence of anti-HD in the general CHB population: a high, intermediate and low HDV endemicity [6]. Low endemicity areas were North America, Northern Europe and Australia where HDV was virtually confined to IDUs; high endemicity areas were poor countries of Africa and South America; intermediate endemicity areas were Eastern Europe, countries facing the Mediterranean Sea, and Taiwan. The clinico-epidemiological analysis showed that in Italy in 1983 the prevalence of

HDV in chronic HBsAg liver disease was 24% [6] with peaks close to 50% in advanced cirrhotic disease; in Taiwan in the early 1990s HDV prevalence was approximately 55% among prostitutes and as high as 91% in IDUs [22].

In the last 25 years, HBV vaccination, public health measures and improvements in hygiene have increasingly controlled HBV infection in the industrialized world, leading to a secondary effect of containment of HDV; formerly intermediate endemicity countries have now been downgraded to low endemicity areas. Vice-versa, the risk of HDV has not changed in the poorest communities of the world where HBV remains uncontrolled.

11.5.1 The Current Clinical Epidemiology in the Developing World

The epidemiological information concerning HDV in the developing world is derived primarily from prevalence rates of total anti-HD, with serum HDV-RNA having been measured in only a few studies. In more recent studies, a distinction has been made between HBsAg carriers recruited at liver clinics and those collected at blood banks, in community surveys, and at healthcare screenings in general medical clinics; the latter were often grouped as a general population comparator. A detailed serological or clinical analysis of patients is usually lacking other than in the case of HDV testing in HIV infection in some series.

The earliest epidemiologic studies in the 1980s were promoted by international agencies which became interested in severe cases of HBsAg-positive hepatitis occurring in the Amazon basin [23], the Central African Republic [24], and the Himalayan foothills [25]. These studies recognized that the liver disease was related to local outbreaks of fulminant hepatitis D in a large number of HBsAg carriers who had acquired HBV infection early in life. Since then, diagnostic facilities have improved in several disadvantaged countries and local reporting has distinctly increased; the following data refer to studies published in the last 15 years.

Replicates of the outbreaks of severe hepatitis D in the 1980s were reported after 2000 in Samara, Russia [26], Greenland [27], and Mongolia [28]; these epidemics occurred through superinfection on a background of high HBV endemicity and affected mainly a young population. HDV infection remains endemic in the Eastern Mediterranean basin [29, 30] and throughout Asia [31]; high prevalence rates have been reported in Russia east of the Urals [32, 33], Pakistan [34], Iran [35], and Tajikistan [16, 35], and in special populations in Vietnam [36, 37], as well as in general in Mongolia [38], with correspondingly high rates of cirrhosis and hepatocellular carcinoma (HCC). Mongolia has the highest prevalence of HDV in the world. In a recent study, as many as 61% of 123 HBsAg-positive patients from the general population were found to have anti-HD using a newly developed sensitive quantitative microarray antibody capture for IgG anti-HD [39].

Using older assays, fragmentary information from India [16, 40, 41] indicates that the prevalence of HDV is low there; a nationwide survey in 2006 concluded that the infection was present in only about 5% of CHB patients [42]. Variable but generally low figures were reported from studies in China [16]; in a recent study in Guangdong, 6.5% of 6604 CHB patients tested positive for IgM anti-HD [43] with the corresponding caveats.

Also irregular is the distribution of HDV in the Pacific area: HDV-RNA was found in 37% of 54 CHB patients in Kiribati, Western Pacific, but in no patient from Tonga, Fiji or Vanuatu; the Kiribati genotype was type 1, clustering with an isolate previously found in Nauru to form a distinct clade of Pacific HDV [44]. Minimal information is available from Indonesia, Malaysia and the Philippines.

Of note, the low seroprevalence reported in India, China and other areas where the endemicity of HBV has been historically high, must be interpreted with caution in the absence of comprehesive and systematic surveys. The striking differences between the low rates of HDV in India and China as opposed to the high rates in neighbouring Pakistan, Mongolia and Vietnam could also depend on lack of screening, thus leading to misinformation that reduces awareness of the HDV issue so that testing is further restricted to only special patients.

Consistent rates of anti-HD in HBsAg carriers with liver disease were reported in sub-Saharan Africa [45], Gabon [46, 47], Cameroon [48, 49], Mauritania [50, 51], Senegal [52], Benin [53], Ghana [54], and Nigeria [55]. In the Central African Republic seroprevalence rates of 50% were reported in 2014 in cirrhotics [45], who were at very high risk to develop hepatocellular carcinoma [56].

In combined samples of blood donors and pregnant women in West and Central Africa HDV seroprevalence rates were 14.9% and 37.8%, respectively. In studies from Mauritania, Nigeria and Senegal, the seroprevalence was three times higher among patients with advanced fibrosis or HCC compared to asymptomatic HBsAg carriers. HDV infection remains highly endemic in the western Amazon Basin [57, 58].

Of note, prevalence estimates in third world countries are sometimes inaccurate, as shown by the bizzarre results between nearby geographical areas [6]. For instance, in Brazil and Saudi Arabia [59], pockets of hyperendemic HDV were found close to areas where the infection was negligible or nonexistent; likewise, north of Mount Kenya, 30% of the HBsAg carriers had anti-HD as opposed to none of 123 patients with HBsAg liver disease south of Mount Kenya [60] and in China anti-HD varied from 20% to 40% in Chongqing to 0% in Wuhan [16].

Conflicting prevalence rates have been reported in other small studies from Africa, suggesting epidemiological patterns based on multiple local independent clusters of the infection. However, many of these studies included small series of patients with disparate demographic and clinical features; discrepancies, therefore, may also be related to biases in the selection of the patients.

11.5.2 Current Clinical–Epidemiological Pattern in the Developed World

With the development of widespread HBV vaccination programs since the 1990s, HDV infection has consistently declined in the developed world [16]. At the end of the 1980s, the prevalence of HDV started to diminish in Europe [61]. In Italy, it diminished from 24% in 1983 to 8% in 1997 [62]. Consistent declines occurred throughout the Mediterranean, in Taiwan, and in areas of Eastern Europe that implemented vaccination. In Taiwan, HDV infection varied widely between groups, with reported prevalence of 74.9% among HIV-infected IDUs, 43.9% among HIV-uninfected IDUs, 11.4% among HIV-infected men who have sex with men, and 11.1% among HIV-infected heterosexuals, but only 4.4% in the general population of HBsAg-positive patients [63]. The reduction was so profound in southern Europe that it led at the end of the 1990s to the assumption that HDV infection was on the way to eradication. This perception reduced awareness of HDV and led to reduced testing, a factor that by itself concealed the true epidemiologic situation. This optimism was premature; hepatitis D is now reviving in Europe, reintroduced by immigrants from areas where HDV remains endemic [64].

The residual burden of hepatitis D in Europe did not decrease further in the last 15 years. In 1386 HBsAg carriers studied in Italy in 2006–2007, the overall prevalence of anti-HD was 8.1% [65] with no further downtrend. In London, the antibody was detected in about 8.5% of HBsAg carriers between 2000 and 2006 [66]. In Hannover, seroprevalences were 8–14% from 1999 onward [67]. In the United Kingdom and in Germany, most patients with hepatitis D come from Eastern Europe, Africa, the Middle East, and Turkey. In France and Spain [68, 69], HDV infection is seen predominantly in people from northern Africa. The proportion of immigrants has also increased in Australia [70]; 71% of 87 HDV patients notified in Victoria in the period 2000–2009 were born overseas.

Recent surveys have acknowledged that in Europe and Taiwan there are still consistent communities of IDUs in which HDV remains endemic [63, 71]. In the United Kingdom, Germany, and Spain more than 70% of the HDV patients born in those countries were injection drug users [72]. In Switzerland, a country with a low general prevalence of HDV infection, a 2011 study reported that 62% of the HDV cases were related to the use of drugs [73]. A consistent proportion of IDUs with HDV also have HCV infection, with as many as 30% of such patients reported in Central Europe [74]. In triple HBV/HDV/HCV infection, HDV is usually the dominant virus [75], inhibiting the expression of serum HCV-RNA as well as of HBV-DNA. However, in a longitudinal study from Italy, viral dominance has changed over time with fluctuating HCV/HBV/HDV virologic profiles [76]. Rates of HDV are high in IDUs with HBV/HIV [77]. In 1319 cases recruited throughout Europe, the prevalence of anti-HD was 14% [16]. In Taiwan, HDV is increasing among individuals with HIV and in recent studies from Taipei and Southern Taiwan 84% to 90% of the HBsAg-positive addicts with HIV were coinfected with HDV [63, 78, 79]; hepatitis D is a major determinant of liver decompensation and death in these patients [80]. Thus, the remaining reservoir of HDV in Europe is maintained by three sources: the historical IDU population, the aging and shrinking residual domestic population that survived the hepatitis D epidemic in the 1970s–1980s, and the expanding population of younger patients immigrating from areas where HDV is endemic.

The lack of proper HDV testing was reported as emblematic in the United States. In the last 25 years attention to HDV waned on the perception that, with the control of HBV, hepatitis D was no longer a problem. Only 8.5% of 25,603 HBsAg patients observed in the US from 1999 to 2013 were tested for anti-HD [81]; therefore, low hepatitis HDV prevalence estimates in the country may be biased due to low testing rates. In the 2003–2004 National Health and Nutrition Examination Survey (NHANES) in the U.S., only 3.6% of the HBsAg carriers were positive for anti-HD [82]. Recent studies are urging reconsideration. In 2005, Bialek and colleagues reported a 34.5% prevalence of HDV infection among 58 drug addicts with acute HBsAg hepatitis [83]. In 2010, Kucirka and colleagues in Baltimore compared the prevalence of anti-HD between 48 IDUs with CHB collected in 1988–1989 and 38 patients collected in 2005–2006; the prevalence of anti-HD increased from 25% in the early cohort to 50% in the recent cohort [84]. In a retrospective review of 1296 CHB patients at California Pacific Medical Center in 2013, 499 were tested for anti-HDV total, and 82 patients were found to be positive (6.3%); 34% were also infected with HCV [85]. Sixty-three percent were born in North America, while most of the others came from Southeast and East Asia and the Middle East; only 23% reported a history of drug use.

In summary, the prevalence of HDV is a dynamic process that is affected by use of the HBV vaccine birth dose as well as by adult vaccination. There is a high risk of death in patients with aggressive liver disease. The most important dynamic currently affecting HDV prevalence in most countries is immigration which may increase or replenish HDV prevalence in a given population even as patients die of HBV/HDV-associated disease or other comorbidities.

11.6 Clinical Changes

The early perception of hepatitis D as a very virulent disease running a swift course to liver failure refers mainly to the epidemic of HDV occurring in the 1970s–1980s in IDUs. The virulence of HDV was attributed to the emergence of more pathogenic strains of HDV through the rapid circulation of the virus in these communities; in retrospect, however, many of these patients had HCV infection as an additional source of liver damage. Although less virulent in non-IDUs, HDV coinfection in the general CHB population correlates with a disease that is more severe and progressive than CHB alone or other forms of viral liver disorders [86]. Patients with chronic hepatitis D are on average one decade younger than those with CHB and the rate of anti-HD increases with the severity of the underlying liver damage.

With the decline of HDV, the clinical scenario of hepatitis D has changed. While most patients with hepatitis D observed in Italy in the 1980s had a florid hepatitis with cirrhosis seen in less than 20% of cases, by the end of the 1990s the proportion of cirrhosis residual to burnt-out inflammation had increased to almost 70% [87]; at the time, patients were classified in retrospective studies into two clinical groups, a larger one in which patients had advanced to cirrhosis and a smaller one in which patients had an asymptomatic non-progressive disease course. In a recent analysis in Torino (A. Smedile, personal communication) the prevalence of chronic hepatitis D among HBsAg-positive patients increased from 6% to 8.4% in the period 2001–2014 due to an increase from 14.5% to 41.6% of HDV-infected immigrants. The finding of cirrhosis was similar (62%) throughout the observation period; patients recruited in the first half had higher levels of ALT and HDV-RNA while liver decompensation and HCC occurred more frequently in the second half. The mean age of the patients was 45 years with no variations during the follow-up. The similar age and percentage of cirrhotics at the end of the 1990s and 15 years later would indicate that the minority of patients originally considered to have a benign disease had instead an indolent but slowly progressive disease that ultimately reached cirrhosis. Similar clinical data were reported from Barcelona [88]. Patients recruited from 1983 to 1995 acquired HDV mainly by coinfection and were often IDUs coinfected by HCV and HIV. In contrast, patients recruited from 1996 to 2008 were older, with a higher proportion of immigrants, most presenting with chronic hepatitis D acquired by superinfection.

In summary, the current clinical scenario of HDV in Europe includes two main clinical features, a disease with a longstanding base that has advanced to cirrhosis in local domestic populations and a more fresh disease in immigrants, recapitulating the florid hepatitis D seen in Europe in the 1970s–1980s.

11.7 HDV and Hepatocellular Carcinoma

The role of HDV in the development of HCC is controversial [89]. In a retrospective multinational European study, HDV infection increased the risk of HCC threefold compared to HBV monoinfection [5]; a comparison of HBV/HDV coinfected patients and HBV monoinfected patients in Sweden indicated that HDV was a strong risk for HCC [90]. However, in a study in England, the risk in the coinfected was not increased compared to the risk seen in the HBV monoinfected although a high death rate in those with HDV infection may have masked the HCC risk [66]. The current impact of HCC in HDV/HBV infections compared to HBV monoinfection should be reconsidered according to the changing natural history of HBV. The latter can now be efficiently treated. Therefore, HCC deaths are increasing in HBV whereas liver failure remains the major cause of death and reason for transplantation in HDV patients.

11.8 Concluding Remarks

Hepatitis D is controlled in industrialized countries with the implementation of universal HBV vaccination in infants and catch up vaccination in adolescents and at risk adults. Residual pools of the infection persist in IDUs and the disease is being reconstituted by immigrants from areas where HDV is endemic. HDV may be returning not only by importation but also by spreading in local populations; immigrants from many parts of the world are often also heavily infected with HBV and circulation of the HBV in their communities might locally restore an HBsAg network providing a fertile terrain for the spreading of HDV. Awareness of hepatitis D was recently resuscitated in the U.S., pointing to IDUs as the major residual pool of HDV in the country.

HDV remains an important public health problem in developing countries where HBV is endemic and not controlled by vaccination. In many areas of Africa and Asia information on the epidemiology of HDV is lacking or incomplete. An important relevant factor that may conceal the true impact of HDV is the lack of testing; this is true not only in the poorest countries of the world, where diagnostic facilities are nevertheless increasing, but also in industrialized countries where testing for a disease incorrectly considered as being on the way to extinction has been neglected in recent years. While efforts are underway in developing countries to improve medical awareness of hepatitis D, more vigilance is needed in the industrialized world to prevent the return of HDV through migratory fluxes.

Control of HDV in superinfected HBsAg carriers remains a challenge. There is no immune prophylaxis to protect the HBsAg carrier from HDV superinfection [91] and the role of therapy is limited. Only a few patients are cured with pegylated interferon, the only therapy for chronic hepatitis D available since the 1990s. New therapeutic strategies are being explored, but the results from preliminary studies have not yet provided evidence of cure [92].

While the prospect of HDV cure in superinfected HBsAg carriers is at present dismal, HBV vaccination offers a simple, cheap and effective protection for the virus-naïves; vaccination campaigns should be implemented with priority in countries and communities where HDV is highly endemic, recognizing that it would take many decades to eliminate the disease globally with a concomitant population at high risk of death from cirrhosis and possibly liver cancer.

Table of Landmark

Reference 6
Comprehensive summary of the knowledge on HDV, and of the prevalence and medical impact of Hepatitis D in the 1980s, when the epidemic of HDV was rampant throughout Southern Europe
Reference 7
Description of the structure of the HDV, its ribozyme and the unique replication strategy through a rolling circle mechanism unknown to human viruses
Reference 12
Classification of the genotypes of HDV; their geographical distribution and medical importance, their potential use in epidemiological analyses
Reference 16
Comprehensive summary of the distribution and prevalence of HDV in the world, derived from 35 years of epidemiological surveys since the discovery of the virus
Reference 20
Establishment of the First International Standard for HDV RNA; will provide the reference for a common molecular approach to diagnosis and monitoring of therapy
Reference 23
The first description of an outbreak of fulminant hepatitis D on the background of high HDV endemicity; a paradigm of other outbreaks that have ravaged poor countries in the third world
Reference 39

Recent recognition that Mongolia is the country with the highest prevalence of HDV in the world, corresponding with the highest incidence of Hepatocellular Carcinoma
Reference 61
Perception of the incipient decline of HDV in Europe in the 1990s; analysis of the factors influencing the decline
Reference 74
Current scenario of hepatitis D in Western Europe; impact of immigration in recapitulating the disease
Reference 77
Comprehensive review of the importance and ominous clinical role of HDV in patients with HIV infection
Reference 85
Raises awareness to the neglected problem of HDV in the US, urging consideration to more extensive testing for hepatitis D
Reference 91
Reports the discouraging results of efforts to develop a HDV vaccine and the reasons why it is difficult to reach immune protection
Given that majority of the landmark literature as it relates to HDV are narrative reviews without a significant amount of original research, the author of this chapter has provided the above take-home messages for key references in place of the landmark table format that is used for other chapters in this book

References

1. Rizzetto M. The delta agent. Hepatology. 1983;3:729–37.
2. Rizzetto M, et al. Epidemiology of hepatitis delta virus: overview. Prog Clin Biol Res. 1991;364:1–20.
3. Rizzetto M, et al. Hepatitis delta virus as a global health problem. Vaccine. 1990;8(Suppl 8):S10–4.
4. Rizzetto M, et al. Chronic hepatitis in carriers of hepatitis B surface antigen, with intrahepatic expression of the delta antigen. An active and progressive disease unresponsive to immunosuppressive treatment. Ann Intern Med. 1983;98:437–41.
5. Fattovich G, et al. Influence of hepatitis delta virus infection on morbidity and mortality in compensated cirrhosis type B. The European Concerted Action on Viral Hepatitis (Eurohep). Gut. 2000;46:420–6.
6. Smedile A, et al. Advances in hepatitis D virus biology and disease. In: Boyer JL, Ockner RK, editors. Progress in liver disease, vol. XII. Philadelphia, PA: WB Saunders; 1994. p. 157–75.
7. Taylor JM. Structure and replication of hepatitis delta virus RNA. Curr Top Microbiol Immunol. 2006;307:1–23.
8. Tseng CH, Lai MM. Hepatitis delta virus RNA replication. Viruses. 2009;1:818–31.
9. Ponzetto A, et al. Titration of the infectivity of hepatitis D virus in chimpanzees. J Infect Dis. 1987;155:72–8.
10. Tamura I, et al. Hepatitis delta virus infection in different time periods in Japan. J Gastroenterol Hepatol. 1990;5:407–10.
11. Kim HS, et al. Prevalence and clinical significance of hepatitis D virus co-infection in patients with chronic hepatitis B in Korea. J Med Virol. 2011;83:1172–7.
12. Le Gal F. Eighth major clade for hepatitis delta virus. Emerg Infect Dis. 2006;12:1447–50.
13. Barros LM, et al. Hepatitis delta virus genotype 8 infection in Northeast Brazil: inheritance from African slaves? Virus Res. 2011;160:333–9.

14. Casey JL, et al. A genotype of hepatitis D virus that occurs in northern South America. Proc Natl Acad Sci U S A. 1993;90:9016–20.
15. Wu JC. Functional and clinical significance of hepatitis D virus genotype II infection. Curr Top Microbiol Immunol. 2006;307:173–86.
16. Rizzetto M, Ciancio A. Epidemiology of hepatitis D. Semin Liver Dis. 2012;32:211–9.
17. Negro F. Hepatitis D virus coinfection and superinfection. In: Seeger C, Locarnini S, editors. The hepatitis B and delta viruses, Cold Spring Harbor perspectives in medicine. Cold Spring Harbor, NY: Cold Spring Harbor Laboratory Press; 2015. p. 329–37.
18. Farci P. Delta hepatitis: an update. J Hepatol. 2003;39(Suppl 1):212–9.
19. Olivero A, Smedile A. Hepatitis delta virus diagnosis. Semin Liver Dis. 2012;32:220–7.
20. Chudy M, et al. Collaborative study to establish a World Health Organization International Standard for Hepatitis D Virus RNA for Nucleic Acid Amplification Technology (NAT)—based assays. WHO Report 2013, WHO/BS/2013.2.227.
21. Le Gal F, et al. First international external quality assessment for hepatitis delta virus RNA quantification in plasma. Hepatology. 2016;64:1483–94.
22. Liaw YF, et al. Hepatitis delta virus infection in Taiwan. Prog Clin Biol Res. 1987;234:479–83.
23. Hadler SC, et al. An epidemic of severe hepatitis due to delta virus infection in Yupca Indians in Venezuela. Ann Intern Med. 1984;100:339–44.
24. Lesbordes JL, et al. Studies on the role of HDV in an outbreak of fulminant hepatitis in Bangui (Central African Republic). Prog Clin Biol Res. 1987;234:451–9.
25. Khuroo MS, et al. An epidemic of hepatitis D in the foothills of the Himalayas in south Kashmir. J Hepatol. 1988;7:151–6.
26. Flodgren E, et al. Recent high incidence of fulminant hepatitis in Samara, Russia: molecular analysis of prevailing hepatitis B and D virus strains. J Clin Microbiol. 2000;38:3311–6.
27. Børresen ML, et al. Hepatitis D outbreak among children in a hepatitis B hyper-endemic settlement in Greenland. J Viral Hepat. 2010;17:162–70.
28. Davaalkham D, et al. Hepatitis delta virus infection in Mongolia: analyses of geographic distribution, risk factors and disease severity. Am J Trop Med Hyg. 2006;75:365–9.
29. Amini N, et al. Prevalence of hepatitis D in the eastern Mediterranean region: systematic review and meta analysis. Hepat Mon. 2013;13:e8210.
30. Degertekin HY, et al. Seropositivity for delta hepatitis in patients with chronic hepatitis B and liver cirrhosis in Turkey: a meta-analysis. Liver Int. 2008;28:494–8.
31. Abbas Z, et al. Hepatitis D: scenario in the Asia-Pacific region. World J Gastroenterol. 2010;16:554–62.
32. Kozhanova TV, et al. [Familial clusters of hepatitis delta in endemic region (republic tyva)]. Eksp Klin Gastroenterol. 2015;(11):15–22.
33. Kozhanova TV, et al. [Viral hepatitis delta. Is there the delta infection problem in the Russian Federation?]. Eksp Klin Gastroenterol. 2014;(12):4–12.
34. Mumtaz K, et al. Virological and clinical characteristics of hepatitis delta virus in South Asia. Virol J. 2011;8:312. https://doi.org/10.1186/1743-422X-8-312.
35. Alavian SM, Alavian SH. Hepatitis D virus infection; Iran, Middle East and Central Asia. Hepat Mon. 2005;5:137–43.
36. Sy BT, et al. High prevalence and significance of hepatitis D virus infection among treatment-naıve HBsAg-positive patients in northern Vietnam. PLoS One. 2013;8:e78094.
37. Hall N, et al. High prevalence of hepatitis delta virus among persons who inject drugs, Vietnam. Emerg Infect Dis. 2015;21:540–3.
38. Inoue J, et al. High prevalence of hepatitis delta virus infection detectable by enzyme immunoassay among apparently healthy individuals in Mongolia. J Med Virol. 2005;76:333–40.
39. Chen X, et al. A novel quantitative microarray antibody capture (Q-MAC) assay identifies an extremely high HDV prevalence amongst HBV infected Mongolians. Hepatology. 2017;66(6):1739–49. https://doi.org/10.1002/hep.28957.

40. Patel FM, Goswami PN. Presence of acute hepatitis D infection in HBsAg positive cancer patients: a preliminary study from west Gujarat. Indian J Med Res. 2016;143:798–800.
41. Jat SL, et al. Prevalence of hepatitis D virus infection among hepatitis B virus-infected individuals in India. Indian J Gastroenterol. 2015;34:164–8.
42. Acharya SK, et al. Viral hepatitis in India. Natl Med J India. 2006;19:203–17.
43. Liao B, et al. Epidemiological, clinical and histological characteristics of HBV/HDV co-infection: a retrospective cross-sectional study in Guangdong, China. PLoS One. 2014;9:e115888.
44. Han M, et al. Molecular epidemiology of hepatitis delta virus in the western Pacific region. J Clin Virol. 2014;61:34–9.
45. Andernach IE, et al. Characterization of hepatitis delta virus in sub-saharan Africa. J Clin Microbiol. 2014;52:1629–36.
46. Makula M, et al. Prevalence and molecular diversity of hepatitis B virus and hepatitis delta virus in urban and rural populations in northern Gabon in Central Africa. J Clin Microbiol. 2009;47:2265–8.
47. Makuwa M, et al. Prevalence and genetic diversity of hepatitis B and delta viruses in pregnant women in Gabon: molecular evidence that hepatitis delta virus clade 8 originates from and is endemic in Central Africa. J Clin Microbiol. 2008;46:754–6.
48. Foupouapouognigni Y, et al. High prevalence and predominance of hepatitis delta virus genotype 1 infection in Cameroon. J Clin Microbiol. 2011;49:1162–4.
49. Birguel J, et al. Viral markers of hepatitis B, C and D and HB vaccination status of a health care team in a rural district of Cameroon. Med Trop. 2011;71:201–2.
50. Mansour W, et al. Virological and epidemiological features of hepatitis delta infection among blood donors in Nouakchott, Mauritania. J Clin Virol. 2012;55:12–6.
51. Mansour W, et al. Prevalence, risk factors, and molecular epidemiology of hepatitis B and hepatitis delta virus in pregnant women and in patients in Mauritania. J Med Virol. 2012;84:1186–98.
52. Vray M, et al. Molecular epidemiology of hepatitis B virus in Dakar, Sénégal. J Med Virol. 2006;78:329–34.
53. De Paschale M, et al. Prevalence of HBV, HDV, HCV, and HIV infection during pregnancy in northern Benin. J Med Virol. 2014;86:1281–7.
54. Asmah RH, et al. Prevalence of hepatitis d infection in patients with hepatitis B virus-related liver diseases in Accra, Ghana. West Afr J Med. 2014;33:32–6.
55. Nwokediuko SC, Ijeoma U. Seroprevalence of antibody to HDV in Nigerians with hepatitis B virus-related liver diseases. Niger J Clin Pract. 2009;12:439–42.
56. Amougou MA, et al. A prominent role of hepatitis D virus in liver cancers documented in Central Africa. BMC Infect Dis. 2016;16:647.
57. Braga WS, et al. Hepatitis D virus infection in the western Brazilian Amazon—far from a vanishing disease. Rev Soc Bras Med Trop. 2012;45:691–5.
58. di Filippo Villa D, et al. Hepatitis D virus and hepatitis B virus infection in Amerindian communities of the Amazonas state, Colombia. Virol J. 2015;12:172. https://doi.org/10.1186/s12985-015-0402-5.
59. Ramia S, et al. Delta agent infection in Riyadh, Saudi Arabia. Trans R Soc Trop Med Hyg. 1987;81:317–8.
60. Greenfield C, et al. Hepatitis delta virus infection in Kenya. Its geographic and tribal distribution. Am J Epidemiol. 1986;123:416–23.
61. Hadziyannis SJ. Decreasing prevalence of hepatitis D virus infection. J Gastroenterol Hepatol. 1997;12:745–6.
62. Gaeta GB, et al. Chronic hepatitis D: a vanishing disease? An Italian multicenter study. Hepatology. 2000;32:824–7.
63. Lin HH, et al. Changing hepatitis D virus epidemiology in a hepatitis B virus endemic area with a national vaccination program. Hepatology. 2015;61:1870–9.
64. Wedemeyer H, et al. Hepatitis D virus infection—not a vanishing disease in Europe! Hepatology. 2007;45:1331–2.

65. Stroffolini T, et al. Evolving clinical landscape of chronic hepatitis B: a multicenter Italian study. J Med Virol. 2009;81:1999–2006.
66. Cross TJ, et al. The increasing prevalence of hepatitis delta virus (HDV) infection in south London. J Med Virol. 2008;80:277–82.
67. Wedemeyer H, Manns MP. Epidemiology, pathogenesis and management of hepatitis D: update and challenges ahead. Nat Rev Gastroenterol Hepatol. 2010;7:31–40.
68. Servant-Delmas A, et al. Increasing prevalence of HDV/HBV infection over 15 years in France. J Clin Virol. 2014;59:126–8.
69. Ordieres C, et al. Prevalence and epidemiology of hepatitis D among patients with chronic hepatitis B virus infection: a report from northern Spain. Eur J Gastroenterol Hepatol. 2017;29:277–83.
70. Shadur B, et al. Hepatitis D virus in Victoria 2000–2009. Intern Med J. 2013;43:1081–7.
71. Rizzetto M, Alavian SM. Hepatitis delta: the rediscovery. Clin Liver Dis. 2013;17:475–87.
72. Rizzetto M. Hepatitis D virus: introduction and epidemiology. Cold Spring Harb Perspect Med. 2015;5(7):a021576.
73. Genné D, Rossi I. Hepatitis delta in Switzerland: a silent epidemic. Swiss Med Wkly. 2011;141:w13176.
74. Heidrich B, et al. Virological and clinical characteristics of delta hepatitis in Central Europe. J Viral Hepat. 2009;16:883–94.
75. Riaz F, et al. An overview of triple infection with hepatitis B, C and D viruses. Virol J. 2011;8:368. https://doi.org/10.1186/1743-422X-8-368.
76. Raimondo G, et al. Longitudinal evaluation reveals a complex spectrum of virological profiles in hepatitis B virus/hepatitis C virus-coinfected patients. Hepatology. 2006;43:100–7.
77. Calle Serrano B, et al. Hepatitis delta and HIV infection. Semin Liver Dis. 2012;32:120–9.
78. Hung CC, et al. Increasing incidence of recent hepatitis D virus infection in HIV-infected patients in an area hyperendemic for hepatitis B virus infection. Clin Infect Dis. 2014;58:1625–33.
79. Hsieh MH, et al. Hepatitis D virus infections among injecting drug users with and without human immunodeficiency virus infection in Taiwan. Kaohsiung J Med Sci. 2016;32:526–30.
80. Fernández-Montero JV, et al. Hepatitis delta is a major determinant of liver decompensation events and death in HIV-infected patients. Clin Infect Dis. 2014;58:1549–53.
81. Kushner T, et al. Delta hepatitis within the Veterans Affairs medical system in the United States: prevalence, risk factors, and outcomes. J Hepatol. 2015;63:586–92.
82. NHANES IV-Hepatitis Laboratory Results: Center for Disease Control 2003–2004.
83. Bialek SR, et al. Risk factors for hepatitis B in an outbreak of hepatitis B and D among injection drug users. J Urban Health. 2005;82:468–78.
84. Kucirka LM, et al. Prevalence, correlates, and viral dynamics of hepatitis delta among injection drug users. J Infect Dis. 2010;202:845–52.
85. Gish RG, et al. Co-infection with hepatitis B and D: epidemiology, prevalence and disease in patients in northern California. J Gastroenterol Hepatol. 2013;28:1521–5.
86. Rizzetto M. Hepatitis D: clinical features and therapy. Dig Dis. 2010;28:139–43.
87. Rosina F, et al. Changing pattern of chronic hepatitis D in southern Europe. Gastroenterology. 1999;117:161–6.
88. Buti M, et al. Clinical outcome of acute and chronic hepatitis delta over time: a long-term follow-up study. J Viral Hepat. 2011;18:434–42.
89. Abbas Z, et al. Hepatitis D and hepatocellular carcinoma. World J Hepatol. 2015;7:777–86.
90. Ji J, et al. A population-based study of hepatitis D virus as potential risk factor for hepatocellular carcinoma. J Natl Cancer Inst. 2012;104:790–2.
91. Roggendorf M. Perspectives for a vaccine against hepatitis delta virus. Semin Liver Dis. 2012;32:256–61.
92. Rizzetto M. Targeting hepatitis D. Semin Liver Dis. 2018;38:66–72. https://doi.org/10.1055/s-0037-1621711. Epub 2018.

12 Clinical Epidemiology of Hepatitis C Virus

Aparna Goel, Aijaz Ahmed, and Imam Waked

Chronic infection with hepatitis C virus (HCV) is a global health challenge with over 75 million people affected globally. The widespread transmission of the virus in the past century has created a large infectious reservoir, especially in low- and middle-income countries (LMICs). There remain 1–2 million new HCV infections worldwide every year.

12.1 Global Prevalence

Over the past decade, several publications have noted a gradual decrease in the estimated global prevalence of HCV [1–5]. In 2005, Hanafiah et al. reported a global HCV antibody-positive (anti-HCV+) prevalence of 180 million persons [1]. Ten years later, Gower et al. reported anti-HCV+ prevalence of 110 million persons globally, with 70–80 million persons with chronic HCV infection (CHC) [4]. The five most populous countries (China, Pakistan, India, Egypt and Russia) account for approximately 50% of the global HCV burden [5].

The decreasing prevalence estimates are attributed to several factors. The older HCV antibody assay was not specific and yielded a high false positive rate, especially in studies performed in Africa. Additionally, many countries reported estimates based on small, regional non-representative samples. For example, the HCV seroprevalence rate in Cameroon was reported as 13.8% in 2002 and

A. Goel · A. Ahmed (✉)
Stanford University School of Medicine, Palo Alto, CA, USA
e-mail: aijazahmed@stanford.edu

I. Waked
National Liver Institute, Shebin El Kom, Egypt
e-mail: iwaked@liver-eg.org

R. J. Wong, R. G. Gish (eds.), *Clinical Epidemiology of Chronic Liver Diseases*,
https://doi.org/10.1007/978-3-319-94355-8_12

corrected to 1.1% in 2016 [6, 7]. In Nigeria, initial estimates reported 7.5 million chronically infected persons but this was corrected to 2.8 million in 2016 [4–6]. Similarly, more recent estimates in south and east Asia corrected the prevalence of CHC from 50 million to 10–14 million [1, 5]. The decrease in estimated prevalence is also a function of time and background mortality of an aging cohort of individuals with chronic infection. This is especially true in LMICs where transmission of HCV occurred in the healthcare setting in the 1960s and 1970s. Lastly, the approval of highly effective direct-acting antivirals (DAAs) for treatment of CHC has resulted in virologic cure of more than 1 million persons in 2015 and 2016 alone [5, 7].

12.2 Genotypes and Genotype Distribution

Hepatitis C virus is a genetically diverse virus with seven known genotypes and regional variations in genotype prevalence [2, 8].

Genotype 1 is the most common worldwide, accounting for nearly 50% of all chronic HCV infections. Genotype 1a is more prevalent in Europe and North America and genotype 1b in Asia. In the United States (U.S.), 75% of all CHC infections are with genotype 1; genotypes 2 and 3 account for the remainder with 10–12% each.

Genotype 2 accounts for 12% of infections globally. It is the predominant genotype in the Sahel region of West Africa, and in eastern parts of South America, representing previous slave trade routes. In Europe, it is more common in countries that had colonial influence in West Africa [9].

Genotype 3 is the second most common genotype globally, accounting for 20% of the infection burden. It is prevalent in South Asia and the Indian subcontinent, where it represents 80–85% of CHC in Bangladesh and Pakistan, 70–75% in east and northeast India, and 40% in central and south India [10–12].

Genotype 4 represents 12–15% of the global HCV burden and is most prevalent in Egypt, the Middle East, and central Sub-Saharan Africa. Egypt is home to 50% of the global HCV genotype 4 population, but its prevalence is increasing in Europe. It accounts for 15% of chronic infections in Belgium, 13.9% in Greece, and 10.1% in Switzerland. Genotype 4 is also over-represented in patients coinfected with both HCV and human immunodeficiency virus (HIV) [10, 13].

Genotype 5 is responsible for 1% or less of the global HCV burden. It is found mainly in South Africa, where it accounts for 40% of all chronic infections. Scattered pockets have been reported in Europe and Syria [2, 10, 14]. Genotype 6 is found predominantly in southeast Asia regions.

Genotype distribution is important in predicting disease progression and was previously important in selecting suitable treatment regimens. Genotype 1a patients had lower SVR rates compared to patients infected with genotype 1b. This was likely due to the higher frequency of mutations at the Q80 position (Q80K) which decreased response to the NS3/4 protease inhibitor simeprevir when combined with pegylated interferon and ribavirin or with sofosbuvir [15]. The Q80K variant is present in more than 30% of patients with genotype 1a infection but in only 0.5% of patients infected with genotype 1b [16]. In addition, NS5A resistance associated variants (RAVs) at positions M28, Q30, L31, and Y93 are found in 5–10% of treatment-naïve patients with genotype 1a and decrease response to NS5A-containing regimens [17]. Genotype 3 is associated with more rapid progression of fibrosis and a higher risk of hepatocellular carcinoma compared to other genotypes [18]. In addition, genotype 3 infection was difficult to treat with the first generation of highly effective DAAs, but now has equal cure rates with subsequent generations of DAAs [19].

HCV variability by Gross National Income (GNI): Low income countries, defined as annual per capita GNI less than $1025, have an estimate of 5.4 million chronically infected persons [20, 21]. Low-middle income countries, with annual per capita GNI $1025 to <$4035, account for an estimated 32.4 million chronically infected persons. High-middle income countries, defined as annual per capita GNI 4035 to <$12,475, are home to approximately 23.3 million persons with CHC. High-income countries, defined as annual per capita GNI ≥ $12,475, account for 16.7 million cases of CHC globally. In total, low and middle income countries account for 78.5% of the global burden of CHC (61.1 million cases) [6, 22, 23]. Unfortunately, many of these countries have limited capacity to diagnose and treat their large burden of chronically infected patients. This calls for a global effort to improve access to HCV treatment where it is needed the most (Table 12.1).

12.3 Incidence

The incidence of new infections has decreased markedly since 1989 [24]. In the United States, there were approximately 300,000 new infections in 1990 compared to 50,000 in 1994 and 20,000 in 2000. However, there has been a recent increase in the number of acute HCV infections in the past decade [25]. This is likely due to the resurgence of intravenous drug use among teenagers and young adults in their 20s [26].

12.4 Acute HCV Infection

While acute hepatitis B virus (HBV) infection becomes a chronic infection in up to 20% of patients, acute HCV infection results in chronic infection in up to 75% of patients (Fig. 12.1).

Table 12.1 HCV Prevalence in Low and Middle Income Countries

Country	Population	% HCV viremia	HCV prevalence	Annual GNI per capita, $, 2015
Low income countries (annual per-capita GNI < 1025)				
Burundi	11,691,348	1.03	120,000	260
Central African Republic	4,426,230	0.61	27,000	330
Malawi	17,307,692	0.26	45,000	340
Liberia	4,500,000	1.2	54,000	380
Niger	20,000,000	1.2	240,000	390
Democratic Republic of the Congo	75,941,176	1.7	1,291,000	410
Madagascar	24,898,144	0.22	55,000	420
The Gambia	2,000,000	1.2	24,000	460
Guinea	12,583,333	1.2	151,000	470
Togo	7,250,000	1.2	87,000	540
Ethiopia	102,166,667	0.6	613,000	590
Guinea Bissau	1,833,333	1.2	22,000	590
Mozambique	27,868,852	0.61	170,000	590
Afghanistan	33,339,406	0.55	183,000	610
Sierra Leone	6,416,667	1.2	77,000	620
Burkina Faso	7,919,747	1.33	105,000	640
Rwanda	10,000,000	0.7	70,000	700
Uganda	40,538,462	1.3	527,000	700
Haiti	11,000,000	0.64	70,400	728
Nepal	28,043,478	0.46	129,000	730
Mali	17,583,333	1.2	211,000	760
South Sudan	12,500,000	0.6	75,000	790
Benin	10,833,333	1.2	130,000	840
Zimbabwe	16,086,957	2.3	370,000	860
Chad	5,359,057	1.12	60,000	880
Tanzania	54,000,000	0.6	324,000	920
Senegal	15,083,333	1.2	181,000	980
Total low income countries	**581,170,549**	**0.93%**	**5,411,400**	**617**
Low-middle income countries (annual per-capita GNI 1025–4035)				
Cambodia	15,944,758	1.59	254,000	1070
Yemen	27,973,856	0.77	214,000	1140
Myanmar	54,084,507	0.71	384,000	1160
Kirghizstan	5,868,421	3.8	223,000	1170
Bangladesh	159,130,435	0.46	732,000	1190
Lesotho	2,090,909	1.1	23,000	1280
Tajikistan	8,461,538	3.77	319,000	1280
Cameroon	23,923,445	0.69	165,000	1320
Kenya	47,379,455	0.24	113,000	1340
Mauritania	4,000,000	1.2	48,000	1370
Cote d'Ivoire	22,666,667	1.2	272,000	1420
Pakistan	211,932,272	3.38	7,172,000	1440
Ghana	27,671,822	1.44	399,000	1480

Table 12.1 (continued)

Country	Population	% HCV viremia	HCV prevalence	Annual GNI per capita, $, 2015
Zambia	16,333,333	0.6	98,000	1490
India	1,285,683,806	0.47	6,026,000	1600
Nicaragua	6,200,000	0.54	33,480	1849
Sudan	41,666,667	0.6	250,000	1920
Moldova	3,500,000	3.30	115,500	1978
Vietnam	94,336,283	1.13	1,066,000	1990
Uzbekistan	30,423,156	4.26	1,297,000	2160
Papua New Guinea	7,779,444	1.2	93,400	2240
Honduras	8,700,000	0.54	46,980	2313
Bhutan	652,174	0.46	3000	2380
Bolivia	11,000,000	0.70	77,000	2393
Nigeria	188,636,028	1.35	2,553,000	2820
Ukraine	42,600,000	3.30	1,405,800	2826
Morocco	31,088,768	0.76	235,000	3030
Guatemala	16,100,000	0.54	86,940	3052
Swaziland	1,181,818	1.1	13,000	3280
Egypt	89,578,947	6.65	5,957,000	3340
Indonesia	261,036,857	0.49	1,289,000	3440
Philippines	103,477,523	0.59	610,000	3550
Guyana	746,000	0.64	4774	3663
Kosovo	1,800,000	0.97	17,460	3796
Sri Lanka	20,704,225	0.71	147,000	3800
Paraguay	6,900,000	0.87	60,030	3823
El Salvador	6,500,000	0.54	35,100	3853
Mongolia	3,011,056	6.38	192,000	3870
Armenia	3,054,054	3.7	113,000	3880
Tunisia	5,905,304	0.95	56,000	3980
Georgia	3,700,000	6.50	240,500	4010
Total low-middle income countries	**2,903,423,530**	**1.12%**	**32,439,964**	**2020**
High-middle income countries (annual per-capita GNI 4035–<12,475)				
Angola	24,588,235	1.7	418,000	4180
Fiji	870,000	0.07	609	4350
Belize	380,000	0.64	2432	4393
Albania	2,800,000	0.32	8960	4543
Jordan	7,643,312	0.31	24,000	4680
Bosnia and Herzegovina	3,500,000	0.97	33,950	4802
Algeria	39,823,529	1.7	677,000	4870
Jamaica	2,700,000	0.64	17,280	5001
Macedonia	2,000,000	1.00	20,000	5094
Namibia	2,363,636	1.1	26,000	5190
Ecuador	16,600,000	0.70	116,200	5367
Serbia	7,000,000	0.97	67,900	5661
Thailand	68,178,450	0.67	460,000	5720

(continued)

Table 12.1 (continued)

Country	Population	% HCV viremia	HCV prevalence	Annual GNI per capita, $, 2015
Iraq	37,861,915	0.22	85,000	5820
Peru	31,000,000	0.70	217,000	5935
South Africa	20,941,176	1.7	356,000	6080
Cuba	11,200,000	0.64	71,680	6157
Belarus	9,500,000	3.30	313,500	6159
Botswana	2,181,818	1.1	24,000	6460
Iran	83,613,445	0.24	199,000	6550
Dominican Republic	10,000,000	0.64	64,000	6553
Azerbaijan	9,863,981	1.93	190,000	6560
Dominica	71,000	0.64	454	6917
Maldives	344,000	0.64	2202	7222
Montenegro	621,000	1.00	6210	7260
Turkmenistan	5,305,040	3.77	200,000	7380
Colombia	50,000,000	0.87	435,000	7448
Bulgaria	7,100,000	1.30	92,300	7612
Lebanon	5,060,729	0.15	7500	7710
China	1,394,000,000	0.7	9,758,000	7930
Grenada	103,000	0.54	556	8391
Suriname	500,000	0.64	3200	9115
Gabon	1,734,694	4.9	85,000	9200
Costa Rica	4,800,000	0.54	25,920	9238
Mexico	122,000,000	0.44	536,800	9511
Romania	19,700,000	2.50	492,500	9531
Mauritius	1,311,475	0.61	8000	9780
Turkey	79,571,664	0.61	483,000	9950
Argentina	44,000,000	0.77	338,800	10,515
Malaysia	31,073,677	1.22	380,000	10,570
Panama	3800,000	0.31	11,780	10,751
Brazil	207,000,000	0.87	1,800,900	11,159
Kazakhstan	24,115,222	2.11	509,000	11,390
Russia	144,774,162	3.28	4,747,000	11,450
Total high-middle income countries	**2,541,595,163**	**0.92%**	**23,316,633**	**8315**
High income countries (annual per-capita GNI ≥ 12,475)				
Norway	5,188,607	1.67	86,650	93,530
Switzerland	8,282,396	1.74	144,114	84,550
Qatar	2,481,539	1.15	28,538	83,990
Luxembourg	569,604	1.56	8886	77,480
Denmark	5,683,483	1.09	61,950	60,270
Australia	23,789,338	2.94	699,407	60,050
Sweden	9,799,186	1.09	106,811	57,900
United States	320,896,618	1.15	3,690,311	55,980
Ireland	4,676,835	1.35	63,137	52,550
Singapore	5,535,002	1.87	103,505	52,090
Iceland	330,815	1.53	5061	50,110
Netherlands	16,939,923	0.96	162,623	48,850

Table 12.1 (continued)

Country	Population	% HCV viremia	HCV prevalence	Annual GNI per capita, $, 2015
Austria	8,633,169	1.70	146,764	47,260
Canada	35,848,610	0.86	308,298	47,250
Finland	5,479,531	1.70	93,152	46,560
Germany	81,686,611	0.93	759,685	45,790
Belgium	11,274,196	1.96	220,974	44,510
Andorra	78,014	1.76	1373	43,270
United Kingdom	65,128,861	1.38	898,778	43,700
Kuwait	3,935,794	1.28	50,378	42,150
France	66,624,068	1.22	812,814	40,710
New Zealand	4,595,700	1.41	64,799	40,020
Japan	127,141,000	1.93	2,453,821	38,840
Brunei	417,542	1.68	7015	38,010
Israel	8,380,100	1.41	118,159	35,770
Italy	60,730,582	2.50	1,518,265	32,830
Spain	46,447,697	1.84	854,638	28,380
South Korea	51,014,947	1.59	811,138	27,450
Greenland	56,114	1.26	707	26,020
Cyprus	1160,985	1.51	17,531	25,810
Malta	431,874	1.66	7169	23,900
Saudi Arabia	31,557,144	0.66	208,277	23,550
Slovenia	2,063,531	1.92	39,620	22,250
Bahamas	386,838	2.24	8665	20,740
Portugal	10,358,076	1.94	200,947	20,470
Greece	10,820,883	1.53	165,560	20,270
Bahrain	1,371,855	1.32	18,108	19,840
Puerto Rico (USA)	3,473,181	2.35	81,620	19,320
Estonia	1,315,407	2.77	36,437	18,320
Czech Republic	10,546,059	1.86	196,157	18,150
Trinidad and Tobago	1,360,092	2.32	31,554	17,640
Slovakia	5,423,801	1.74	94,374	17,570
Oman	4,199,810	1.62	68,037	16,910
Uruguay	3,431,552	1.45	49,758	15,720
Lithuania	2,904,910	2.45	71,170	15,080
Latvia	1,977,527	2.80	55,371	14,990
Seychelles	93,419	2.85	2662	14,680
Barbados	284,217	2.49	7077	14,510
Chile	17,762,681	0.98	174,074	14,100
Virgin Islands (USA)	103,574	2.61	2703	13,660
Poland	37,986,412	1.55	588,789	13,310
Antigua and Barbuda	99,923	2.19	2188	13,270
Hungary	9,843,028	1.86	183,080	12,970
Equatorial Guinea	1,175,389	3.42	40,198	12,820
Croatia	4,203,604	1.49	62,634	12,760
Total high income countries	**1,145,981,654**	**1.75%**	**16,695,511**	**34,518**

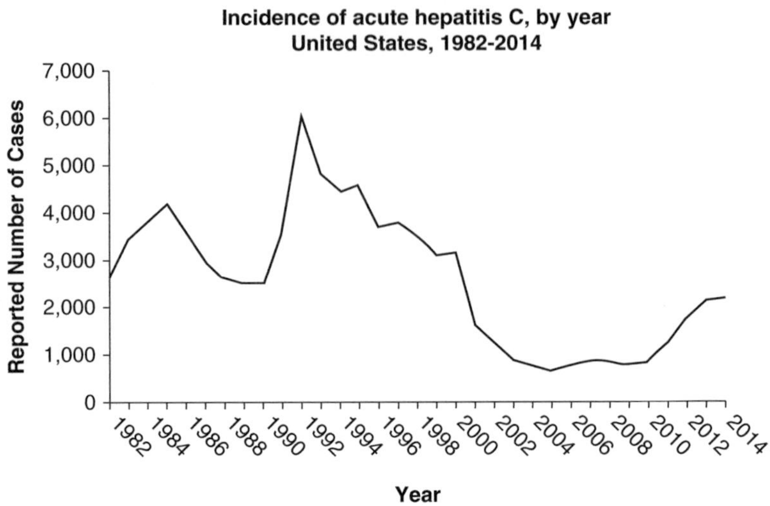

Fig. 12.1 Reported cases of acute HCV in the USA (CDC data) [29]

12.5 HCV Transmission

HCV is transmitted mainly by blood or blood products. The sexual transmission rate is low and it is not transmitted by casual contact (hugging, kissing), sharing of utensils (drinking glasses, food plates, spoons) or towels [27]. The risk of infection following needle stick for HCV is 1.8% (compared to 6–30% for HBV, and 0.3% for HIV) [28]. Iatrogenic transmission is an important method in low-middle income countries with areas of high prevalence. Patient-to-patient transmission can occur from contaminated multi-dose vials and sharing of needles and syringes.

In areas of high prevalence, unsafe injections and nosocomial transmission are the most important routes of spread. On the other hand, in areas of low prevalence, recreational injection drug use is the most common route of transmission [29]. In a lower prevalence country such as the U.S., 60% of HCV infections are transmitted through injection drug use, 15% by sexual transmission, and 10% due to blood transfusions before 1992 [30]. In higher prevalence countries such as Egypt, 50% of infections are attributed to unsafe healthcare vaccination and treatment regimens including the mass use of anti-schistosomal medications in the 1960s–1980s [31].

HCV in Egypt is a prototypical example of parenteral transmission due to widespread use of unsafe injections [32]. Between 1960 and 1980, mass treatment for schistosomiasis was advocated by the Egyptian government with support of the World Health Organization in an effort to eliminate the disease. A series of six to nine daily intravenous injections were the standard treatment at that time. There were over 2 million injections annually in approximately 250,000 patients totaling 36 million injections for over 6 million persons during the time period. Almost all of these treatments utilized shared, poorly sterilized syringes and needles. Using cohort specific exposure indices for anti-schistosomal treatment and HCV prevalence rates, there is a clear association between the transmission of HCV and schistosomiasis therapy [33].

The role of unsafe injections in transmission of HCV is also noted in Cameroon. In urban communities where healthcare facilities and vaccination were present with unsafe practices between 1950 and 1970, the age specific HCV seroprevelance rate was 30–40% in those who were older than 40 years in 2005. In contrast, in Yokaduma, a jungle community where health services were almost non-existent and vaccination was not introduced, the HCV seroprevalence rate in the same age cohort is much lower [34].

HCV can survive on environmental surfaces at room temperature for 16–72 hours. In a recent report, HCV was detected for up to 6 weeks in syringes, swabs and drug sharing equipment. Among injection drug users (IDUs), sharing drug preparation equipment (cookers, cotton, compresses, etc.) can transmit infection, and distributing clean needles and syringes is insufficient to interrupt transmission [35]. In a study from the U.S., the greatest risk factor for HCV acquisition was a history of intravenous drug use with an odds ratio of 149 (45–494) [36]. HCV seroprevalence rates of 60–90% have been reported among IDUs in Moscow [37], Bulgaria [38], Amsterdam [39], New York [40], New Zealand [41], and Alexandria (Egypt) [42].

The age-related HCV seroprevalence rates in a community are related to the prevalent method of transmission. In LMICs where unsafe healthcare injections play an important role in transmission (as in Egypt [43], Pakistan [44], Turkey [45], Mongolia [46], and parts of China [47]), HCV seroprevalence rates continuously increase with age (Fig. 12.2). On the other hand, in regions where injection drug use is the main source of transmission, the age-related prevalence curve is usually bell-shaped, with a peak around the age equivalent to the time when drug use was most common in each community: 1950–1970 in the USA [48], 1960–1980 in Australia [49], and 1970–1990 in the UK [49] and Russia [49] (Fig. 12.2).

In an effort to diagnose patients with HCV, the Centers for Disease Control and Prevention (CDC) identified individuals at risk as those who were exposed to blood products before the availability of HCV testing, individuals who intermittently used or continue to use intravenous drugs or inhale cocaine, individuals with chronic renal failure on dialysis, incarcerated individuals, those occupationally exposed to blood products, individuals who received organ or tissue grafts from HCV-positive donors, and individuals who have had body piercing and tattooing [50].

Although an increased risk of HCV infection has been reported in individuals with multiple sexual partners, there is no evidence of transmission in monogamous relationships. A study of 776 serodiscordant spouses who were followed for an average of 10 years did not show transmission through sexual intercourse. Individuals in these partnerships had regular intercourse without using barrier protection. Only three new HCV infections were detected (incidence: 0.37/1000 person-years), and the infecting strain in the partner was different from the strain in the HCV-infected spouse, indicating the low risk of HCV transmission by sexual intercourse [49].

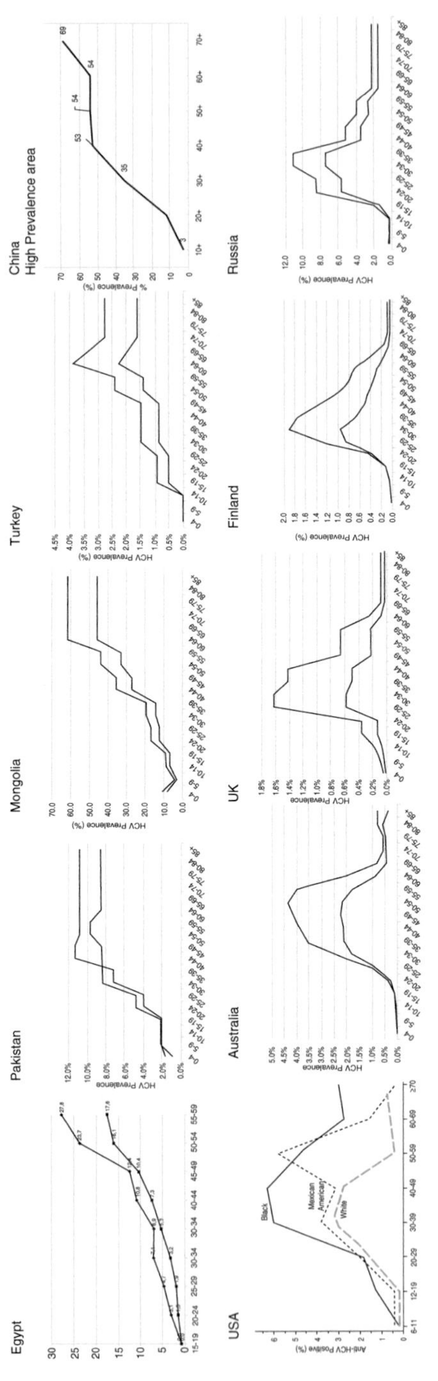

Fig. 12.2 Changes in HCV prevalence with increasing age

12.6 Clinical Manifestations

Although the majority of patients with CHC are asymptomatic, approximately 37% have symptoms, of which the most common is fatigue. CHC can significantly impair quality of life. Compared to controls and patients with HBV infection, CHC patients had more profound impairment of all aspects of the short form-36 (SF-36) quality of life questionnaire, especially social functioning, energy and fatigue [51].

HCV can have extrahepatic manifestations, mostly induced by immune mechanisms. These extrahepatic manifestations can on occasion be the only sign of the infection and, at times, can be more troubling than the liver disease [52]. Nearly any organ system may be involved including hematologic, dermatologic, renal, endocrine, salivary, ocular, vascular, and neuromuscular systems [53]. The spectrum of extrahepatic manifestations includes glomerulonephritis, diabetes, thyroiditis, seronegative arthritis/arthralgia, aplastic anemia, porphyria cutanea tarda, autoimmune phenomena including Sjogren syndrome, granulomas, presence of autoantibodies, and CREST syndrome (calcinosis cutis, Raynaud's phenomenon, esophageal dysfunction, sclerodactyly, telangiectasia).

Cryoglobulins (immune complexes of polyclonal IgG, monoclonal IgM, complement component C1q and HCV) form cold precipitate plasma complexes that bind to endothelial C1q receptors and deposit in small and medium-sized blood vessels. They cause inflammation in skin, kidney and other tissues, and are detected in 50% of patients with CHC [54, 55]. The clinical syndrome of essential mixed cryoglobulinemia affects 1–2% of CHC patients, and presents with rash, digital ischemia and ulcers, arthralgia and neuropathy. Pulmonary fibrosis and pulmonary vasculitis may occasionally be manifestations of CHC-associated cryoglobulinemia [56].

12.7 Prognosis of HCV

Acute HCV infection results in a chronic infection in 65–70% of people, where it follows a slowly progressive course. The rate of progression is variable, but most patients have either no progression or slowly progressive liver disease. Over 20 years, only 10–20% of those chronically infected will develop cirrhosis, and of those, 1–4% per year progress to develop severe hepatic decompensation or hepatocellular carcinoma (HCC) [57].

An estimated 15–30% of chronically infected persons will never develop liver fibrosis or cirrhosis, and the HCV infection will not significantly impact life expectancy. Another 20% to 30% of patients develop rapidly progressive fibrosis with cirrhosis, decompensated cirrhosis, and liver cancer within 20–25 years of exposure. The remaining 50–65% of patients develop fibrosis progression to cirrhosis, but at variable rates ranging from 25 years to more than 40 years [58].

The progression of HCV infection was demonstrated in a series of liver biopsies performed 17 years after acquisition of HCV through anti-D immune globulin in 363 women in Ireland during 1977 and 1978 [56]. Almost half (49%) had no fibrosis; 34% had early fibrosis; 15% had advanced fibrosis with bridging; and only 7 (2%) had established cirrhosis (two of whom reported excessive alcohol intake). The most common symptom was fatigue (66%); and liver enzymes were normal in 45%.

12.8 Factors Affecting Rate of Progression of Fibrosis

Several factors have been found to impact the rate of fibrosis progression in patients with CHC.

- *Initial fibrosis*: The present level of fibrosis helps predict progression rate over the following years. For individuals who do not have any evidence of fibrosis on an initial biopsy, the risk of developing cirrhosis over the next 20 years is 25–30%. If a patient has fibrosis on initial biopsy, he/she will develop progressive fibrosis and eventually cirrhosis. All patients with portal fibrosis develop cirrhosis over 18–20 years. Individuals with more advanced fibrosis on initial biopsy will develop cirrhosis in only 8–10 years [59].
- *Alcohol use*: Patients with chronic HCV who drink alcohol on a regular basis (>30 g/day in males, >20 g/day in females) have a higher fibrosis score compared with individuals who do not drink alcohol [60].
- *Age at initial infection*: Patients who acquire HCV when they are greater than 40 years of age have more advanced fibrosis regardless of how long they have had the disease, compared with individuals who are infected at a younger age [61, 62]. Only 40 of 1667 HCV-positive young IDUs developed end-stage liver disease or HCC over a 14-year follow-up (2.4%) [63], while end-stage liver disease developed over 9 years in 12% of patients older than 58 who contracted HCV through blood transfusion [64].
- *Degree of steatosis*: Patients with higher degrees of steatosis have more fibrosis and develop cirrhosis at a faster rate. At 6 years follow-up, fibrosis progressed in 6% of those who had less than 5% steatosis, and in 33% of those who had more than 30% steatosis [65].
- *Other factors*: Family history of advanced liver disease [62], coinfection with HBV or HIV [66, 67], and/or insulin resistance and the metabolic syndrome [68, 69] also increase the rate of progression of liver disease.

12.9 Complications from HCV Cirrhosis

Patients with well-compensated cirrhosis have a 10-year survival close to 80%. By contrast, individuals who have moderate to severe liver dysfunction or hepatic decompensation have a 10-year survival of 30%. The rate at which patients with cirrhosis develop decompensated liver disease is approximately 3–5% per year. The rate at which individuals develop HCC is on the average about 1–4% per year, varying by ethnicity and region [70]. The 5-year calculated cumulative incidence of HCC in patients with HCV-associated cirrhosis was 30% in Japanese patients and

17% in European and American patients. This is higher than the 5-year cumulative rates from other causes of cirrhosis including HBV-associated cirrhosis and alcoholic cirrhosis [71].

Benvegnù et al. [72] followed patients with compensated cirrhosis for a decade in Italy. Most HCV monoinfected patients did not develop complications (69%), while 31% developed at least one complication. The most frequent complication was HCC, which occurred in 21% of cases, followed by ascites (19%), gastrointestinal bleeding (4.5%), and encephalopathy (2%). Death from liver disease occurred in 19%, mostly due to HCC, indicating that, in this population, HCC was the most frequent and life threatening complication.

HCV infection increases mortality from liver disease and from extrahepatic causes. In a community-based long-term prospective cohort study involving 23,800 adults over a 16.2 years follow-up (REVEAL-HCV study), the mortality rates over the duration of the study due to hepatic diseases was 12.8% for patients who had chronic HCV infection, 1.6% for those who were HCV seropositive but with undetectable HCV RNA, and 0.7% for seronegative individuals. Mortality rates from extrahepatic causes were 19.8% for patients who had CHC, 12.2% for HCV seropositive individuals, and 11.0% for seronegative individuals [73].

12.10 Effect of Treatment Outcome

A sustained virologic response (SVR) to treatment is associated with improved outcome and significantly less progression of liver disease. Veldt et al. showed that in patients with advanced fibrosis-cirrhosis the 5-year incidence of liver related mortality was 4.4% (CI: 0–12.9%) in patients who achieved SVR with interferon-based therapy vs. 12.9% (CI: 7.7–18.0%) in patients who failed to achieve an SVR. Additionally, the 5-year rate of liver failure was 0% in those who achieved an SVR and 3.3% (CI: 8.4–18.2%) in those who did not [74].

In addition, an SVR is associated with reduced all-cause mortality. van der Meer et al. followed patients with advanced fibrosis/cirrhosis treated with an IFN-based regimen from 1990 to 2003, and found that the 10-year cumulative rate of all-cause mortality was close to 26.0% in patients who failed to achieve an SVR and 8.9% in patients who achieved an SVR. The 10-year incidence of liver-related death or transplant was 1.9% in patients with an SVR and 27.4% without SVR; the 10-year cumulative rate of HCC was 5.1% vs. 21.8%, respectively [75].

12.11 Future Trends and Prospects

Although the prevalence of HCV is decreasing globally and has the potential to decrease further over the next few years with highly effective DAA therapies, the burden of the disease will probably increase over the coming years as the population with chronic infection ages, especially in LMICs. As the infected cohorts age, a greater fraction will have HCV infection for sufficient periods of time to develop cirrhosis, complications from end-stage liver disease and HCC. Infected populations

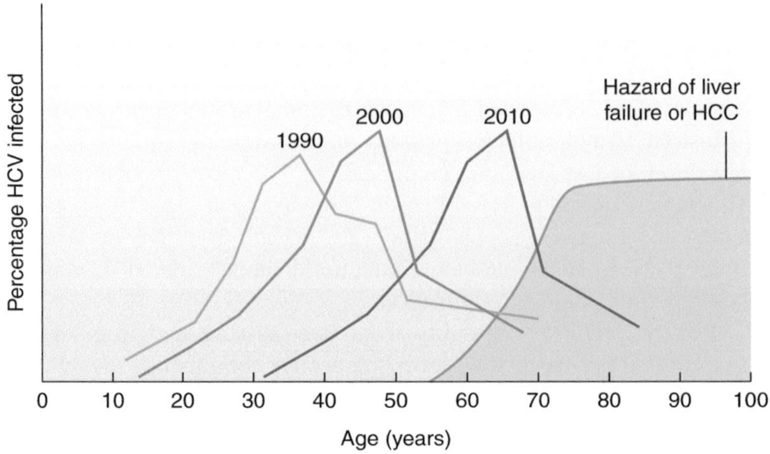

Fig. 12.3 Dynamic course of HCV infection in the US. As the cohort born between 1945 and 1965 ages, a greater fraction will have HCV infection for sufficient time at old-enough ages to develop liver failure and HCC [3]

in LMICs, where infection is mainly concentrated in older ages, have already reached this threshold, and complications of HCV infection are increasing. In Egypt, the age standardized rate (ASR)/100,000 for HCC has been gradually increasing over the past three decades. The ASR was 5.2 in the 1980s, and has reached 25.6 in 2012, representing the massive infections that occurred more than 35 years ago [76]. The increase in HCC incidence in Egypt will be mirrored in other countries with a similar pattern of transmission history although at a much lower rate. The ASR for HCC has also more than doubled over the period from 1980 to 2012 in countries where intravenous drug use was the main cause of transmission of HCV (e.g., in the USA from 3 to 6.1, and in Australia from 2 to 4.2) [77, 78]. The infected population in these countries acquired HCV in the 1970s and 1980s and is now approaching the threshold of developing complications from liver disease (Fig. 12.3).

The global burden of disease (GBD) study has shown that the relative impact of viral hepatitis (including HCV) on global mortality has increased over the last 20 years. In 1993, viral hepatitis was the 10th leading cause of global mortality, and the 5th leading cause of mortality due to infectious diseases. By 2013, viral hepatitis had become the 7th leading cause of global mortality and the 2nd leading cause of mortality due to infections disease (following lower respiratory infections), with the relative impact of other infectious diseases decreasing (diarrheal disorders from 4th to 12th, TB from 6th to 11th, and infections in preterm infants from 7th to 19th) [79].

Second and third generation DAAs have high cure rates in clinical trials and in real-life treatment [78, 80–87]. Achieving SVR in patients who have not developed advanced fibrosis or cirrhosis will reverse the natural history of the disease and prevent further development of complications [80, 81]. However, in patients with advanced fibrosis/cirrhosis, the natural history may not be completely reversed. The rate of progression to end-stage liver disease and HCC will decrease, but will not be abolished among patients with cirrhosis who successfully clear infection [88, 89].

Furthermore, whether patients with end-stage liver disease will benefit from successful treatment is not confirmed, and the need for liver transplantation, development of HCC and mortality will continue in this group.

To change the increasing trend in global burden of HCV, global treatment access and uptake must increase rapidly, especially in low-middle income countries, and must be available to patients with all stages of fibrosis. Treating patients with no fibrosis or with early stages of fibrosis will prevent progression to cirrhosis and its complications, and treating patients with advanced fibrosis/cirrhosis has the potential to decrease the rate of developing complications. However, unless global access is increased soon, the impact of DAAs on the burden of disease will not be seen in the near future.

In 2016, the 69th World Health Assembly approved the Global Health Sector Strategy to eliminate hepatitis infection by 2030, and the WHO introduced global targets for all countries to be met by 2030 for the care and management of HCV including "a 90% reduction in new cases of chronic hepatitis C, a 65% reduction in hepatitis C deaths, and treatment of 80% of eligible people with chronic hepatitis C infections."

With the advent of newer generations of highly effective DAAs, HCV has the potential to become the first chronic viral infection to be eradicated with treatment. The ability to cure HCV calls for a global effort to increase access and make treatment available for all.

Summary Table of Landmark Literature—HCV

Study title and authors	Study design	Summary results	Main limitations
Mohd Hanafiah K, Groeger J, Flaxman AD, Wiersma ST. Hepatology. 2013;57:1333–42	Systematic review of Medline, Embase, and Cinahl from 1980–2007 to update the global epidemiology of hepatitis C virus (HCV), which included pooled estimates from 232 articles	• Global prevalence and number of people with anti-HCV has increased from 2.3% to 2.8% and from >122 to >185 million between 1990 and 2005 • Central and East Asia and North Africa/Middle East are estimated to have high prevalence (>3.5%); South and Southeast Asia, sub-Saharan Africa, Andean, Central, and Southern Latin America, Caribbean, Oceania, Australasia, and Central, Eastern, and Western Europe have moderate prevalence (1.5–3.5%); whereas Asia Pacific, Tropical Latin America, and North America have low prevalence (<1.5%)	• Estimates are limited to available literature and some regions without robust HCV epidemiology data may have inaccurate estimates • Prevalence data included studies through 2007, which precedes major efforts to improve HCV screening, linkage to care, and treatment

Study title and authors	Study design	Summary results	Main limitations
Blach S, Zeuzem S, Manns M, Altraif I, Duberg AS, Muljono DH, Waked I, Alavian SM, The Polaris Observatory HCV Collaborators. Lancet Gastroenterology Hepatology. 2017;2(3):161–176	Systematic review followed by a country-level disease burden models using data from manuscripts published after 2013	• Study provided updated prevalence data in the more recent era • The global prevalence of chronic HCV is estimated to be 1.0% (95% uncertainty interval 0.8–1.1) in 2015, corresponding to 71.1 million (62.5–79.4) individuals • Genotypes 1 and 3 were the most common cause of infections (44% and 25%, respectively)	• Estimates are limited to available literature and some regions without robust HCV epidemiology (especially in sub-Saharan Africa), data may have been less accurate • Inherent limitations of assumptions made by the model design may have affected the estimates that were generated
Riou J, Aït Ahmed M, Blake A, Vozlinsky S, Brichler S, Eholié S, Boëlle PY, Fontanet A, HCV Epidemiology in Africa Group. Journal of Viral Hepatitis. 2016;23:244–55	Systematic review with meta-analysis of HCV seroprevalence data among adults in African countries via 2000–2014 structured search of MEDLINE, AJOL, and grey literature, which included 262 studies	• Among North Africa region, HCV seroprevalence was high in Egypt at 14.7% and lowest in Libya at 1.2% • In West Africa region, highest HCV seroprevalence was in Burkina Faso at 6.1% and lowest in Senegal at 1.0% • In Middle Africa region, highest HCV seroprevalence was seen in Cameroon and Gabon at 4.9% and lowest in the Democratic Republic of Congo at 2.1% • In East Africa region, highest HCV seroprevalence was seen in Ethiopia at 2.7% and lowest in Mozambique at 1.3% • In South Africa region, overall prevalence was low overall ranging from 1.1% to 1.6%	• Estimates are limited to available literature and some regions without robust HCV epidemiology data may have inaccurate estimates

References

1. Mohd Hanafiah K, Groeger J, Flaxman AD, Wiersma ST. Global epidemiology of hepatitis C virus infection: new estimates of age-specific antibody to HCV seroprevalence. Hepatology. 2013;57:1333–42.
2. Thrift AP, El-Serag HB, Kanwal F. Global epidemiology and burden of HCV infection and HCV-related disease. Nat Rev Gastroenterol Hepatol. 2017;14:122–32. https://doi.org/10.1038/nrgastro.2016.176.
3. Thomas DL. Global control of hepatitis C: where challenge meets opportunity. Nat Med. 2013;19:850–8.
4. Gower E, Estes C, Blach S, Razavi-Shearer K, Razavi H. Global epidemiology and genotype distribution of the hepatitis C virus infection. J Hepatol. 2014;61(1 Suppl):S45–57.
5. Blach S, Zeuzem S, Manns M, Altraif I, Duberg AS, Muljono DH, Waked I, Alavian SM, The Polaris Observatory HCV Collaborators. Global prevalence and genotype distribution of hepatitis C virus infection in 2015: a modelling study. Lancet Gastroenterol Hepatol. 2017;2(3):161–76. https://doi.org/10.1016/S2468-1253(16)30181-9.
6. Riou J, Aït Ahmed M, Blake A, Vozlinsky S, Brichler S, Eholié S, Boëlle PY, Fontanet A, HCV Epidemiology in Africa Group. Hepatitis C virus seroprevalence in adults in Africa: a systematic review and meta-analysis. J Viral Hepat. 2016;23:244–55.
7. Foster GR. Chronic hepatitis C: less of a problem than first thought? Lancet Gastroenterol Hepatol. 2016;2:146–7. https://doi.org/10.1016/S2468-1253(16)30209-6.
8. Messina JP, Humphreys I, Flaxman A, Brown A, Cooke GS, Pybus OG, Barnes E. Global distribution and prevalence of hepatitis C virus genotypes. Hepatology. 2015;61:77–87.
9. Markov PV, van de Laar TJ, Thomas XV, Aronson SJ, Weegink CJ, van den Berk GE, et al. Colonial history and contemporary transmission shape the genetic diversity of hepatitis C virus genotype 2 in Amsterdam. J Virol. 2012;86:7677–87.
10. Germer JJ, Mandrekar JN, Bendel JL, Mitchell PS, Yao JD. Hepatitis C virus genotypes in clinical specimens tested at a national reference testing laboratory in the United States. J Clin Microbiol. 2011;49:3040–3.
11. Christdas J, Sivakumar J, David J, Daniel HD, Raghuraman S, Abraham P. Genotypes of hepatitis C virus in the Indian sub-continent: a decade-long experience from a tertiary care hospital in South India. Indian J Med Microbiol. 2013;31:349–53.
12. Attaullah S, Khan S, Ali I. Hepatitis C virus genotypes in Pakistan: a systemic review. Virol J. 2011;8:433. https://doi.org/10.1186/1743-422X-8-433.
13. Alberti A, Lacoin L, Morais E, Lefevre C, Abogunrin S, Iheanacho I. Literature review of the distribution of hepatitis C virus genotypes across Europe. J Med Virol. 2016;88:2157–69.
14. Smith DB, Bukh J, Kuiken C, Muerhoff AS, Rice CM, Stapleton JT, Simmonds P. Expanded classification of hepatitis C virus into 7 genotypes and 67 subtypes: updated criteria and genotype assignment web resource. Hepatology. 2014;59:318–27.
15. Lawitz E, Matusow G, DeJesus E, Yoshida EM, Felizarta F, Ghalib R, Godofsky E, Herring RW, Poleynard G, Sheikh A, Tobias H, Kugelmas M, Kalmeijer R, Peeters M, Lenz O, Fevery B, De La Rosa G, Scott J, Sinha R, Witek J. Simeprevir plus sofosbuvir in patients with chronic hepatitis C virus genotype 1 infection and cirrhosis: a phase 3 study (OPTIMIST-2). Hepatology. 2016;64:360–9.
16. Sarrazin C, Lathouwers E, Peeters M, Daems B, Buelens A, Witek J, Wyckmans Y, Fevery B, Verbinnen T, Ghys A, Schlag M, Baldini A, De Meyer S, Lenz O. Prevalence of the hepatitis C virus NS3 polymorphism Q80K in genotype 1 patients in the European region. Antivir Res. 2015;116:10–6.
17. Wyles DL, Gutierrez JA. Importance of HCV genotype 1 subtypes for drug resistance and response to therapy. J Viral Hepat. 2014;21:229–40.
18. Nkontchou G, Ziol M, Aout M, Lhabadie M, Baazia Y, Mahmoudi A, Roulot D, Ganne-Carrie N, Grando-Lemaire V, Trinchet JC, Gordien E, Vicaut E, Baghad I, Beaugrand M. HCV geno-

type 3 is associated with a higher hepatocellular carcinoma incidence in patients with ongoing viral C cirrhosis. J Viral Hepat. 2011;18:e516–22.
19. Buti M, Esteban R. Hepatitis C virus genotype 3: a genotype that is not 'easy-to-treat'. Expert Rev Gastroenterol Hepatol. 2015;9:375–85.
20. https://datahelpdesk.worldbank.org/knowledgebase/articles/906519-world-bank-country-and-lending-groups.
21. http://databank.worldbank.org/data/download/site-content/CLASS.xls.
22. Madhava V, Burgess C, Drucker E. Epidemiology of chronic hepatitis C virus infection in sub-Saharan Africa. Lancet Infect Dis. 2002;2:293–302.
23. http://polarisobservatory.org/polaris/hepC.htm.
24. https://www.cdc.gov/hepatitis/statistics/incidencearchive.htm.
25. https://www.cdc.gov/hepatitis/statistics/.
26. Zibbell JE, Iqbal K, Patel RC, et al. Increases in hepatitis C virus infection related to injection drug use among persons aged ≤30 years—Kentucky, Tennessee, Virginia, and West Virginia, 2006–2012. MMWR Morb Mortal Wkly Rep. 2015;64:453–8.
27. https://www.cdc.gov/hepatitis/hcv/hcvfaq.htm#section2.
28. CDC. Infect Control. https://www.cdc.gov/oralhealth/infectioncontrol/faq/bloodborne_exposures.htm.
29. Paintsil E, He H, Peters C, Lindenbach BD, Heimer R. Survival of hepatitis C virus in syringes: implication for transmission among injection drug users. J Infect Dis. 2010;202:984–90.
30. Alter MJ. Epidemiology of hepatitis C virus infection. World J Gastroenterol. 2007;13:2436–41.
31. Sievert W, Altraif I, Razavi HA, Abdo A, Ahmed EA, Alomair A, Amarapurkar D, Chen CH, Dou X, El Khayat H, Elshazly M, Esmat G, Guan R, Han KH, Koike K, Largen A, McCaughan G, Mogawer S, Monis A, Nawaz A, Piratvisuth T, Sanai FM, Sharara AI, Sibbel S, Sood A, Suh DJ, Wallace C, Young K, Negro F. A systematic review of hepatitis C virus epidemiology in Asia, Australia and Egypt. Liver Int. 2011;31(Suppl 2):61–80.
32. Elgharably A, Gomaa AI, Crossey MME, Norsworthy PJ, Waked I, Taylor-Robinson SD. Hepatitis C in Egypt—past, present, and future. Int J Gen Med. 2017;10:1–6. https://doi.org/10.2147/IJGM.S119301.
33. Frank C, Mohamed MK, Strickland GT, Lavanchy D, Arthur RR, Magder LS, El Khoby T, Abdel-Wahab Y, Aly Ohn ES, Anwar W, Sallam I. The role of parenteral antischistosomal therapy in the spread of hepatitis C virus in Egypt. Lancet. 2000;355:887–91.
34. Nerrienet E, Pouillot R, Lachenal G, Njouom R, Mfoupouendoun J, Bilong C, Mauclere P, Pasquier C, Ayouba A. Hepatitis C virus infection in cameroon: a cohort-effect. J Med Virol. 2005;76:208–14.
35. Thibault V, Bara JL, Nefau T, Duplessy-Garson C. Hepatitis C transmission in injection drug users: could swabs be the main culprit? J Infect Dis. 2011;204:1839–42.
36. Armstrong GL, Wasley A, Simard EP, McQuillan GM, Kuhnert WL, Alter MJ. The prevalence of hepatitis C virus infection in the United States, 1999 through 2002. Ann Intern Med. 2006;144:705–14.
37. Rhodes T, Platt L, Maximova S, Koshkina E, Latishevskaya N, Hickman M, Renton A, Bobrova N, McDonald T, Parry JV. Prevalence of HIV, hepatitis C and syphilis among injecting drug users in Russia: a multi-city study. Addiction. 2006;101:252–66.
38. Vassilev ZP, Hagan H, Lyubenova A, Tomov N, Vasilev G, Krasteva D, Des Jarlais DC. Needle exchange use, sexual risk behaviour, and the prevalence of HIV, hepatitis B virus, and hepatitis C virus infections among Bulgarian injection drug users. Int J STD AIDS. 2006;17:621–6.
39. van den Hoek JA, van Haastrecht HJ, Goudsmit J, de Wolf F, Coutinho RA. Prevalence, incidence, and risk factors of hepatitis C virus infection among drug users in Amsterdam. J Infect Dis. 1990;162:823–6.
40. Des Jarlais DC, Perlis T, Arasteh K, Torian LV, Hagan H, Beatrice S, Smith L, Wethers J, Milliken J, Mildvan D, Yancovitz S, Friedman SR. Reductions in hepatitis C virus and HIV infections among injecting drug users in New York City, 1990–2001. AIDS. 2005;19(Suppl 3):S20–5.

41. Kemp R, Miller J, Lungley S, Baker M. Injecting behaviours and prevalence of hepatitis B, C and D markers in New Zealand injecting drug user populations. N Z Med J. 1998;111:50–3.
42. El-Ghazzawi E, Drew L, Hamdy L, El-Sherbini E, Sadek S-D, Saleh E. Intravenous drug addicts: a high risk group for infection with human immunodeficiency virus, hepatitis viruses, cytomegalo virus and bacterial infections in Alexandria Egypt. J Egypt Public Health Assoc. 1995;70:127–50.
43. Egypt Health Issues Survey 2015 [FR313]—The DHS Program: Ministry of Health, Egypt, El-Zanaty and Associates, Egypt, ICF International. Egypt Health Issues Survey. Cairo: Ministry of Health and ICF International; 2015.
44. Liakina V, Hamid S, Tanaka J, Olafsson S, Sharara AI, Alavian SM, Gheorghe L, El Hassan ES, Abaalkhail F, Abbas Z, Abdou A, Abourached A, Al Braiki F, Al Hosani F, Al Jaberi K, Al Khatry M, Al Mulla MA, Al Quraishi H, Al Rifai A, Al Serkal Y, Alam A, Alashgar HI, Alawadhi S, Al-Dabal L, Aldins P, Alfaleh FZ, Alghamdi AS, Al-Hakeem R, Aljumah AA, Almessabi A, Alqutub AN, Alswat KA, Altraif I, Alzaabi M, Andrea N, Assiri AM, Babatin MA, Baqir A, Barakat MT, Bergmann OM, Bizri AR, Blach S, Chaudhry A, Choi MS, Diab T, Djauzi S, El Khoury S, Estes C, Fakhry S, Farooqi JI, Fridjonsdottir H, Gani RA, Ghafoor Khan A, Goldis A, Gottfredsson M, Gregorcic S, Hajarizadeh B, Han KH, Hasan I, Hashim A, Horvath G, Hunyady B, Husni R, Jafri W, Jeruma A, Jonasson JG, Karlsdottir B, Kim DY, Kim YS, Koutoubi Z, Lesmana LA, Lim YS, Löve A, Maimets M, Makara M, Malekzadeh R, Matičič M, Memon MS, Merat S, Mokhbat JE, Mourad FH, Muljono DH, Nawaz A, Nugrahini N, Priohutomo S, Qureshi H, Rassam P, Razavi H, Razavi-Shearer D, Razavi-Shearer K, Rozentale B, Sadik M, Saeed K, Salamat A, Salupere R, Sanai FM, Sanityoso Sulaiman A, Sayegh RA, Schmelzer JD, Sibley A, Siddiq M, Siddiqui AM, Sigmundsdottir G, Sigurdardottir B, Speiciene D, Sulaiman A, Sultan MA, Taha M, Tarifi H, Tayyab G, Tolmane I, Ud Din M, Umar M, Valantinas J, Videčnik-Zorman J, Yaghi C, Yunihastuti E, Yusuf MA, Zuberi BF, Gunter J. Historical epidemiology of hepatitis C virus (HCV) in select countries—volume 3. J Viral Hepat. 2015;22(Suppl 4):4–20.
45. Bruggmann P, Berg T, Øvrehus AL, Moreno C, Brandão Mello CE, Roudot-Thoraval F, Marinho RT, Sherman M, Ryder SD, Sperl J, Akarca U, Balık I, Bihl F, Bilodeau M, Blasco AJ, Buti M, Calinas F, Calleja JL, Cheinquer H, Christensen PB, Clausen M, Coelho HS, Cornberg M, Cramp ME, Dore GJ, Doss W, Duberg AS, El-Sayed MH, Ergör G, Esmat G, Estes C, Falconer K, Félix J, Ferraz ML, Ferreira PR, Frankova S, García-Samaniego J, Gerstoft J, Giria JA, Gonçales FL Jr, Gower E, Gschwantler M, Guimarães Pessôa M, Hézode C, Hofer H, Husa P, Idilman R, Kåberg M, Kaita KD, Kautz A, Kaymakoglu S, Krajden M, Krarup H, Laleman W, Lavanchy D, Lázaro P, Marotta P, Mauss S, Mendes Correa MC, Müllhaupt B, Myers RP, Negro F, Nemecek V, Örmeci N, Parkes J, Peltekian KM, Ramji A, Razavi H, Reis N, Roberts SK, Rosenberg WM, Sarmento-Castro R, Sarrazin C, Semela D, Shiha GE, Sievert W, Stärkel P, Stauber RE, Thompson AJ, Urbanek P, van Thiel I, Van Vlierberghe H, Vandijck D, Vogel W, Waked I, Wedemeyer H, Weis N, Wiegand J, Yosry A, Zekry A, Van Damme P, Aleman S, Hindman SJ. Historical epidemiology of hepatitis C virus (HCV) in selected countries. J Viral Hepat. 2014;21(Suppl 1):5–33.
46. Saraswat V, Norris S, de Knegt RJ, Sanchez Avila JF, Sonderup M, Zuckerman E, Arkkila P, Stedman C, Acharya S, Aho I, Anand AC, Andersson MI, Arendt V, Baatarkhuu O, Barclay K, Ben-Ari Z, Bergin C, Bessone F, Blach S, Blokhina N, Brunton CR, Choudhuri G, Chulanov V, Cisneros L, Croes EA, Dahgwahdorj YA, Dalgard O, Daruich JR, Dashdorj NR, Davaadorj D, de Vree M, Estes C, Flisiak R, Gadano AC, Gane E, Halota W, Hatzakis A, Henderson C, Hoffmann P, Hornell J, Houlihan D, Hrusovsky S, Jarčuška P, Kershenobich D, Kostrzewska K, Kristian P, Leshno M, Lurie Y, Mahomed A, Mamonova N, Mendez-Sanchez N, Mossong J, Nurmukhametova E, Nymadawa P, Oltman M, Oyunbileg J, Oyunsuren T, Papatheodoridis G, Pimenov N, Prabdial-Sing N, Prins M, Puri P, Radke S, Rakhmanova A, Razavi H, Razavi-Shearer K, Reesink HW, Ridruejo E, Safadi R, Sagalova O, Sanduijav R, Schréter I, Seguin-Devaux C, Shah SR, Shestakova I, Shevaldin A, Shibolet O, Sokolov S, Souliotis K, Spearman CW, Staub T, Strebkova EA, Struck D, Tomasiewicz K, Undram L, van der Meer AJ, van

Santen D, Veldhuijzen I, Villamil FG, Willemse S, Zuure FR, Silva MO, Sypsa V, Gower E. Historical epidemiology of hepatitis C virus (HCV) in select countries—volume 2. J Viral Hepat. 2015;22(Suppl 1):6–25.
47. Lu WP, Lin GX, Shi S, Dong JH. Simultaneously high prevalences of hepatitis B and C virus infections in a population in Putian County, China. J Clin Microbiol. 2012;50:2142–4.
48. McQuillan GM, Kruszon-Moran D, Denniston MM, Hirsch R. Viral hepatitis. NCHS data brief, no. 27. Hyattsville, MD: National Center for Health Statistics; 2010.
49. Vandelli C, Renzo F, Romanò L, Tisminetzky S, De Palma M, Stroffolini T, Ventura E, Zanetti A. Lack of evidence of sexual transmission of hepatitis C among monogamous couples: results of a 10-year prospective follow-up study. Am J Gastroenterol. 2004;99:855–9.
50. https://www.cdc.gov/hepatitis/hcv/hcvfaq.htm#a6.
51. Foster GR, Goldin RD, Thomas HC. Chronic hepatitis C virus infection causes a significant reduction in quality of life in the absence of cirrhosis. Hepatology. 1998;27:209–12.
52. Recommendations for prevention and control of hepatitis C virus (HCV) infection and HCV-related chronic disease. Centers for Disease Control and Prevention. MMWR Recomm Rep. 1998;47(RR-19):1–39.
53. Hadziyannis SJ. Skin diseases associated with hepatitis C virus infection. J Eur Acad Dermatol Venereol. 1998;10:12–21.
54. Liakina V, Speiciene D, Irnius A, Naraskeviciene J, Barakauskiene A, Semuchiniene T. Prevalence of cryoglobulinemia in patients with chronic HCV infection. Med Sci Monit. 2002;8:CR31–6.
55. Cicardi M, Cesana B, Del Ninno E, Pappalardo E, Silini E, Agostoni A, Colombo M. Prevalence and risk factors for the presence of serum cryoglobulins in patients with chronic hepatitis C. J Viral Hepat. 2000;7:138–43.
56. Kenny-Walsh E. Clinical outcomes after hepatitis C infection from contaminated anti-D immune globulin. Irish Hepatology Research Group. N Engl J Med. 1999;340:1228–33.
57. Alberti A, Chemello L, Benvegnù L. Natural history of hepatitis C. J Hepatol. 1999;31(Suppl 1):17–24.
58. Thein H-H, Yi Q, Dore GJ, et al. Estimation of stage-specific brosis progression rates in chronic hepatitis C virus infection: a meta-analysis and meta-regression. Hepatology. 2008;48:418–31.
59. Yano M, Kumada H, Kage M, Ikeda K, Shimamatsu K, Inoue O, Hashimoto E, Lefkowitch JH, Ludwig J, Okuda K. The long-term pathological evolution of chronic hepatitis C. Hepatology. 1996;23:1334–40.
60. Poynard T, Bedossa P, Opolon P. Natural history of liver fibrosis progression in patients with chronic hepatitis C. The OBSVIRC, METAVIR, CLINIVIR, and DOSVIRC Groups. Lancet. 1997;349:825–32.
61. Ryder SD, Irving WL, Jones DA, Neal KR, Underwood JC, Trent Hepatitis C Study Group. Progression of hepatic fibrosis in patients with hepatitis C: a prospective repeat liver biopsy study. Gut. 2004;53:451–5.
62. Akuta N, Chayama K, Suzuki F, et al. Risk factors of hepatitis C virus-related liver cirrhosis in young adults: positive family history of liver disease and transporter associated with antigen processing 2(TAP2)*0201 allele. J Med Virol. 2001;64:109–16.
63. Thomas DL, Astemborski J, Rai RM, Anania FA, Schaeffer M, Galai N, Nolt K, Nelson KE, Strathdee SA, Johnson L, Laeyendecker O, Boitnott J, Wilson LE, Vlahov D. The natural history of hepatitis C virus infection: host, viral, and environmental factors. JAMA. 2000;284:450–6.
64. Di Bisceglie AM, Goodman ZD, Ishak KG, Hoofnagle JH, Melpolder JJ, Alter HJ. Long-term clinical and histopathological follow-up of chronic posttransfusion hepatitis. Hepatology. 1991;14:969–74.
65. Fartoux L, Chazouillères O, Wendum D, Poupon R, Serfaty L. Impact of steatosis on progression of fibrosis in patients with mild hepatitis C. Hepatology. 2005;41:82–7.
66. Ragni MV, Belle SH. Impact of human immunodeficiency virus infection on progression to end-stage liver disease in individuals with hemophilia and hepatitis C virus infection. J Infect Dis. 2001;183:1112–5.

67. Benhamou Y, et al. Liver fibrosis progression in human immunodeficiency virus and hepatitis C virus coinfected patients. The Multivirc Group. Hepatology. 1999;30:1054–8.
68. D'Souza R, Sabin CA, Foster GR. Insulin resistance plays a significant role in liver fibrosis in chronic hepatitis C and in the response to antiviral therapy. Am J Gastroenterol. 2005;100:1509–15.
69. Muzzi A, et al. Insulin resistance is associated with liver fibrosis in non-diabetic chronic hepatitis C patients. J Hepatol. 2005;42:41–6.
70. Fattovich G, Giustina G, Degos F, Tremolada F, Diodati G, Almasio P, Nevens F, Solinas A, Mura D, Brouwer JT, Thomas H, Njapoum C, Casarin C, Bonetti P, Fuschi P, Basho J, Tocco A, Bhalla A, Galassini R, Noventa F, Schalm SW, Realdi G. Morbidity and mortality in compensated cirrhosis type C: a retrospective follow-up study of 384 patients. Gastroenterology. 1997;112:463–72.
71. Fattovich G, Stroffolini T, Zagni I, Donato F. Hepatocellular carcinoma in cirrhosis: incidence and risk factors. Gastroenterology. 2004;127:S35–50.
72. Benvegnù L, Gios M, Boccato S, Alberti A. Natural history of compensated viral cirrhosis: a prospective study on the incidence and hierarchy of major complications. Gut. 2004;53:744–9.
73. Lee MH, Yang HI, Lu SN, Jen CL, You SL, Wang LY, Wang CH, Chen WJ, Chen CJ, R.E.V.E.A.L.-HCV Study Group. Chronic hepatitis C virus infection increases mortality from hepatic and extrahepatic diseases: a community-based long-term prospective study. J Infect Dis. 2012;206:469–77.
74. Veldt BJ, Heathcote EJ, Wedemeyer H, Reichen J, Hofmann WP, Zeuzem S, Manns MP, Hansen BE, Schalm SW, Janssen HL. Sustained virologic response and clinical outcomes in patients with chronic hepatitis C and advanced fibrosis. Ann Intern Med. 2007;147:677–84.
75. van der Meer AJ, Veldt BJ, Feld JJ, Wedemeyer H, Dufour JF, Lammert F, Duarte-Rojo A, Heathcote EJ, Manns MP, Kuske L, Zeuzem S, Hofmann WP, de Knegt RJ, Hansen BE, Janssen HL. Association between sustained virological response and all-cause mortality among patients with chronic hepatitis C and advanced hepatic fibrosis. JAMA. 2012;308:2584–93.
76. WHO. International Agency for Research on Cancer (IARC). Globocan: Cancer Today. http://gco.iarc.fr/today/online-analysis-table?mode=population&mode_population=world&population=900&sex=0&cancer=7&type=0&statistic=0&prevalence=0&color_palette=default.
77. WHO. Globocan. http://globocan.iarc.fr/old/FactSheets/cancers/liver-new.asp.
78. Curry MP, O'Leary JG, Bzowej N. Sofosbuvir and velpatasvir for HCV in patients with decompensated cirrhosis. N Engl J Med. 2015;373:2618–28.
79. Stanaway JD, Flaxman AD, Naghavi M, Fitzmaurice C, Vos T, Abubakar I, Abu-Raddad LJ, Assadi R, Bhala N, Cowie B, Forouzanfour MH, Groeger J, Mohd Hanafiah K, Jacobsen KH, James SL, MacLachlan J, Malekzadeh R, Martin NK, Mokdad AA, Mokdad AH, Murray CJ, Plass D, Rana S, Rein DB, Richardus JH, Sanabria J, Saylan M, Shahraz S, So S, Vlassov VV, Weiderpass E, Wiersma ST, Younis M, Yu C, El Sayed Zaki M, Cooke GS. The global burden of viral hepatitis from 1990 to 2013: findings from the Global Burden of Disease Study 2013. Lancet. 2016;388:1081–8.
80. Feld JJ, Jacobson IM, Hezode C. Sofosbuvir and velpatasvir for HCV genotype 1,2,4,5, and 6 infection. N Engl J Med. 2015;373:2599–607.
81. Foster GR, Afdhal N, Roberts SK. Sofosbuvir and velpatasvir for HCV genotype 2 and 3 infection. N Engl J Med. 2015;373:2608–17.
82. Gane E, Poordad F, Wang S, Asatryan A, Kwo PY, Lalezari J, Wyles DL, Hassanein T, Aguilar H, Maliakkal B, Liu R, Lin CW, Ng TI, Kort J, Mensa FJ. High efficacy of ABT-493 and ABT-530 treatment in patients with HCV genotype 1 or 3 infection and compensated cirrhosis. Gastroenterology. 2016;151:651–9.
83. Jacobson IM, Lawitz E, Kwo PY, Hézode C, Peng CY, Howe AY, Hwang P, Wahl J, Robertson M, Barr E, Haber BA. Safety and efficacy of elbasvir/grazoprevir in patients with hepatitis C virus infection and compensated cirrhosis: an integrated analysis. Gastroenterology. 2017;152:1372–1382.e2. https://doi.org/10.1053/j.gastro.2017.01.050. pii: S0016-5085(17)30150-6.

84. Brown A, Hezode C, Zuckerman E, et al. P0771: C-SCAPE: efficacy and safety of 12 weeks of grazoprevir ± elbasvir ± ribavirin in patients with HCV GT2, 4, 5 or 6 infection. J Hepatol. 2015;62:S619.
85. Kwo P, Gane EJ, Peng CY, Pearlman B, Vierling JM, Serfaty L, Buti M, Shafran S, Stryszak P, Lin L, Gress J, Black S, Dutko FJ, Robertson M, Wahl J, Lupinacci L, Barr E, Haber B. Effectiveness of elbasvir and grazoprevir combination, with or without ribavirin, for treatment-experienced patients with chronic hepatitis C infection. Gastroenterology. 2017;152:164–75.
86. Elsharkawy A, Fouad R, El Akel W, El Raziky M, Hassany M, Shiha G, Said M, Motawea I, El Demerdash T, Seif S, Gaballah A, El Shazly Y, Makhlouf MAM, Waked I, Abdelaziz AO, Yosry A, El Serafy M, Thursz M, Doss W, Esmat G. Sofosbuvir-based treatment regimens: real life results of 14 409 chronic HCV genotype 4 patients in Egypt. Aliment Pharmacol Ther. 2017;45:681–7. https://doi.org/10.1111/apt.13923.
87. Eletreby R, Elakel W, Said M, El Kassas M, Seif S, Elbaz T, El Raziky M, Abdel Rehim S, Zaky S, Fouad R, Gamal Eldeen H, Abdo M, Korany M, Yosry A, El Serafy M, El-Sayed MH, ElShazly Y, Waked I, Doss W, Esmat G. Real life Egyptian experience of efficacy and safety of Simeprevir/Sofosbuvir therapy in 6211 chronic HCV genotype IV infected patients. Liver Int. 2016;37:534–41. https://doi.org/10.1111/liv.13266.
88. Aleman S, Rahbin N, Weiland O, Davidsdottir L, Hedenstierna M, Rose N, Verbaan H, Stål P, Carlsson T, Norrgren H, Ekbom A, Granath F, Hultcrantz R. A risk for hepatocellular carcinoma persists long-term after sustained virologic response in patients with hepatitis C-associated liver cirrhosis. Clin Infect Dis. 2013;57:230–6.
89. Di Marco V, Calvaruso V, Ferraro D, Bavetta MG, Cabibbo G, Conte E, Cammà C, Grimaudo S, Pipitone RM, Simone F, Peralta S, Arini A, Craxì A. Effects of eradicating hepatitis C virus infection in patients with cirrhosis differ with stage of portal hypertension. Gastroenterology. 2016;151:130–9.

Enteric Hepatitis Viruses: Hepatitis A Virus and Hepatitis E Virus

13

Mohammad Sultan Khuroo, Mehnaaz S. Khuroo, and Naira S. Khuroo

Abstract

Hepatitis A is an infectious disease of the liver caused by hepatitis A virus. Hepatitis A has a global distribution with endemicity inversely proportional to higher socioeconomic conditions and standards of sanitation and hygiene. Hepatitis A virus infection is predominantly spread directly from one person to another through orofecal transmission and through contaminated food and water. The clinical outcome is strongly correlated with age, being mostly subclinical in young children and symptomatic in older children and adults. Hepatitis A vaccine is safe, highly immunogenic and protective against clinical hepatitis A.

Hepatitis E is an infectious disease of the liver caused by the hepatitis E virus. Hepatitis E is the most common cause of large-scale waterborne epidemics of jaundice in developing countries. In addition, around a third to a half of endemic acute viral hepatitis in these countries is caused by hepatitis E. The disease has high incidence and severity in pregnant women. Recently, hepatitis E is being recognized as an important clinical problem in the industrialized world that is related to unique zoonotic foodborne transmission. Hepatitis E in these countries has particular relevance to the solid organ transplant population due to risk of progression of infection to chronic hepatitis E and cirrhosis with liver failure and death in such patients. Hepatitis E causes a number of extrahepatic manifestations

M. S. Khuroo
Department of Medicine, Sher-I-Kashmir Institute of Medical Sciences, Srinagar, Kashmir, India

King Faisal Specialist Hospital and Research Centre, Riyadh, Saudi Arabia

Digestive Diseases Centre, Dr. Khuroo's Medical Clinic, Srinagar, Kashmir, India

M. S. Khuroo (✉)
Department of Pathology, Govt. Medical College Srinagar, Srinagar, Kashmir, India

N. S. Khuroo
Dr. Khuroo's Medical Clinic, Srinagar, Kashmir, India

R. J. Wong, R. G. Gish (eds.), *Clinical Epidemiology of Chronic Liver Diseases*,
https://doi.org/10.1007/978-3-319-94355-8_13

including a wide spectrum of neurological syndromes. Hepatitis E virus can be transmitted through blood and blood component transfusions, and donor screening is being done in many countries. There has been a significant advance in drug treatment of chronic hepatitis E and the availability of hepatitis E vaccine promises control of the hepatitis E burden in future.

13.1 Introduction

Viral hepatitis is an infection which involves predominantly the liver [1]. As of today, five unrelated hepatotropic pathogens, hepatitis A virus (HAV), hepatitis B virus (HBV), hepatitis C virus (HCV), hepatitis D virus (HDV) and hepatitis E virus (HEV) are recognized to cause almost all cases of viral hepatitis [2]. A few more parenterally-transmitted agents have been identified that were suspected to cause hepatitis including human pegivirus (HPgV) (formerly known as GBV-C/HGV), TT virus (TTV) and other TTV-related viruses (SANYAN, YONBON, SEN viruses and TTV-like Mini-virus). None of these are known to cause hepatitis in humans as of today [3, 4]. There have been "new kids on the block" about whom we have more to learn. Two more novel agents in the pegivirus genera of the family Flaviviridae have been identified and named as human hepagivirus 1 (HHpgV-1) [5] and human pegivirus 2 (HPgV-2) [6]. A number of other systemic viral infections that may involve the liver and cause hepatitis include Epstein-Barr virus (EBV), cytomegalovirus (CMV), herpes simplex virus (HSV), varicella zoster virus (VZV) and Severe Acute Respiratory Syndrome [3].

Viral hepatitis is a global health problem. Hepatitis viruses play a significant role in the story of global disease and death and pose a colossal health challenge [7]. The Global Burden of Disease (GBD) Study 2013 revealed, unlike most communicable diseases, a significant increase in the mortality and morbidity for acute hepatitis, cirrhosis and liver cancer from 1990 to 2013 [8]. The deaths rose from 0.89 to 1.45 million; years of life lost (YLLs) from 31.0 to 41.6 million; years lived with disability (YLDs) from 0.65 to 0.87 million and disability-adjusted life-years (DALYs) from 31.7 to 42.5 million. Viral hepatitis ranked as the seventh leading cause of death in 2013, an increase from tenth in 1990.

The 2014 World Health Assembly requested the World Health Organization (WHO) to examine the feasibility of eliminating viral hepatitis by 2030. Recently, WHO published an advocacy brief on "Combating Hepatitis B and C to reach Elimination by 2030" [9]. It was proposed that the viral hepatitis response should reach five prevention and treatment service coverage targets by 2030. These include increases in (1) three-dose hepatitis B vaccine coverage from 82% to 90%, (2) prevention of mother-to-child transmission of HBV from 38% to 90%, (3) blood and injection safety coverage from 89% to 100%, (4) safe syringe set distribution for injection drug users (IDUs) from 20 to 300 per person per year and (5) diagnosis and treatment coverage for HBV and HCV from 5% to 90% and from <1% to 80%, respectively. This will reduce incidence of HBV and HCV by 90% and mortality by 65%. As 90% of deaths are caused by HBV and HCV, the advocacy brief did not elaborate on how to reduce the impact of HAV and HEV by 2030.

Hepatitis viruses are broadly divided into two distinct groups, based on the mode of transmission and ability to cause persistent infection. Three viruses (HBV, HCV and HDV) are transmitted either by parenteral, sexual or mother-to-baby routes and can cause persistent viremia, chronic hepatitis, cirrhosis and hepatocellular carcinoma. In contrast, the other two hepatitis viruses (HAV and HEV) share an enteric route of transmission and a self-limiting course and do not contribute to liver cirrhosis and liver cancer [10]. In this chapter we cover the historical background, morphology, replication, global epidemiology, clinical manifestations, laboratory features, and diagnosis, treatment and global control of the two enteric hepatitis viruses HAV and HEV.

13.2 Hepatitis A Virus

Hepatitis A is an infection of the liver etiologically related to HAV. Hepatitis A has global distribution with endemicity proportional to socioeconomic conditions and standards of sanitation and hygiene. It is estimated that HAV infected 117 million people with 31 million symptomatic illnesses and 30,283 deaths in 1990, with an increase to 126 million infections with 35,245 deaths in 2005 [8]. The mortality had increased over the years in the age groups 2–12 years and above 35 years of age. HAV infection is predominantly spread from one person to another through the orofecal route or by contaminated food and water. The clinical outcome is strongly correlated with age, being mostly subclinical in children ≤6 years and symptomatic in older children and adults. Hepatitis A vaccine is safe, highly immunogenic and protective against clinical hepatitis A [11].

13.2.1 Historical Background

Viral hepatitis had a devastating effect on the military population during World War II [12]. Early volunteer studies principally among prisoners led to recognition of two types of hepatitis differing in the primary route of transmission and period of incubation. In 1947 McCallum et al. termed infectious and serum hepatitis as hepatitis A and hepatitis B, respectively [13]. Studies on the existence of two types of viral hepatitis were confirmed and extended in volunteer studies in mentally-challenged children at the Willowbrook State School in New York [14]. The two infectious sera, namely MS-1 and MS-2 (obtained from serum of patient M.S. during his first and second bout of hepatitis) played a crucial role in subsequent studies on the two forms of viral hepatitis. Studies on humans and marmosets characterized HAV as a small virus resistant to ether and heat, transmitted through feces and distinct from HBV. However, HAV could not be cultivated or identified [15]. In 1973 HAV was identified by Feinstone et al. using immune electron microscopy to examine stool specimens taken from a prison volunteer infected with the Willowbrook MS-1 infectious sera [16]. Further studies led to a serological test for HAV, isolation of the virus in cell culture and development of the HAV vaccine [17, 18].

13.2.2 Morphology

HAV is classified in the *hepatovirus* genus of the *Picornaviridae* family [1, 11]. HAV exists only as a single serotype, with three genotypes (I–III) that circulate in humans and three additional genotypes (IV–VI) recognized in non-human primates [19, 20]. Humans are the only natural host for HAV. The virus is heat-stable and an acid/ether resistant RNA virus [17]. The virion is a non-enveloped, symmetrical, small 27-nm, spherical particle. The capsid of the virus is icosahedral in symmetry. The icosahedron is a three-dimensional figure with 20-faces resembling a soccer ball. The capsid is made of subunits called capsomeres. Each capsomere is made of five protomers. Each protomer of HAV is made of three capsid proteins namely VP1 (ID), VP2 (IB) and VP3 (IC). VP4 (IA) does not seem to be incorporated into the virion. Thus, the HAV capsid is made from 60 densely-packed protomers, each consisting of three major structural proteins. The HAV genome is about 7.5 kb and is divided in to three parts: a long untranslated region (UTR) at the 5′ end which contains a type III internal ribosome entry site (IRES), a single open reading frame and a short UTR at the 3′ polyadenylated end. The HAV genome is organized into three regions, namely P1, P2 and P3, and encodes 11 genes. The P1 region encodes four capsid proteins and the P2 and P3 regions encode a series of non-structural proteins [1, 10, 11] (Fig. 13.1).

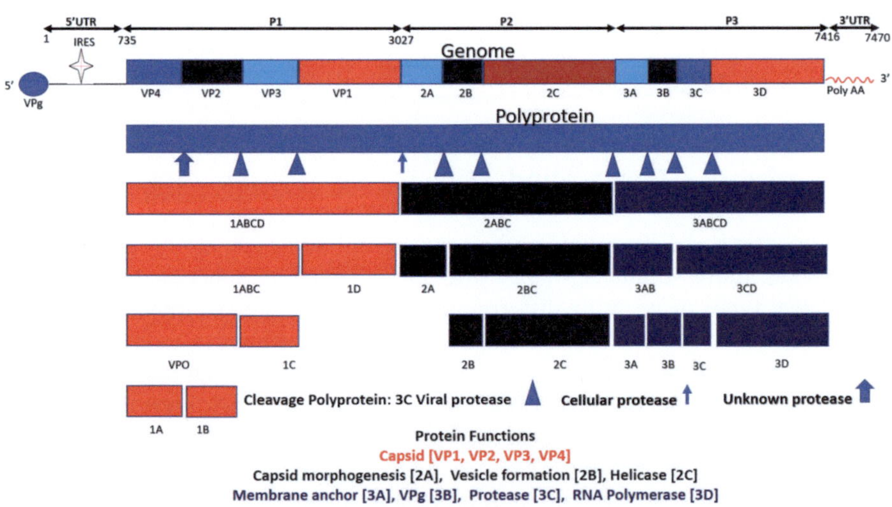

Fig. 13.1 Hepatitis A virus genome and gene expression. The genome is 7.470 kb and is divided in to three parts: long UTR (nucleotide 1–734) at 5′ end which contains IRES, a single ORF (nucleotide 735–7416) and short UTR (nucleotides 7416–7470) at 3′ polyadenylated end. HAV genome is organized in to three regions namely P1, P2 and P3 and encodes 11 genes (shown by colors in genome bar). ORF is translated in to a polyprotein of 2227 amino acids. This polyprotein is cleaved posttranslationally at 10 specific sites (shown by arrows). The function of proteins is delineated (Author's original work) [*UTR* untranslated region, *ORF* open reading frame, *IRES* type III internal ribosome entry site, *VPg* viral protein genome]

13.2.3 Replication

Replication of HAV RNA starts with attachment of the virus to receptors on the cell wall with endocytosis of the virus into the hepatocytes [21]. In the cell, VP4 is released, which in turn opens a hole in the host endosomal membrane, allowing viral genome into the host cytoplasm. The genome (ORF, 6681 nucleotides), under influence of IRES, is translated into a polyprotein (2227 amino acids). This polyprotein is cleaved post-translationally at ten specific sites to release four capsid proteins and seven non-structural proteins. The cleavage occurs at eight specific sites by unique 3C viral protease, at one site by a cellular protease and at another site by an unknown protease. Four structural proteins [VP1 (ID), VP2 (IB), VP3 (IC) and VP4 (IA)] correspond to the P1 segment of the genome, while P2 and P3 segments represent a series of nonstructural proteins. The structural proteins (VP1, VP2 and VP3) form the procapsid (Fig. 13.1). A negative-sense RNA replicon is formed within vesicles derived from the ER, with the binding of non-structural proteins to the 3′ end of the genomic RNA. Subsequent to this, multiple copies of positive-sense RNA are synthesized and packed in to the procapsid, forming the virion. Virion is egressed from the hepatocytes after cell lysis [1, 11].

13.2.4 Global Epidemiology

The understanding of the epidemiology of hepatitis A is based on population-based seroprevalence (IgG anti-HAV) studies. The world is divided into three zones, the very-high endemic zone, the high-to-intermediate endemic zone and the low endemic zone [22] (Table 13.1). In addition, the morbidity and mortality of HAV infection depends upon the age of exposure to infection. HAV infection is usually asymptomatic or subclinical in children below 6 years of age. In contrast, clinical disease with jaundice occurs in older children and adults [23, 24].

The very-high endemic zone includes resource-poor countries of Southeast Asia and Sub-Saharan Africa. In such countries, poor sanitary conditions, overcrowding, and contaminated water and food promotes universal exposure to HAV infection in children soon after weaning. The age at the midpoint of population immunity (50%) is in childhood at around age 5 years. The majority of these infections are subclinical and seroconversion is usually asymptomatic. Seroprevalence data reveal that ≥90% of children seroconvert before 10 years of age and adults have protective IgG anti-HAV. HAV circulation in the community is ubiquitous, but clinical hepatitis E disease occurs in only a small percentage of children and is of mild severity. HAV infections in adults are reported infrequently in such countries [25].

The high-to-intermediate endemic zone for HAV comprises the developing countries of Asia, Latin America, Eastern Europe, and the Middle East [26–28]. In these countries, there is recent continued improvement in sanitary conditions and access to safe water, with reduced exposure of children to HAV infection. The

Table 13.1 Global epidemiology of hepatitis A virus

Endemicity zones	Very high	High to intermediate	Low
Socio-economic status	Low-resource	Developing	Developed
Countries	Sub-Saharan Africa, south-east Asia	Asia, Latin America, Eastern Europe, Middle East	Western Europe, Australia, New Zealand, Canada, USA, Japan, Korea, Singapore
Age at midpoint of population immunity (50%)	<5 years	High 5–14 years, Intermediate 15–34 years	>35 years
Ig anti-HAV	>90%	<50%	<50%
Childhood infections	Universal	Uncommon	Nil
Immunity	High	Low	Very low
HAV circulation in community	Very common	Common	Negligible
Adult infections	Not seen	Common (paradoxical)	Not seen
Disease load	Negligible	Adolescents and adults	Special groups (Travelers); schools; camps
Outbreaks	Not seen	Person-to-person, foodborne	Food borne outbreaks (imported)

age at the midpoint of population immunity (50%) is from 5 to 14 years (high endemic zone) and 15 to 34 years (intermediate endemic zone). HAV circulation in the community is common. There is exposure to HAV infection in older children and adolescents and most of these infections are symptomatic. Person-to-person and foodborne outbreaks of HAV infection are common. Thus, paradoxically, such regions of the world have high occurrence of clinical hepatitis A in young adults.

The low endemic zone of HAV spreads over the developed world, including Western Europe, Australia, New Zealand, Canada, the United States, Japan, Korea, and Singapore. HAV circulation in the community is negligible. Exposure to children in these countries is infrequent and anti-HAV seropositivity increases slowly throughout early childhood. The age at the midpoint of population immunity (50%) is after 35 years of age. The seroprevalence of IgG anti-HAV is high in older age groups as a result of past exposure to HAV during childhood (cohort effect). A high proportion of children and adults are susceptible to HAV infection. However, clinical disease in these age groups is not encountered as there is negligible circulation of the virus in the community. However, HAV infections are reported in travellers to endemic countries and in crowded situations with suboptimum sanitary conditions like schools, prisons and camps. Outbreaks and large-scale epidemics of HAV have been traced to contaminated foods and fruits, imported from endemic zones [29–32]. It is estimated that there was a significant increase in morbidity and mortality from hepatitis A over the years from 1990 to 2005 [33].

13.2.5 Mode of Transmission

Humans are the lone hosts and source of spread and transmission for HAV. HAV infection is spread directly from one person to another through the orofecal route. Large quantities of virus (up to $>10^8$ infectious particles per milliliter) are shed in feces from the late incubation period until the first week of clinical disease. The infectious period starts 1–3 weeks before and lasts for 1–8 days after onset of jaundice. The transmission is supported by low hygiene, overcrowded families, and close contact and occurs among international travellers, prisoners and military forces and in day-care centers, schools, and institutions with the mentally challenged. Endemicity of HAV in developing countries is maintained by person-to-person spread from subclinical HAV infections in children once they are weaned from breastfeeding and exposed to a contaminated environment and low hygiene standards.

Contaminated food and water can transmit HAV infection. Foods of a diverse nature including dairy products, shellfish, and produce can be contaminated [30, 34, 35]. Shellfish can become contaminated with HAV in sea water contaminated with human fecal material, and are a particular risk for transmission of the virus because certain shellfish, including oysters, are often eaten raw [35]. Outbreaks and large-scale epidemics of hepatitis A have been traced to consumption of raw or partially cooked bivalve mollusks including mussels, oysters, and clams [36, 37]. Bivalve mollusks concentrate HAV over 100-fold from contaminated sea water [38]. The Shanghai epidemic of 1988, causing more than 300,000 cases, was caused by contaminated clams [39]. Fresh produce can be contaminated by irrigation water that contains human fecal material. Infected food handlers may also contaminate foodstuffs and beverages and result in outbreaks of HAV [40]. The risk of transmission of HAV occurs from virus shedding during the incubation period. Contaminated food includes uncooked food items or cooked foods handled after cooking by infectious food workers. It is important to be aware that although the level of infectious HAV in foodstuffs generally declines over time, the length of time over which infectious virus remains varies widely between foods and levels may remain high even after lengthy periods of refrigeration (up to a month or more) or freezing (for several months) in some food items [35]. Researchers have found that the length of time over which HAV remains infectious on produce (green onions, lettuce, peppers, and spinach in one study) refrigerated at a cold temperature (<10 °C) exceeds the average shelf life of those foods [35]. Frozen foods are another area of concern. Both shellfish and berries that had been frozen for several months have been associated with HAV outbreaks, with studies showing that when food has been contaminated prior to being frozen, a substantial percentage of hepatitis A viruses will still be infectious even after lengthy frozen storage [35]. Water is also a risk for transmitting HAV infection to western unvaccinated tourists [41]. HAV can be transmitted to a traveller through contaminated drinking water, ice and water-based drinks, fruits and salads washed with contaminated water, milk products, contaminated shellfish, and swimming in polluted water.

Bloodborne transmission of HAV infection has been reported [42], but occurs rarely. Outbreaks of HAV infection occurring in Injection Drug Users (IDUs) may be caused by sharing infected needles [43]; however, such source of spread has not been conclusively proved in view of the confounding potential of fecal-oral transmission. HAV infection does also spread among men having sex with men [44].

13.2.6 Clinical Manifestations

Acute hepatitis A disease passes through four phases including incubation period (15–45 days), prodromal symptoms (1–7 days), icteric period (2–6 weeks) and convalescence (up to 6 weeks) (Fig. 13.2). The clinical outcome is strongly correlated with age. HAV infection in children below 6 years of age is either asymptomatic or subclinical, while older children and adults commonly experience symptomatic disease [45]. Acute hepatitis A presentation resembles disease caused by other hepatitis viruses and may vary from mild short-lasting icteric disease to acute liver failure. During the incubation period the patient is asymptomatic, but sheds the virus in the stools in large quantities and is infectious. The prodromal stage lasts for 1–7 days and precedes onset of jaundice. Patients develop constitutional symptoms which include anorexia, nausea and vomiting, abdominal discomfort, diarrhea, fatigue, malaise, arthralgia, myalgia, and headache. Patients often complain of altered taste and aversion to fat and smoking. Low grade fever between 38 and 39 °C (100–102 °F) lasts for several days but subsides with the onset of jaundice. The icteric phase starts with dark urine and light colored stools; within 1–5 days patients develop icterus of the sclera and skin. Within days, patients develop varying degree of pruritus, which lasts for a variable period related to the severity of cholestasis.

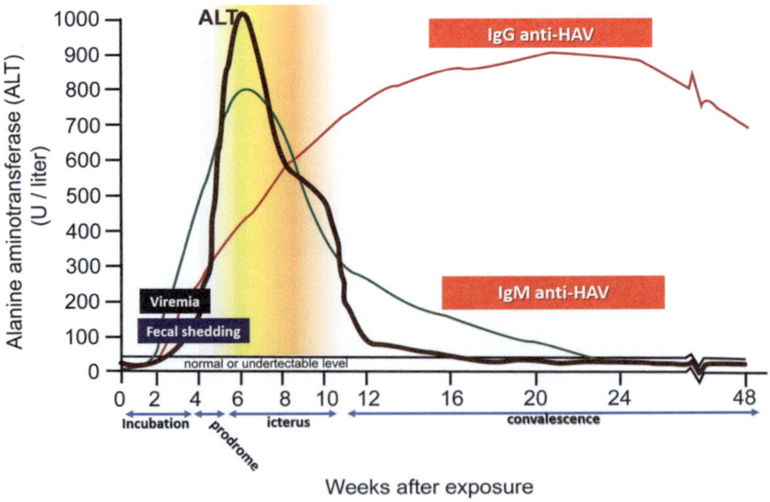

Fig. 13.2 Clinical course of hepatitis A (Author's original work)

With the appearance of jaundice, there is significant abatement of systemic symptoms. Physical examination reveals icterus and tender hepatomegaly. Splenomegaly and cervical lymphadenopathy is detected in 10–20% of patients. Rarely, a few spider angioma may appear which disappear during convalescence. The icteric phase lasts for up to 4–6 weeks and patients convalesce over several weeks. Patients complain of fatigue and weight loss of 2.5–5 kg. Clinical examination is unremarkable except for mild tender hepatomegaly. Complete clinical and biochemical recovery occurs in almost all patients [46].

A small percentage of patients may present with an unusual variant called cholestatic hepatitis A [47]. Patients have a protracted clinical course lasting for 12–18 weeks that is dominated by severe cholestasis with deep jaundice, dark urine, clay stools and severe itching, resembling large bile duct obstruction. All patients show clearance of the virus and clinical recovery. Occasionally, HAV disease relapses in some patients after recovery from the acute illness [48]. Relapse is characterized by reappearance of jaundice and other symptoms of hepatitis with abnormalities of liver tests and fecal viral shedding [49]. All patients eventually recover.

Fulminant hepatitis A occurs in 1:1000 cases of acute hepatitis A and may be fatal [50]. The disease can be recognized early on by worsening prothrombin time, significant reduction in liver size (detected on percussion for liver dullness), irritability, and alteration in sleep rhythm. The risk for fulminant hepatitis increases with patient age and is particularly high in patients above 30 years [51]. HAV superinfection in patients with compensated chronic liver disease are at higher risk for fulminant hepatitis A [52].

Rare complications of acute hepatitis A include joint pains, cutaneous vasculitis, cryoglobulinemia, pancreatitis, myocarditis, atypical pneumonia, aplastic anemia, red cell aplasia, and neurologic syndrome such as Guillain–Barre, myelopathy, mononeuritis and meningoencephalitis [53, 54]. Rarely, autoimmune hepatitis can be triggered by a self-limited acute hepatitis A [55].

13.2.7 Laboratory Features and Diagnosis

During the incubation period patients with hepatitis A have no abnormality in laboratory tests. However, there is short-term viremia and significant fecal shedding of the virus. Alanine transaminase (ALT) and aspartate transaminase (AST) are elevated during the prodromal phase, while serum bilirubin remains within normal limits. Peak levels may vary and can reach from 400 to 4000 IU or more. The serum enzymes show a progressive decline during convalescence and eventually return to normal. The magnitude of rise in serum enzymes has no prognostic significance. Serum alkaline phosphatase may be normal or show mild elevation. However, patients with cholestatic hepatitis A depict marked elevation of serum alkaline phosphatase and GGT. Serum albumin levels stay unchanged in most patients [56].

Serum bilirubin rises above 2.5 mg/dL during the icteric phase of disease. Serum bilirubin rises to levels ranging from 5 to 20 mg/dL. Hyperbilirubinemia is biphasic, with rise of both conjugated and unconjugated bilirubin. Deep jaundice with serum bilirubin levels of 20 mg/dL are associated with severe disease. HAV infection in patients with glucose 6-phosphatase deficiency or sickle cell anemia, can induce acute hemolytic crises leading to extremely high levels of serum bilirubin (≥30 mg/dL). This is not necessarily associated with a poor prognosis.

HAV infection is associated with several abnormalities in blood counts including transient neutropenia and lymphopenia followed by relative lymphocytosis and atypical lymphocytes (2–20%). The INR has prognostic significance and increased values occur in patients with severe hepatic synthetic defect which signifies extensive hepatocellular necrosis. Hypoglycemia occurs occasionally and is related to inadequate intake with underlying poor hepatic glycogen reserves. IgM anti-HAV is detectable during early clinical disease and stays reactive for 4–6 months and is the gold standard for diagnosis of acute HAV infection [57–59]. IgG anti-HAV are detected during acute phase and persist for life. IgG anti-HAV are used to evaluate seroprevalence of HAV. Stool HAV RNA is rarely employed for diagnosis of acute hepatitis A [60].

13.2.8 Treatment

Patients with acute hepatitis A need supportive treatment [56]. No specific antiviral therapy is available. During the prodromal period, nausea and vomiting may require treatment with antiemetics. A few patients will require a short hospital stay to manage dehydration. Intravenous alimentation is rarely needed, most commonly in patients who have persistent vomiting and cannot maintain oral intake. Patients often need bed rest with bathroom privileges during prodromal and icteric disease. At a later stage patients should be advised to restrict activity and not resume working until disease recovery ensues. Restriction of diet has no proven benefit. A high calorie diet is advisable. A low-fat, high-carbohydrate diet is often enforced. However, apart from being palatable this regimen has no added advantage. Alcohol and hepatotoxic drugs should be avoided. Acetaminophen may be administered if needed to a maximum dose of 2–4 g/day in adults. Patients with cholestasis may benefit from bile salt sequestering resin cholestyramine and/or ursodeoxycholic acid (UDCA) [61]. Corticosteroid therapy has no role, even in severe cases, unless there is evidence for autoimmune hepatitis.

At the outset, it is not possible to predict the course of disease and all patients need to be watched carefully for severe disease and impending acute liver failure. Patients with rapidly shrinking liver size, high INR, rapid rise in serum bilirubin and ascites with confusion, altered sleep pattern and disorientation should be identified early and admitted to intensive care for management of acute liver failure. Liver transplantation has been done in patients with progressive liver failure [50, 62].

13.2.9 Global Control

Global control of hepatitis A is dependent upon improved socioeconomic status and improvement in living standards, which in turn reduce virus transmission in the community and disease burden, independent of other measures. Another important measure is to supply safe potable drinking water and ensure proper sewage disposal to reduce person-to-person transmission of HAV infection. We need to target personal hygiene practices like regular hand washing, especially in restaurants, schools, offices, homes for the mentally challenged etc., in order to help reduce the risk of infection. Western tourists should be discouraged from ingestion of uncooked or inadequately cooked foods, salads, untreated tap water and ice creams.

Both passive and active immunization are playing a major role in global control of hepatitis A [25, 63, 64]. Fortunately, all preparations of immune serum globulin (IG) contain HAV antibodies in sufficient concentrations to impart effective protection [65]. IG, administered 0.02 mL/kg, prevents clinically apparent hepatitis A when administered before exposure as in international travelers or following exposure as in intimate contacts. HAV vaccine is safe, immunogenic and effective in preventing hepatitis A [66, 67]. Vaccine is safe above 1 year of age and protects 4 weeks after a primary inoculation [68]. National immunization programs with good coverage rates in children have dramatically declined incidence rates of HAV infections in Italy, Spain, and, most strikingly, in the U.S. [69]. Targeted HAV vaccine, especially in travelers to endemic regions and in other high risk groups, is effective and needs to be enforced [70]. If travel is imminent, concomitant IG (0.02 mL/kg) should be administered along with the first dose of vaccine. Developing countries have implemented a single dose of inactivated HAV vaccine to improve coverage and reduce costs; this has been successful to control HAV epidemics in Argentina and Chile [66, 71–73].

A number of HAV vaccines are available (Table 13.2). These include three monovalent inactivated HAV vaccines [HAVRIX (GSK), Vaqta (Merck) and Avaxim

Table 13.2 Hepatitis A vaccines

Vaccine	Age yr.	Dose (mL)	Antigen quantity	Schedule
Monovalent inactivated HAV vaccines				
Havrix (GSK) Junior	2–16	0.5	720 ELISA units inactivated HAV antigen	0, 6–12 mon
Havrix (GSK) 1440	>16	1	1440 ELISA units inactivated HAV antigen	0, 6–12 mon
Vaqta (Merck) Paed	1–18	0.5	25 units inactivated protein	0, 6–18 mon
Vaqta (Merck) Adult	>18	1	50 units inactivated protein	0, 6–18 mon
Avaxim (Sanofi)	>2	0.5	160 ELISA units of inactivated HAV antigen	0, 6–12 mon
Combined HAV-HBV vaccine				
Twinirix (GSK) Junior	1–16	0.5	360 ELISA units HAV and 10 μg recombinant HBsAg protein	0, 1, 6 mon
Twinirix (GSK) 720/20	2–16	1	720 ELISA units HAV and 20 μg recombinant HBsAg protein	0, 1, 6 mon
Combined HAV-typhoid vaccine				
Vivaxim (Sanofi)	>16	1	160 ELISA units HAV antigen	0, 6–36 mon
Live attenuated HAV vaccine (Chinese)				
H2-strain	>1	1	$10^{5.50}$ $TCID_{50}$ given subcutaneously (tissue culture infective dose)	Single dose
L-A-1-strain	>1	1	$10^{5.50}$ $TCID_{50}$ given subcutaneously (tissue culture infective dose)	Single dose

(Sanofi)], two combined vaccines [Twinirix (GSK) and Vivaxim (Sanofi)] and two Chinese live attenuated vaccines [H2-strain and L-A-1-strain] [25, 74]. Based on the global epidemiology and hepatitis A disease pattern, WHO has put forward recommendations for global pre-exposure prophylaxis. These include:

1. HAV vaccination programs are not recommended in very high endemic zones. In such countries, there is universal exposure to HAV infection in children below 5 years of age, and thus the population is "protected" from HAV infection.
2. Countries with improving socioeconomic status and with high to intermediate endemicity have high rate of HAV infection in adults. It is recommended that an HAV vaccination program should be incorporated into the national immunization schedule for children over 1 year of age. This decision should be individualized for each country based on incidence of acute infections, the magnitude of change from high to intermediate endemicity and cost considerations. This algorithm causes a striking decrease in incidence of new and symptomatic HAV infections [75–78].
3. In low endemic zones, HAV circulation is negligible and HAV are rarely reported in adults. Thus, mass vaccination is not recommended. However, most of the adult population lacks anti-HAV and is susceptible to HAV infection. Thus, targeted vaccination in selected groups who are at increased risk of infection is recommended. These include: (1) travelers to intermediate and high endemic zones; (2) people needing life-long blood products; (3) men who have sex with men; (4) IDUs; (5) patients with cirrhosis, as they run a risk of a severe clinical disease course.
4. HAV vaccine is now being recommended for western travelers to endemic areas and for contacts of patients with acute HAV infection [79].
5. HAV vaccine has been successfully used to control community wide outbreaks. Vaccination should be initiated early on during the epidemic. Supplemental health education and improved sanitation needs to be enforced.

13.3 Hepatitis E Virus

Hepatitis E is an infectious disease of the liver etiologically related to HEV. Hepatitis E is the most common cause of massive outbreaks of jaundice in resource-poor countries. In addition, around a third to a half of endemic acute viral hepatitis in such regions is caused by HEV. In 2005, the hepatitis E worldwide disease burden was computed in 9 of the 21 GBD 2010 regions, representing 71% of the world's population. It was estimated that around 20 million cases of incident HEV infection had occurred, with an estimated 3.4 million cases causing around 70,000 deaths and 3000 stillbirths [80]. Pregnant women are highly susceptible to HEV infection with concomitant high death rates. Recently, HEV infections have been reported in many industrialized countries related to unique zoonotic foodborne transmission. Hepatitis E in these countries has particular relevance to organ transplant populations due to an increased risk of progression of acute infection to chronic hepatitis E and cirrhosis, liver failure and death. HEV infection targets body organs other than the liver and causes a number of manifestations and several syndromes affecting the nervous system, including Bell's palsy, encephalitis, brachial neuropathy, peripheral neuropathy and Guillain–Barre syndrome. Transfusion-associated HEV infections are known to occur and can be prevented by donor screening using NAT testing. There has been a significant advance in antiviral treatment of chronic hepatitis E and the availability of recombinant vaccine promises control of the hepatitis E burden in future [81].

13.3.1 Historical Background

Hepatitis E was discovered in Kashmir, India, in 1978 during studies on an epidemic of hepatitis which resulted in 52,000 icteric cases with 1700 deaths. The ingenious field studies leading to its discovery had remarkable human interest stories related to the hard weather, primitive healthcare and remote region of the world [82] (www.drkhuroo.in). The disease had several unique features which now are fundamental to description of the disease [83]. The epidemic was water borne and the epidemic curve was highly compressed lasting for around 7 weeks. No secondary cases were reported following the epidemic [84]. The disease affected young adults and selectively spared children [85, 86]. Pregnant women were highly susceptible to HEV infection with high death rates [87, 88] and there was high propensity for vertical transmission with fetal and perinatal morbidity and mortality [89, 90]. The disease was self-limited and chronic viremia, chronic hepatitis and cirrhosis did not occur following HEV infection [91]. A disease with similar characteristics was described to cause around half of endemic disease in this region [92].

In 1983, Dr. Mikhail Balayan identified virus-like-particles (VLP) from his own stool samples collected during an episode of hepatitis which occurred following his self-ingestion of nine stools collected from Soviet soldiers who had developed an outbreak of non-A hepatitis in Afghanistan from August to September 1981 [93]. The disease was transmitted to several primates and VLP were characterized [94–96]. However, the virus could not be cloned and sequenced due to paucity of VLP in stools. Finally, it was observed that bile samples of infected cynomolgus macaques had large quantities of VLP. Reyes et al. (1990) reported on partial cloning of HEV [97]. Later, a full length genome (7.6 kb) was cloned [98] and an enzyme immunoassay developed for detection of antibodies to HEV [99].

13.3.2 Morphology

HEV has marked heterogeneity and is widely distributed in the animal kingdom [100] (Fig. 13.3). HEV has been classified in the family *Hepeviridae* with two genera: *Orthohepevirus* with four species A–D and *Piscihepevirus* with one isolate infecting Cutthroat trout [101]. *Orthohepevirus A* species comprises seven HEV isolates (genotype HEV-1 to HEV-7). These include two isolates involving human alone (genotypes HEV-1 and HEV-2), two isolates prevalent in pigs, boar, deer and

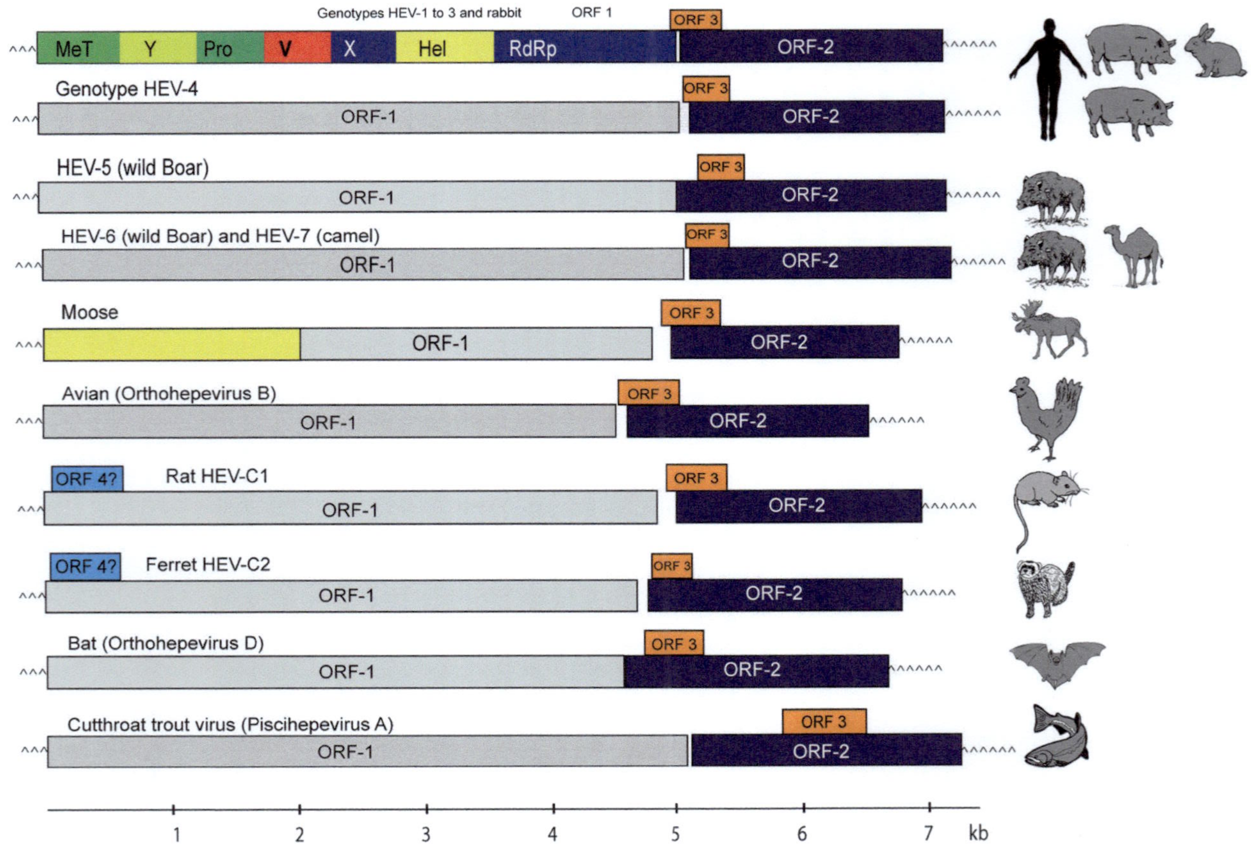

Fig. 13.3 Hepatitis E virus distribution in animal kingdom. The genomic structure, with open reading frames of various isolates of HEV have been drawn. The distribution of each isolate in various animals is shown. Refer to text for detailed classification of hepatitis E viruses (Khuroo MS, Khuroo MS, Khuroo NS. Hepatitis E: discovery, global impact, control and cure. World J Gastroenterol. 2016;22(31):7030–45)

infecting humans (HEV-3 and HEV-4), two isolates infecting wild boar in Japan (HEV-5 and HEV-6) and one isolate identified in dromedaries from Dubai, which also infected a liver transplant patient (HEV-7). *Orthohepevirus B* includes HEVs infecting chicken with three different genotypes (avian HEV-1, avian HEV-2 and avian HEV-3). *Orthohepevirus C* includes HEVs infecting rats (HEV-C1) and ferrets (HEV-C2) and *orthohepevirus D* includes HEV isolate infecting the bat.

HEV is a non-enveloped, spherical, icosahedral particle of 27–30 nm in size. The surface of the virus has spikes [96]. The virus resists acid and mild alkaline media and does not get inactivated by chloroform and ether [102]. The genome of the virus is a single-stranded RNA of ~7.2 kb, with a 7-methylguanine cap (m^7G) at its 5′ end. It is polyadenylated at its 3′ end. HEV RNA replicons express genomic RNA and only one bicistronic 2.2 kb subgenomic RNA. The genome has three partially overlapping ORF (open reading frames). ORF1encodes a non-structural polyprotein (pORF1); ORF2 encodes the major viral capsid protein (pORF2); and ORF3 encodes a small phosphoprotein (pORF3) which is associated with the cytoskeleton and microtubules. This phosphoprotein is also involved in HEV egress from hepatocytes [103] (Fig. 13.4).

13.3.3 Replication

The life cycle of HEV has not been studied in detail. The gut is the primary site of entry of virion into the body and viral replication occurs in the hepatocytes. The virus concentrates and binds on the surface of hepatocytes and is internalized. On entry, the virus uncoats itself and releases the HEV genome. The HEV genome in turn replicates into a negative-sense transcript which becomes the template for full length positive-sense genomic RNA and a subgenomic RNA (2.2 kb). The subgenomic RNA translates into ORF2 and ORF3 proteins. ORF2 protein packages the genomic RNA leading to formation of the virion. ORF3 protein along with lipids envelop the virion which in turn is egressed from the cell [104, 105].

13.3.4 Global Epidemiology

HEV has a global distribution [106] (Fig. 13.5). There are several global epidemiological disease patterns, determined by several factors including socioeconomic status, quality of drinking water, sanitary conditions, prevalent HEV genotypes in humans (Fig. 13.6) and regional occurrence of HEV infection in animals [107].

Hyperendemic zone. Hyperendemic disease presents as massive water borne outbreaks of hepatitis which hit such regions on periodic intervals [108] (Table 13.3). Around half of endemic disease in such regions is caused by hepatitis E. HEV-1 is prevalent in regions of southern, central and southeast Asia, north, east and southern Africa, Latin America, and northwest China (Xinjiang Uyghur) [109, 110]. HEV-2 has been reported to cause hyperendemic disease in central America (Mexico) and west Africa.

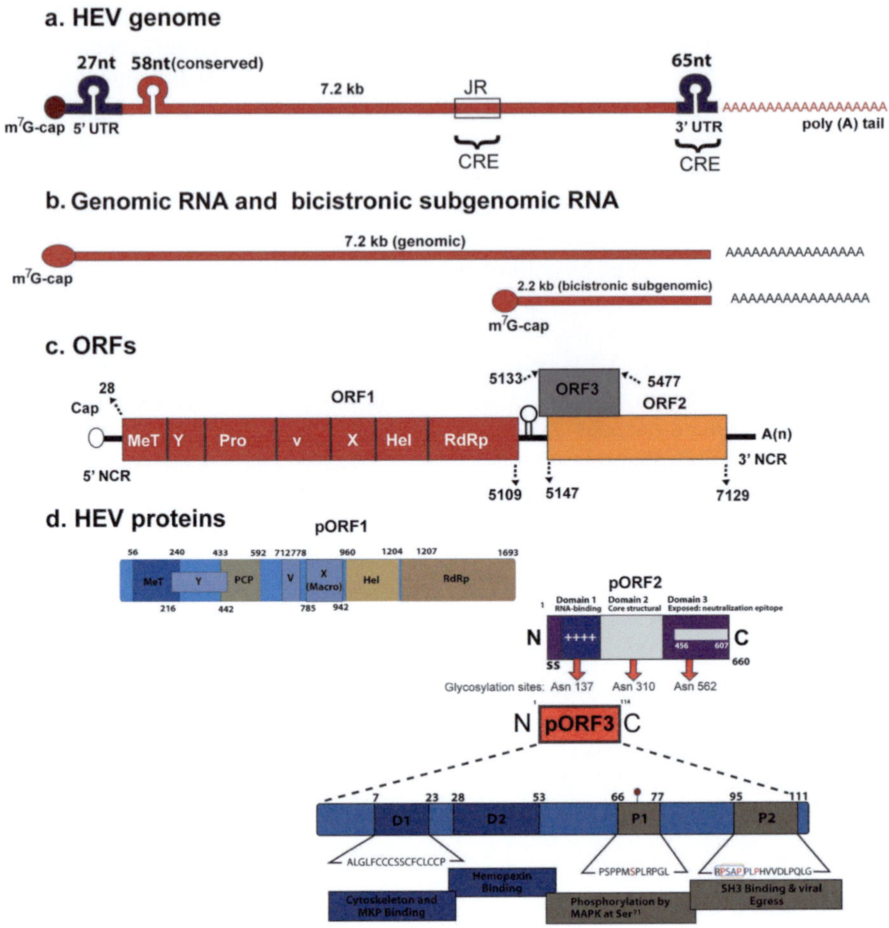

Fig. 13.4 Hepatitis E virus genome and gene expression. The genome ~7.2 kb, with a 7-methylguanine cap (m^7G) at its 5′ end and a poly (A) at its 3′ end. The genome has short UTRs at 5′ end (27 nucleotides) and at 3′ end (65 nucleotides) and a conserved 58-nucleotide stretch near its 5′ end region within ORF1; these elements fold into conserved stem-loop and hairpin structures. HEV RNA replicons express genomic RNA and bicistronic 2.2 kb subgenomic RNA. The genome contains three partially overlapping ORFs-which encode three proteins: pORF1 (693 aa, non-structural protein), pORF2 (660 aa, capsid protein), pORF3 (114 aa, cytoskeleton protein) (Khuroo MS, Khuroo MS. Hepatitis E: an emerging global disease—from discovery towards control and cure. J Viral Hepat. 2016;23(2):68–79) [*UTR* untranslated region, *ORF* open reading frame, *aa* amino acids]

Endemic zone. Hepatitis E in an endemic zone accounts for nearly one-fourth of sporadic acute viral hepatitis. No epidemics of hepatitis E are reported in these regions. This zone includes several countries in the Middle East, southeast Asia, Taiwan and central and eastern China. The socioeconomic status of these regions has shown recent improvement and with access to better sanitation and safer water sources there has been a fall in disease incidence. The disease is etiologically related

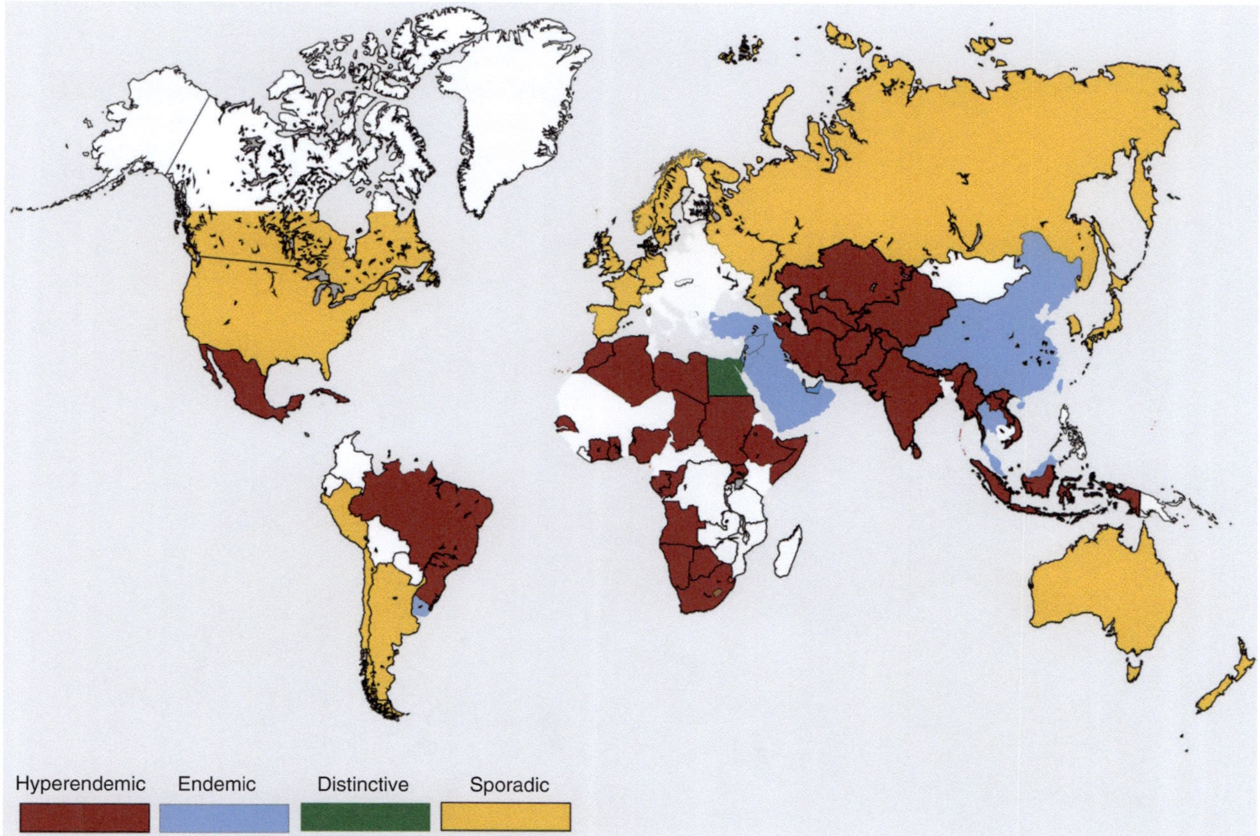

Fig. 13.5 Global distribution of hepatitis E according to patterns of endemicity. The definitions of various zones is given in text (Khuroo MS, Khuroo MS, Khuroo NS. Hepatitis E: Discovery, global impact, control and cure. World J Gastroenterol. 2016;22(31):7030–45)

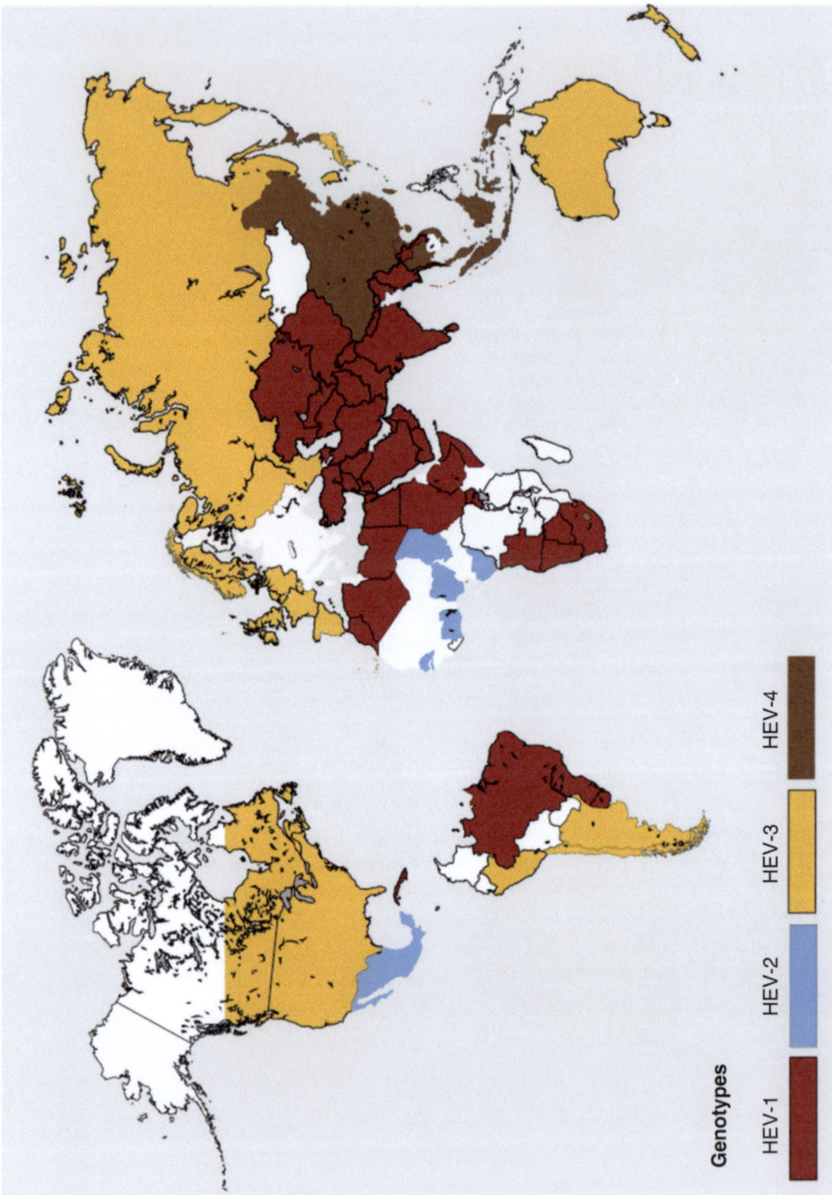

Fig. 13.6 Geographic distribution of HEV genotypes 1–4 (Khuroo MS, Khuroo MS, Khuroo MS, Khuroo NS. Hepatitis E: discovery, global impact, control and cure. World J Gastroenterol. 2016;22(31):7030–45)

Table 13.3 Account of 10 periodic epidemics recorded in Kashmir, India from 1978 to 2013

Place	Year	Population exposed	Icteric cases	Deaths
Gulmarg	1978–79	600,000	20,083	600
Sopore	1979–80	200,000	6000	200
Handwara	1980–81	400,000	11,500	400
Jammu Army Camp	1981–82	845	206	0
Kupwara	1981–82	500,000	15,000	550
Jammu	1983–84	176,833	518	2
Pinglina	1993–94	10,000	156	2
Shopian	1994–95	60,000	1500	17
Maharajpora, Sopore	2007–2008	720	21	2
Pattan, Gulmarg	2012–13	20,000	600	2
Total	**1978–2013**	**1,968,398**	**55,563**	**1775**

Khuroo MS, Khuroo MS, Khuroo NS. Transmission of hepatitis E virus in developing countries. Viruses. 2016;8(9). pii: E253

to HEV-1 in the Middle East, while HEV-4 is the predominant prevalent genotype in Taiwan, China and southeast Asia [111, 112].

Distinctive zone. A distinctive hepatitis E zone is limited to Egypt [113]. Young children in this community are exposed to HEV infection and most of such infections are asymptomatic or subclinical. Adults have a high seroprevalence of anti-HEV, resembling hepatitis A seroepidemiology. Epidemics of hepatitis E do not occur and a small percentage of endemic hepatitis in adults is etiologically related to HEV infection. The phenomenon of higher death rates in pregnant women is not encountered. HEV-1 is a predominant cause of disease with distinct isolates not encountered in endemic zones [114].

Sporadic zone. Autochthonous sporadic HEV infections are present as isolated case reports or small outbreaks of HEV infection in developed countries. These infections are spread through food-borne zoonotic transmission; however, some cases may be transfusion-associated. The sporadic zone includes most of the industrialized regions including North America, western Europe, some countries of South America, Russia, Japan, South Korea, Australia and New Zealand. The disease is generally caused by HEV-3 in all these countries; however, HEV-4 contributes to disease in Japan and a few European countries [115–118].

13.3.5 Mode of Transmission

Waterborne transmission. Hepatitis E in developing countries causes large-scale epidemics, involving hundreds to thousands of cases [95, 108, 119, 120] (Fig. 13.7). The disease is etiologically related to HEV-1 and HEV-2. The majority of these epidemics are caused by gross fecal contamination of public water supplies. There are several settings by which the public water sources become fecally contaminated. These include (1) heavy rains causing flooding and reversal of flow of fecally contaminated river water into the drinking water sources upstream; (2) cracks in water

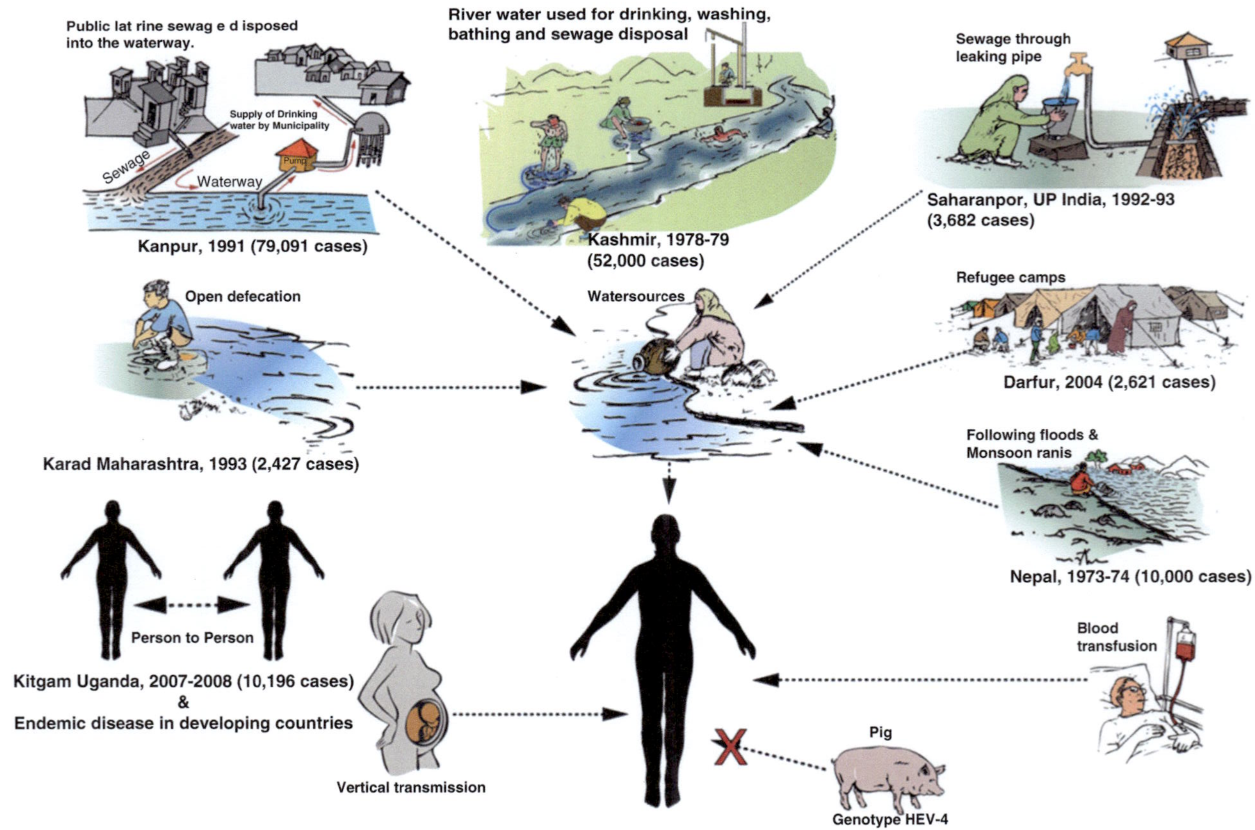

Fig. 13.7 Mode of transmission of HEV genotypes 1 and 2 in developing countries. The setting of contamination of drinking water has been drawn in sketches, with epidemics reported in each case (Khuroo MS, Khuroo MS, Khuroo NS. Transmission of hepatitis E virus in developing countries. Viruses. 2016;8(9). pii: E253)

pipes laid within the sewage channels with consequent fecal contamination; (3) raw sewage contaminating open drinking water sources; and (4) crowded refugee camps with poor sewage disposal and unsafe water supplies. Understanding the circumstances of contamination of public water sources is useful in planning control of epidemics.

Person-to-person transmission. Transmission of hepatitis E from one person to another has been documented during an epidemic of hepatitis E [121]. The epidemic, with 10,196 icteric cases and 160 deaths, occurred in northern Uganda from October 2007 through June 2008 [121]. Risk factors for transmission of HEV infection included attending the funeral, close contact with the index patient and practice of washing hands in the family basin prior to meals. Person-to-person transmission has been suspected in some epidemics of hepatitis E showing multiple epidemic peaks over a protracted period [120].

Endemic hepatitis E disease in developing countries is possibly transmitted from one person to another. This is supported by the observation that around a third of these infections were in close contact with another case of hepatitis E [88, 92]. Also, one-third of the close contacts develop evidence of HEV infection several weeks after onset of disease in the index case [122]. This pointed to a spread of HEV infection from one person to another rather than infections occurring simultaneously. However, intrafamilial spread of sporadic HEV infection was reported to occur infrequently in another study [123].

Zoonotic transmission. Hepatitis E is a zoonotic disease [100]. HEV-3 and HEV-4 are ubiquitous in domestic pigs, wild boar and sicca deer and show cross-transmission of infection from one animal species to another. The common practice of eating the parboiled flesh or liver of game animals can cause autochthonous isolated cases and small outbreaks of hepatitis E [124] (Fig. 13.8). Pig liver in the supermarket and Corsican figatelli sausage in several industrialized countries are infected with live HEV and consumptions of these food items can cause human infections [125–127]. Another risk factor for HEV transmission is vocational exposure of veterinarians and workers on pig farms to pig manure and pig sewage. Several agricultural products like raspberries, strawberries and some vegetables can become contaminated infected from pig slurry used as a pasture fertilizer and can transmit hepatitis E. Similarly, surface run-off of the pig slurry can contaminate surface water, which in turn can contaminate produce like fruits and vegetables. These run-offs can also contaminate coastal waters, fish and shellfish, which are risk factors for spread of hepatitis E. HEV infection is prevalent in several animal species in India including domestic pigs, sheep, goat and buffalo [128, 129]. However, these infections are not transmitted to humans in this population. All human infections in India are caused by HEV-1, while animals are infected with HEV-4 and unrelated to human infections [129].

A distinct isolate named HEV-7 (Camelid HEV) has been found in dromedaries in Dubai and caused chronic hepatitis E in a liver transplant patient. This patient had the habit of consuming camel meat and milk [130]. Recently, evidence of past hepatitis E infection has been documented in around half of dromedaries from several countries [131]. Around 2% of such animals were either viremic or showed

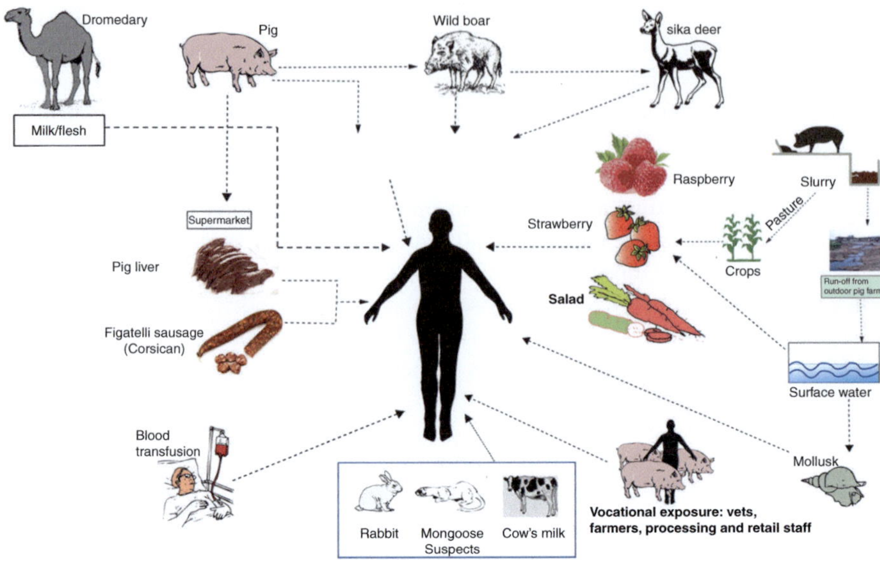

Fig. 13.8 Zoonotic transmission of HEV genotype 3 and 4 in developed and many developing countries (Khuroo MS, Khuroo MS, Khuroo NS. Transmission of hepatitis E virus in developing countries. Viruses. 2016;8(9). pii: E253)

shedding of virus in stools. Thus, camel meat and/or milk is a potential source of transmission of camelid HEV-7 in these countries. The epidemiology of hepatitis E in China has been complex and in continuous transformation [132, 133]. Hepatitis E was hyperendemic all over China in the past. However, over the years, HEV-4 has been introduced in northeast China and at present is the dominant genotype in this community.

Parenteral transmission. Transfusion-associated hepatitis E caused by HEV-1 was documented in Kashmir in 1995 [134]. Subsequent to this, transfusion-associated HEV infections were reported from several countries including Japan and the United Kingdom [135–137]. Recently, healthy donors from several industrialized countries were found to be viremic, lasting for up to 45 days [138–141]. Extrapolating data from such studies, the number of transfusion-associated HEV infections per year amounted to 80,000–100,000 in England and 1600–5900 in Germany. Blood and blood products are often required in pregnant women, patients with chronic liver disease, solid organ transplant patients, HIV+ patients, and patients with hematological neoplasm. HEV infections are known to cause either severe disease or run a complicated protracted course in these clinical conditions. In view of the above, there is urgent need to conduct donor screening programs for HEV in many industrialized countries using NAT testing.

Vertical transmission. Vertical transmission from HEV-infected mother to fetus and neonates is known to occur frequently [89]. Intrauterine fetal and neonatal HEV infections cause significant perinatal morbidity and mortality [90]. Occurrence and severity of fetal HEV infections correlate with severity of liver disease in the mother

[142]. HEV is known to replicate in many body tissues including the placenta, and placental infections correlate with fetal and maternal mortality [143]. In view of the above data, it has been postulated that severe intrauterine infections may produce toxins which overwhelm maternal circulation and cause severe liver disease and systemic disease.

Transmission of HEV through milk. Colostrum from infected mothers is often positive for HEV RNA [144]. As viral titers are low, breastfeeding is an unlikely route of transmission for neonatal HEV infections. Camelid HEV-7 infection can be transmitted from camel milk as reported in a liver transplant patient from Dubai [145]. Recently, HEV-4 in high titers was detected in cow's milk in a mixed farm from Dali, Yunnan, China. Raw and pasteurized milk samples were infectious to rhesus monkeys. In contrast, a short spell of boiling inactivated the virus and did not transmit the disease to rhesus monkeys [146]. These findings point to cow's milk as a potential source of transmission of hepatitis E in endemic regions of the World.

Nosocomial transmission. Healthcare workers are not particularly at high risk for contracting HEV infections [147]. However, HEV is known to spread in hemodialysis units and small outbreaks have been reported in inpatient populations and healthcare workers [148–150].

Sexual transmission. Sexual contact is not a high risk for spread of HEV infection. High seroprevalence of IgG antibodies in men who have sex with men and in HIV-infected patients has been reported [151, 152].

13.3.6 Clinical Manifestations

The clinical manifestations of acute hepatitis E resemble those of acute hepatitis A, including an incubation period (15–45 days), prodromal symptoms (1–7 days), icteric period (2–6 weeks) and convalescence (up to 6 weeks) [84, 153]. HEV infection can present from subclinical infection to typical acute viral hepatitis, to acute liver failure [50, 85, 154]. Most of the patients with epidemic or endemic hepatitis E in developing countries are young adults (15–45 years) (Table 13.4). Cholestatic features occur in around 20% of patients and are more pronounced [84]. Disease runs a severe clinical course in pregnant women, with maternal mortality of over 44.4% in the third trimester [87, 88]. The clinical profile of acute liver failure during pregnancy is dramatic with severe encephalopathy, gastrointestinal bleeding, cerebral edema and cerebellar coning developing in a matter of a few days. HEV infections can superinfect patients with well-compensated liver cirrhosis and culminate in rapid hepatic decompensation and death [155–158]. HEV superinfection occurs in approximately 21% of cirrhotic patients in India, with a rapid worsening in liver synthetic function, causing rapidly progressive liver failure and culminating in 30-day mortality of 34%. Almost all cases of hepatitis E in developing countries are self-limiting unless patients are immune suppressed. However, there may be relapse of clinical and biochemical disease activity in an occasional patient and a small percentage of patients present with prolonged cholestasis as seen in hepatitis A [159].

Table 13.4 Human hepatitis E virus infections: genotypes and clinical-epidemiological characteristics

HEV genotype	Disease pattern	Geographical distribution	Mode of transmission	Age distribution	Severe disease in pregnancy	Chronicity	Disease severity	Death rate (%)
1	Hyperendemic (epidemic, endemic)	Asia, Africa	Water borne Person-to-person	Young adults (21–30 years)	Yes	No	Modest	4% α
	Endemic	Africa	Person-to-person µ	Young adults (21–30 years)	Yes	No	Modest	4% α
	Distinctive	Egypt	Person-to-person µ	Children (<10 years)	No	No	Low	Negligible
2	Hyperendemic (epidemic, endemic)	Central America, Africa	Water borne	Young adults (21–30 years)	Yes	No	Modest	4% α
3	Sporadic	Asia, America, Europe, Oceania	Food borne zoonotic Transfusion-associated	Older males (35–86 years)	No	Yes (organ transplant patients)	High	8% ß
4	Sporadic, small outbreaks	Asia	Food borne zoonotic Transfusion-associated	Older males (35–86 years)	No	No	Very high	11% ß
7	Sporadic	UAE	Camel flesh and milk	Elderly	No	Yes (liver transplant patient)	–	–

µ—Data on person-to-person transmission of HEV infections in endemic areas are conflicting; α—deaths reported mostly in pregnant women; ß—mortality very high in patients with chronic liver disease, approaching 70%

Hepatitis E in industrialized countries is seen as an autochthonous infection caused by HEV-3 and HEV-4 and mostly related to zoonotic food-borne transmission or following blood transfusion [124, 135, 136, 160–162]. Disease occurs in higher age groups and has more severe clinical manifestations than disease in endemic zones. Hepatic and extrahepatic complications are reported in around 15% of such patients and acute liver failure occurs in 8–11% of patients. HEV superinfection in chronic alcoholic patients with cirrhosis in these countries leads to rapid hepatic decompensation and high mortality. Hepatitis E in such regions does not cause high mortality in pregnant women.

Most HEV infections run a self-limiting course with eventual clinical, biochemical and virologic recovery. However, a subset of immunocompromised patients with solid-organ transplant, HIV and hematological neoplasm infected with HEV-3 can develop chronic hepatitis E and cirrhosis [160, 163, 164]. The diagnostic criteria of chronic hepatitis E include persistent viremia using PCR in blood and stool and modest liver abnormalities lasting beyond 3 months. Acute HEV disease usually is asymptomatic with isolated liver enzyme abnormality resembling drug toxicity. However, a subgroup of patients run a rapid downhill course with progressive liver fibrosis and cirrhosis and culminating in end-stage liver disease in a 2 to 3-year period. Use of tacrolimus, low platelets and low CD4s in HIV-infected patients are associated with high risk for development of liver fibrosis [165].

Hepatitis E can present with a wide range of extrahepatic manifestations, including cryoglobulinemia with skin rashes, glomerulonephritis, autoimmune thyroiditis, thrombocytopenia, aplastic anemia, myositis and acute pancreatitis [166–171]. A small percentage of infected patients present with a broad group of manifestations involving the nervous system. These include Guillain–Barre syndrome, brachial neuropathy, peripheral neuropathy, and Bell's palsy [166, 172–175]. Extrahepatic hepatitis E disease has a global distribution, is independent of genotype, and has variable clinical outcome. The pathogenesis of HEV-related manifestations of the nervous system may be multifactorial. HEV may trigger immune reactions and induce antiganglioside antibodies through molecular mimicry [176]. Also, HEV replicates in many body tissues and shows significant neurotropism which may cause disease.

13.3.7 Laboratory Manifestations and Diagnosis

Laboratory abnormalities in acute hepatitis E resemble those seen in acute hepatitis caused by other hepatitis viruses and have been described above (HAV). Diagnosis of acute hepatitis E is primarily based on detection of IgM antibody to HEV [177]. The test becomes positive within 2 weeks of infection and stays detectable for up to 5 months. There have been major issues concerning the sensitivity and specificity of this assay. The test results may vary based on HEV genotype in the sample tested. The test shows especially poor performance in immunocompromised patients. Several related viral infections may cross-react in such a test system [178]. Two assays namely Wantai HEV-IgM ELISA based on improved mu-capture (Beijing

Wantai Biological Pharmacy) and Assure HEV IgM rapid chromatographic test (Genelabs Diagnostics) have shown improved performance and diagnostic positivity of over 90% in immunocompetent patients. [179–182]. In view of the above, IgM antibody to HEV is the recommended diagnostic test for HEV infection in an immunocompetent host. IgG antibody to HEV is useful for seroprevalence studies. Antibody levels have also been employed to assess protective antibody levels during vaccine trials. IgG anti-HEV levels of 2.5 WHO units and above are believed to be protective [170, 183]. HEV RNA detection in serum and stools have a role in diagnosing HEV infections in immunocompromised patients who often show negative IgM anti-HEV tests [184, 185]. The test is also useful in the diagnosis of chronic HEV-3 infection. Such patients continue to be viremic and show fecal viral shedding beyond 3 months. Serial HEV RNA testing is essential to document response to antiviral drug therapy [183, 186, 187]. Another NAT test, the loop-mediated isothermal amplification (LAMP) assay is a one-step, single-tube isothermal amplification of HEV RNA. The assay can be performed quickly and needs no special equipment and is recommended for resource limited areas [188] (Table 13.5).

13.3.8 Treatment

Patients with acute hepatitis E need supportive care as in acute hepatitis A (see above). HEV infection in pregnant women requires a careful combined approach between the hepatologist and the obstetrician [88]. Such patients are at high risk of acute liver failure. Patients with impending signs of acute liver failure need intensive care management. Termination of pregnancy and its beneficial effects on liver disease in the mother is debatable [142]. Vertical HEV transmission to fetus causes

Table 13.5 Diagnosis of hepatitis E virus infection

Test	Method	Uses	Comments
IgM anti-HEV	ELISA ICT (POCT)	Acute infection	Assays vary in performance, issue of genotype applicability, poor performance in immune disorders, cross-reactive with other viral infections
IgG anti-HEV	ELISA ICT (POCT)	Seroprevalence Acute infection Natural protection Vaccine efficacy	Assays vary in performance
HEV RNA	NAT	Acute infection Confirm chronicity Anti-viral response Donor screening	Viremia short-lasting, in-house assays vary in performance, advantage immune disorders
HEV antigen	EIA	Acute infection	81% concordance with HEV RNA

Khuroo MS, Khuroo MS. Hepatitis E: an emerging global disease—from discovery towards control and cure. J Viral Hepat. 2016;23(2):68–79

ICT immunochromatographic test, *POCT* point of care test, *NAT* nucleic acid test, *EIA* enzyme immunoassay

Table 13.6 Effect of drugs on HEV replication and their use and impact on immunosuppressant therapy during chronic HEV infection in solid organ transplant patients

Class	Drug	Effect on HEV replication	Clinical use
Calcineurin inhibitors	Cyclosporine, tacrolimus	Stimulates HEV replication with increase in HEV load and promotes HEV persistence	Reduce dose
mTOR inhibitors	Rapamycin, everolimus	Stimulates HEV replication with increase in HEV load	Reduce dose
Antimetabolite immunosuppressant	Mycophenolate mofetil	Inhibits HEV replication and helps HEV clearance	Continue the drug
Guanosine analog	Ribavirin	Inhibits HEV replication and causes HEV clearance	Primary drug for therapy
Cytokines	PEGylated interferon α	Inhibits HEV replication and causes HEV clearance	Indicated if ribavirin therapy fails
Nucleotide analog	Sofosbuvir	Inhibits HEV replication in vitro	Unclear, clinical trials indicated

Khuroo MS, Khuroo MS, Khuroo NS. Hepatitis E: discovery, global impact, control and cure. World J Gastroenterol. 2016;22(31):7030–45

intrauterine deaths and high perinatal morbidity and mortality [89, 90]. Neonates born to such mothers need neonatal intensive care management.

HEV superinfection in compensated chronic liver disease presents as rapid acute on chronic hepatic decompensation. Patients need active management of complications of liver failure, namely ascites, encephalopathy, variceal bleed and renal failure. Such patients may benefit from ribavirin therapy against HEV infection [189].

Immunosuppressed patients with chronic hepatitis E are successfully managed with antiviral therapy and selective reduction in immunosuppressant therapy (Table 13.6). Ribavirin in a dose of 600 mg per day is the drug of choice and clears the virus within a few weeks of therapy; most such patients maintain a sustained virologic response [183]. Calcineurin inhibitors and mTOR inhibitors enhance replication of HEV and may lead to incremental increases in viral levels in blood and stool and persistence of HEV RNA [190]. These immunosuppressants need to be reduced in dose for virus clearance. In contrast, mycophenolic acid inhibits HEV RNA replication and promotes clearance of the virus. Recently, sofosbuvir has been shown to inhibit HEV replication and may be useful in selected patients [191].

13.3.9 Global Control

Control of hepatitis E in developing countries is a challenging task and requires clean drinking water, good sanitation, and proper personal hygiene [192]. Western travelers to such regions should avoid drinking contaminated water or beverages and avoid eating uncooked shellfish [193]. Patients with solid organ transplant need to eat properly-cooked pork and deer meat. Patients should abstain from eating raw or undercooked pork liver from supermarkets. Intake of Corsican figatelli sausage is a high risk for HEV infection and should be avoided [194]. Development of a hepatitis E vaccine has been a major breakthrough in control of hepatitis E [195]. The Chinese vaccine HEV-239 has been derived from a HEV-1 Chinese isolate. It is a particulate vaccine, consists of truncated ORF2 protein (368–606 amino acids) and has been expressed in *Escherichia coli*. The vaccine induces a healthy T-cell dependent immune response. HEV-239 marketed as Hecolin in China is administered as 30 μg doses at 0, 1 and 6 months. The vaccine is highly immunogenic and efficacious [196, 197]. HEV-239 has been shown to give cross protective efficacy against HEV-4. It is imperative that hepatitis E vaccine be made available in other countries for trials and use [198]. To do so, we need to extend vaccine safety data in the pediatric age group, the elderly and pregnant women. Post-marketing phase IV studies need to be done once the vaccine is available globally. Studies of the cost effectiveness of the vaccine program for prevention of hepatitis E need to be done [170].

13.4 Summary

Viral hepatitis is a global disease that causes approximately 1.45 million deaths per year, of which hepatitis A contributes to over 35,000 deaths and hepatitis E to approximately 70,000 deaths and 3000 stillbirths. Hepatitis A has global distribution, with endemicity proportional to socioeconomic conditions and clinical disease correlating with age of occurrence of infection. Paradoxically, of late, clinical disease is being encountered more often in the adult population in developing countries with recent improvement in sanitary conditions and safer water supplies. Epidemics of hepatitis A continue to occur in industrialized countries, including the U.S., due of consumption of polluted fruits imported from developing countries. Hepatitis A vaccine has a major role to play in global control of hepatitis A.

Hepatitis E is being recognized as a disease of reemerging importance. Hepatitis E viruses have several animal reservoirs with complex ecology and genetic heterogeneity. Originally reported as a major health problem in resource-poor countries, zoonotic hepatitis E is now recognized as an important clinical problem in the industrialized world. Hepatitis E virus can be transmitted through blood and blood component transfusions, and donor screening is being done in many countries. Recently, major strides have been made in the management of the disease. Furthermore, an effective vaccine is available that promises better control of the hepatitis E burden.

Acknowledgments The work was supported by "Dr. Khuroo's Medical Trust" a non-profit organization which supports academic activities, disseminates medical education and helps poor patients for medical treatment.

Disclosure: All authors have nothing to disclose.

Summary Table of Landmark Literature

Publication	Topic/study design	Summary	Main limitations
Berg MG, et al. Discovery of a novel human pegivirus in blood associated with hepatitis C virus co-infection. PLoS Pathog. 2015;11(12):e1005325 [6]	Metagenomic next-generation sequencing and the sequence-based ultra-rapid pathogen identification bioinformatics pipeline were used for pathogen detection in an HCV-infected patient who died from sepsis and multi-organ failure. Serological assays were then used to screen for the newly identified pathogen human pegivirus 2 in 2440 plasma samples from patients infected with HIV, HBV, or HCV and volunteer blood donors testing negative for all of those	A new member of the family Flaviviridae, a second human pegivirus, was identified: human pegivirus 2 (HPgV-2) Phylogenetic, PCR, and serological analyses confirmed that HPgV-2 is a novel blood-borne virus infectious to humans. HPgV-2 viremia was found in 1.1% of 742 HCV-infected individuals; none of the 1458 non-HCV infected samples were HPgV-2 RNA positive	Samples all originated from the U.S.; ongoing studies will be needed to determine global prevalence of HPgV-2 and the full extent of its sequence diversity
Feinstone SM, et al. Hepatitis A: detection by immune electron microscopy of a viruslike antigen associated with acute illness. Science. 1973;182(4116):106–8 [16]	Stool specimens from patients with hepatitis A were examined for virus-like antigens using immune electron microscopy	A virus-like particle serologically associated with hepatitis A infection was detected. A serologic technique was developed with which antibody to hepatitis A can be detected, providing for the first time a means of diagnosing and studying hepatitis A	
Khuroo MS. Study of an epidemic of non-A, non-B hepatitis. Possibility of another human hepatitis virus distinct from post-transfusion non-A, non-B type. Am J Med. 1980;68(6):818–24 [84]	A team survey of every household in the Baramulla district of Kashmir, India was carried out to assess a hepatitis epidemic using a questionnaire and physical examination to look for jaundice. Blood samples were collected from those with suspected hepatitis and their contacts with serum assays carried out to test for hepatitis A and B	Among 16,620 inhabitants, 275 viral hepatitis cases were found (1.65% incidence). Tests of samples from the drinking water source (a local stream) found a coliform reaction in all samples, suggesting fecal contamination and a waterborne source of the hepatitis epidemic. This was the important first large study that identified the virus later known as hepatitis E	

Publication	Topic/study design	Summary	Main limitations
Khuroo MS et al. Hepatitis E: discovery, global impact, control and cure. World J Gastroenterol. 2016;22(31):7030–45 [81]	This is a recent major review of hepatitis E that covers its discovery, taxonomy and classification, genetic organization, replication, animal reservoirs, global distribution, mode of transmission, diagnosis, vaccine, and treatment	This review gives updates on all aspects of hepatitis E, with important information on the contrasting epidemiological and disease patterns in developing and industrialized countries, approaches to control in developing countries, the best assays for diagnosis, treatment requirements, and the risks associated with hepatitis E in the immunocompromised and pregnant women	

References

1. Zuckerman AJ. Hepatitis viruses. In: Baron S, editor. Medical microbiology. 4th ed. Galveston, TX: University of Texas Medical Branch at Galveston; 1996. p. 1–169.
2. Krugman S. The Gordon Wilson Lecture. The ABC's of viral hepatitis. Trans Am Clin Climatol Assoc. 1992;103:145–56.
3. Heathcote E, Feld J. Hepatitis caused by other viruses. In: Feldman M, Friedman LS, Brandt LJ, editors. Sleisinger & Fordtran's gastrointestinal and liver disease. 8th ed. Philadelphia, PA: Saunders; 2006. p. 1719–29.
4. Khuroo MS. Discovery of hepatitis G virus. Ann Saudi Med. 1997;17(2):209–16.
5. Kapoor A, Kumar A, Simmonds P, Bhuva N, Singh Chauhan L, Lee B, et al. Virome analysis of transfusion recipients reveals a novel human virus that shares genomic features with hepaciviruses and pegiviruses. mBio. 2015;6(5):e01466-15.
6. Berg MG, Lee D, Coller K, Frankel M, Aronsohn A, Cheng K, et al. Discovery of a novel human pegivirus in blood associated with hepatitis C virus co-Infection. PLoS Pathog. 2015;11(12):e1005325.
7. Wood NJ. Viral hepatitis: progress and promise. Nat Rev Gastroenterol Hepatol. 2011;8(5):239.
8. Stanaway JD, Flaxman AD, Naghavi M, Fitzmaurice C, Vos T; Abubakar I; Abu-Raddad LJ, et al. The global burden of viral hepatitis from 1990 to 2013: findings from the Global Burden of Disease Study 2013. Lancet. 2016;388:1081–8.
9. WHO. Combating hepatitis B and C to reach elimination by 2030. Advocacy brief. Switzerland, May 2016. p. 1–20. www.who.int/hepatitis/publications.
10. Tahaei SM, Mohebbi SR, Zali MR. Enteric hepatitis viruses. Gastroenterol Hepatol Bed Bench. 2012;5(1):7–15.
11. Lemon SN. Type A viral hepatitis: epidemiology, diagnosis and prevention. Clin Chem. 1997;43(8(B)):1494–9.
12. Purcell RH. The discovery of the hepatitis viruses. Gastroenterology. 1993;104(4):955–63.
13. MacCallum FO. Homologous serum jaundice. Lancet. 1947;250(6480):691–2.
14. Krugman S, Giles JP, Hammond J. Infectious hepatitis. Evidence for two distinctive clinical, epidemiological, and immunological types of infection. JAMA. 1967;200(5):365–73.

15. Dienstag JL, Purcell RH. Recent advances in the identification of hepatitis viruses. Postgrad Med J. 1977;53(621):364–73.
16. Feinstone SM, Kapikian AZ, Purcell RH. Hepatitis A: detection by immune electron microscopy of a viruslike antigen associated with acute illness. Science. 1973;182(4116):1026–8.
17. Provost PJ, Wolanski BS, Miller WJ, Ittensohn OL, McAleer WJ, Hilleman MR. Physical, chemical and morphologic dimensions of human hepatitis A virus strain CR326 (38578). Proc Soc Exp Biol Med. 1975;148(2):532–9.
18. Martin A, Lemon SM. Hepatitis A virus: from discovery to vaccines. Hepatology. 2006;43(2 Suppl 1):S164–72.
19. Purcell RH. Hepatitis viruses: changing patterns of human disease. Proc Natl Acad Sci U S A. 1994;91(7):2401–6.
20. Nainan OV, Xia G, Vaughan G, Margolis HS. Diagnosis of hepatitis a virus infection: a molecular approach. Clin Microbiol Rev. 2006;19(1):63–79.
21. Siegl G. Replication of hepatitis A virus and processing of proteins. Vaccine. 1992;10(Suppl 1):S32–5.
22. Gust ID. Epidemiological patterns of hepatitis A in different parts of the world. Vaccine. 1992;10(Suppl 1):S56–8.
23. Jacobsen KH, Wiersma ST. Hepatitis A virus seroprevalence by age and world region, 1990 and 2005. Vaccine. 2010;28(41):6653–7.
24. WHO. The global prevalence of hepatitis A virus infection and susceptibility: a systematic review. Gęneva: World Health Organization, Department of Immunization, Vaccines and Biologicals; 2009.
25. WHO. WHO position papers on HAV vaccines, June 2012. Weekly Epidemiological Record; 2012.
26. Kim YJ, Lee HS. Increasing incidence of hepatitis A in Korean adults. Intervirology. 2010;53(1):10–4.
27. Munne MS, Vladimirsky S, Moreiro R, Ciocca M, Cuarterolo M, Otegui L, et al. Molecular characterization of hepatitis A virus in children with fulminant hepatic failure in Argentina. Liver Int. 2008;28(1):47–53.
28. Santos DC, Martinho JM, Pacheco-Moreira LF, Araujo CC, Oliveira BC, Lago BV, et al. Fulminant hepatitis failure in adults and children from a Public Hospital in Rio de Janeiro, Brazil. Braz J Infect Dis. 2009;13(5):323–9.
29. Collier MG, Khudyakov YE, Selvage D, Adams-Cameron M, Epson E, Cronquist A, et al. Outbreak of hepatitis A in the USA associated with frozen pomegranate arils imported from Turkey: an epidemiological case study. Lancet Infect Dis. 2014;14(10):976–81.
30. Wheeler C, Vogt TM, Armstrong GL, Vaughan G, Weltman A, Nainan OV, et al. An outbreak of hepatitis A associated with green onions. N Engl J Med. 2005;353(9):890–7.
31. Centers for Disease C, Prevention. Hepatitis A outbreak associated with green onions at a restaurant—Monaca, Pennsylvania, 2003. MMWR Morb Mortal Wkly Rep. 2003;52(47):1155–7.
32. Centers for Disease C, Prevention. Foodborne transmission of hepatitis A—Massachusetts, 2001. MMWR Morb Mortal Wkly Rep. 2003;52(24):565–7.
33. Mohd Hanafiah K, Jacobsen KH, Wiersma ST. Challenges to mapping the health risk of hepatitis A virus infection. Int J Health Geogr. 2011;10:57.
34. Fiore AE. Hepatitis A transmitted by food. Clin Infect Dis. 2004;38(5):705–15.
35. Sanchez G. Processing strategies to inactivate hepatitis A virus in food products: a critical review. Compr Rev Food Sci Food Saf. 2015;14(6):771–84.
36. Halliday ML, Kang LY, Zhou TK, Hu MD, Pan QC, Fu TY, et al. An epidemic of hepatitis A attributable to the ingestion of raw clams in Shanghai, China. J Infect Dis. 1991;164(5):852–9.
37. Hansman GS, Oka T, Li TC, Nishio O, Noda M, Takeda N. Detection of human enteric viruses in Japanese clams. J Food Prot. 2008;71(8):1689–95.
38. Amri I, Hmaied F, Loisy F, Lebeau B, Barkallah I, Saidi M, et al. [Hepatitis A virus detection in shellfish from Tunisia by reverse transcription-nested PCR—investigation of a correlation between viral and bacterial contamination]. Pathol Biol (Paris). 2011;59(4):217–21.

39. Cooksley WG. What did we learn from the Shanghai hepatitis A epidemic? J Viral Hepat. 2000;7(Suppl 1):1–3.
40. Chironna M, Lopalco P, Prato R, Germinario C, Barbuti S, Quarto M. Outbreak of infection with hepatitis A virus (HAV) associated with a foodhandler and confirmed by sequence analysis reveals a new HAV genotype IB variant. J Clin Microbiol. 2004;42(6):2825–8.
41. Behrens RH, Collins M, Botto B, Heptonstall J. Risk for British travellers of acquiring hepatitis A. BMJ. 1995;311(6998):193.
42. Hollinger FB, Khan NC, Oefinger PE, Yawn DH, Schmulen AC, Dreesman GR, et al. Posttransfusion hepatitis type A. JAMA. 1983;250(17):2313–7.
43. O'Donovan D, Cooke RP, Joce R, Eastbury A, Waite J, Stene-Johansen K. An outbreak of hepatitis A amongst injecting drug users. Epidemiol Infect. 2001;127(3):469–73.
44. Corey L, Holmes KK. Sexual transmission of hepatitis A in homosexual men: incidence and mechanism. N Engl J Med. 1980;302(8):435–8.
45. Lankarani KB, Mahmoodi M, Honarvar B, Nematollahi P, Zamiri N, Ghaffarpasand F. Determinants of poor outcome in patients with hepatitis A infection: a four-year retrospective study in Shiraz, Southern Iran. Arch Virol. 2014;159(8):1901–7.
46. Ciocca M. Clinical course and complications of hepatitis A infection. Vaccine. 2000;18(Suppl 1):S71–S4.
47. Gordon SC, Reddy KR, Schiff L, Schiff ER. Prolonged intrahepatic cholestasis secondary to acute hepatitis A. Ann Intern Med. 1984;101(5):635–7.
48. Glikson M, Galun E, Oren R, Tur-Kaspa R, Shouval D. Relapsing hepatitis A. Review of 14 cases and literature survey. Medicine (Baltimore). 1992;71(1):14–23.
49. Sjogren MH, Tanno H, Fay O, Sileoni S, Cohen BD, Burke DS, et al. Hepatitis A virus in stool during clinical relapse. Ann Intern Med. 1987;106(2):221–6.
50. Khuroo MS. Acute liver failure in India. Hepatology. 1997;26(1):244–6.
51. Brown GR, Persley K. Hepatitis A epidemic in the elderly. South Med J. 2002;95(8):826–33.
52. Vento S, Garofano T, Renzini C, Cainelli F, Casali F, Ghironzi G, et al. Fulminant hepatitis associated with hepatitis A virus superinfection in patients with chronic hepatitis C. N Engl J Med. 1998;338(5):286–90.
53. Willner IR, Uhl MD, Howard SC, Williams EQ, Riely CA, Waters B. Serious hepatitis A: an analysis of patients hospitalized during an urban epidemic in the United States. Ann Intern Med. 1998;128(2):111–4.
54. Ilan Y, Hillman M, Oren R, Zlotogorski A, Shouval D. Vasculitis and cryoglobulinemia associated with persisting cholestatic hepatitis A virus infection. Am J Gastroenterol. 1990;85(5):586–7.
55. Tagle Arrospide M, Leon Barua R. [Viral hepatitis A as a triggering agent of autoimmune hepatitis report of a case and review of literature]. Rev Gastroenterol Peru. 2003;23(2):134–7.
56. Dienstag JL. Acute viral hepatitis. In: Fauci AS, Braunwald E, Kasper DL, Hauser SL, Longo DL, Jameson JL, Loscalzo JL, editors. Harrison's principles of internal medicine. 17th ed. New York, NY: McGraw-Hill Companies Inc.; 2008. p. 1932–49.
57. Kao HW, Ashcavai M, Redeker AG. The persistence of hepatitis A IgM antibody after acute clinical hepatitis A. Hepatology. 1984;4(5):933–6.
58. Liaw YF, Yang CY, Chu CM, Huang MJ. Appearance and persistence of hepatitis A IgM antibody in acute clinical hepatitis A observed in an outbreak. Infection. 1986;14(4):156–8.
59. Hoofnagle JH, Di Bisceglie AM. Serologic diagnosis of acute and chronic viral hepatitis. Semin Liver Dis. 1991;11(2):73–83.
60. Yotsuyanagi H, Iino S, Koike K, Yasuda K, Hino K, Kurokawa K. Duration of viremia in human hepatitis A viral infection as determined by polymerase chain reaction. J Med Virol. 1993;40(1):35–8.
61. Coppola N, Genovese D, Pisaturo M, Taffon S, Argentini C, Pasquale G, et al. Acute hepatitis with severe cholestasis and prolonged clinical course due to hepatitis A virus Ia and Ib coinfection. Clin Infect Dis. 2007;44(9):e73–7.
62. William R. Classification, etiology and considerations of outcome in acute liver failure. Semin Liver Dis. 1996;16:343.

63. Fiore A, Baxter LC, Bell BP, Hershow R, Passaro D, Twiddy S, et al. Hepatitis A 2004 vaccination in children: methods and findings of a survey in two states. Am J Prev Med. 2007;33(4):346–52.
64. Advisory Committee on Immunization P, Fiore AE, Wasley A, Bell BP. Prevention of hepatitis A through active or passive immunization: recommendations of the Advisory Committee on Immunization Practices (ACIP). MMWR Recomm Rep. 2006;55(RR-7):1–23.
65. Prevention of hepatitis A through active or passive immunization: recommendations of the Advisory Committee on Immunization Practices (ACIP). MMWR Recomm Rep. 1996;45(RR-15):1–30.
66. Abarca K, Ibanez I, Perret C, Vial P, Zinsou JA. Immunogenicity, safety, and interchangeability of two inactivated hepatitis A vaccines in Chilean children. Int J Infect Dis. 2008;12(3):270–7.
67. Demicheli V, Tiberti D. The effectiveness and safety of hepatitis A vaccine: a systematic review. Vaccine. 2003;21(19–20):2242–5.
68. Aristegui J, Morales JL, Dal-Re R, Gonzalez A, Gallego MS, Garrote E. Safety and immunogenicity of an inactivated hepatitis A vaccine in children 2 to 5 years old. Infection. 1995;23(5):334–8.
69. Arnal JM, Frisas O, Garuz R, Antonanzas F. Cost effectiveness of hepatitis A virus immunisation in Spain. Pharmacoeconomics. 1997;12(3):361–73.
70. Wolfe MS. Hepatitis A and the American traveler. J Infect Dis. 1995;171(Suppl 1):S29–32.
71. Blanco Fernandez MD, Torres C, Riviello-Lopez G, Poma HR, Rajal VB, Nates S, et al. Analysis of the circulation of hepatitis A virus in Argentina since vaccine introduction. Clin Microbiol Infect. 2012;18(12):E548–51.
72. Briem H, Safary A. Immunogenicity and safety in adults of hepatitis A virus vaccine administered as a single dose with a booster 6 months later. J Med Virol. 1994;44(4):443–5.
73. Van Damme P, Mathei C, Thoelen S, Meheus A, Safary A, Andre FE. Single dose inactivated hepatitis A vaccine: rationale and clinical assessment of the safety and immunogenicity. J Med Virol. 1994;44(4):435–41.
74. Mao JS, Chai SA, Xie RY, Chen NL, Jiang Q, Zhu XZ, et al. Further evaluation of the safety and protective efficacy of live attenuated hepatitis A vaccine (H2-strain) in humans. Vaccine. 1997;15(9):944–7.
75. Belmaker I, Dukhan L, Yosef Y, Leventhal A, Dagan R. Elimination of hepatitis a infection outbreaks in day care and school settings in southern Israel after introduction of the national universal toddler hepatitis a immunization program. Pediatr Infect Dis J. 2007;26(1):36–40.
76. Fangcheng Z, Xuanyi W, Mingding C, Liming J, Jie W, Qi J, et al. Era of vaccination heralds a decline in incidence of hepatitis A in high-risk groups in China. Hepat Mon. 2012;12(2):100–5.
77. Dagan R, Leventhal A, Anis E, Slater P, Ashur Y, Shouval D. Incidence of hepatitis A in Israel following universal immunization of toddlers. JAMA. 2005;294(2):202–10.
78. Hanna JN, Warnock TH, Shepherd RW, Selvey LA. Fulminant hepatitis A in indigenous children in north Queensland. Med J Aust. 2000;172(1):19–21.
79. Victor JC, Monto AS, Surdina TY, Suleimenova SZ, Vaughan G, Nainan OV, et al. Hepatitis A vaccine versus immune globulin for postexposure prophylaxis. N Engl J Med. 2007;357(17):1685–94.
80. Rein DB, Stevens GA, Theaker J, Wittenborn JS, Wiersma ST. The global burden of hepatitis E virus genotypes 1 and 2 in 2005. Hepatology. 2012;55(4):988–97.
81. Khuroo MS, Khuroo MS, Khuroo NS, Hepatitis E. Discovery, global impact, control and cure. World J Gastroenterol. 2016;22(31):7030–45.
82. Khuroo MS. Discovery of hepatitis E—the untold story. JK-Practitioner. 2004;11(3):291–4.
83. Khuroo MS, Kamili S, Khuroo MS, Al Ashgar H. Hepatitis E. In: Al Knawy B, Shiffman ML, Wiesner RL, editors. Hepatology: a practical approach. Amsterdam: Elsevier B.V.; 2004.
84. Khuroo MS. Study of an epidemic of non-A, non-B hepatitis. Possibility of another human hepatitis virus distinct from post-transfusion non-A, non-B type. Am J Med. 1980;68(6):818–24.

85. Khuroo MS, Rustgi VK, Dawson GJ, Mushahwar IK, Yattoo GN, Kamili S, et al. Spectrum of hepatitis E virus infection in India. J Med Virol. 1994;43(3):281–6.
86. Khuroo MS, Khuroo MS. Seroepidemiology of a second epidemic of hepatitis E in a population that had recorded first epidemic 30 years before and has been under surveillance since then. Hepatol Int. 2010;4(2):494–9.
87. Khuroo MS, Teli MR, Skidmore S, Sofi MA, Khuroo MI. Incidence and severity of viral hepatitis in pregnancy. Am J Med. 1981;70(2):252–5.
88. Khuroo MS, Kamili S. Aetiology, clinical course and outcome of sporadic acute viral hepatitis in pregnancy. J Viral Hepat. 2003;10(1):61–9.
89. Khuroo MS, Kamili S, Jameel S. Vertical transmission of hepatitis E virus. Lancet. 1995;345(8956):1025–6.
90. Khuroo MS, Kamili S, Khuroo MS. Clinical course and duration of viremia in vertically transmitted hepatitis E virus (HEV) infection in babies born to HEV-infected mothers. J Viral Hepat. 2009;16(7):519–23.
91. Khuroo MS, Saleem M, Teli MR, Sofi MA. Failure to detect chronic liver disease after epidemic non-A, non-B hepatitis. Lancet. 1980;2(8185):97–8.
92. Khuroo MS, Duermeyer W, Zargar SA, Ahanger MA, Shah MA. Acute sporadic non-A, non-B hepatitis in India. Am J Epidemiol. 1983;118(3):360–4.
93. Balayan MS, Andjaparidze AG, Savinskaya SS, Ketiladze ES, Braginsky DM, Savinov AP, et al. Evidence for a virus in non-A, non-B hepatitis transmitted via the fecal-oral route. Intervirology. 1983;20(1):23–31.
94. Jameel S, Durgapal H, Habibullah CM, Khuroo MS, Panda SK. Enteric non-A, non-B hepatitis: epidemics, animal transmission, and hepatitis E virus detection by the polymerase chain reaction. J Med Virol. 1992;37(4):263–70.
95. Kane MA, Bradley DW, Shrestha SM, Maynard JE, Cook EH, Mishra RP, et al. Epidemic non-A, non-B hepatitis in Nepal. Recovery of a possible etiologic agent and transmission studies in marmosets. JAMA. 1984;252(22):3140–5.
96. Bradley DW, Balayan MS. Virus of enterically transmitted non-A, non-B hepatitis. Lancet. 1988;1(8589):819.
97. Reyes GR, Purdy MA, Kim JP, Luk KC, Young LM, Fry KE, et al. Isolation of a cDNA from the virus responsible for enterically transmitted non-A, non-B hepatitis. Science. 1990;247(4948):1335–9.
98. Tam AW, Smith MM, Guerra ME, Huang CC, Bradley DW, Fry KE, et al. Hepatitis E virus (HEV): molecular cloning and sequencing of the full-length viral genome. Virology. 1991;185(1):120–31.
99. Yarbough PO, Tam AW, Fry KE, Krawczynski K, McCaustland KA, Bradley DW, et al. Hepatitis E virus: identification of type-common epitopes. J Virol. 1991;65(11):5790–7.
100. Pavio N, Meng XJ, Renou C. Zoonotic hepatitis E: animal reservoirs and emerging risks. Vet Res. 2010;41(6):46.
101. Smith DB, Simmonds P, International Committee on Taxonomy of Viruses Hepeviridae Study G, Jameel S, Emerson SU, Harrison TJ, et al. Consensus proposals for classification of the family Hepeviridae. J Gen Virol. 2014;95(Pt 10):2223–32.
102. Emerson SU, Arankalle VA, Purcell RH. Thermal stability of hepatitis E virus. J Infect Dis. 2005;192(5):930–3.
103. Ahmad I, Holla RP, Jameel S. Molecular virology of hepatitis E virus. Virus Res. 2011;161(1):47–58.
104. Reyes GR, Huang CC, Tam AW, Purdy MA. Molecular organization and replication of hepatitis E virus (HEV). Arch Virol Suppl. 1993;7:15–25.
105. Cao D, Meng XJ. Molecular biology and replication of hepatitis E virus. Emerg Microbes Infect. 2012;1(8):e17.
106. Khuroo MS, Khuroo MS. Hepatitis E: an emerging global disease—from discovery towards control and cure. J Viral Hepat. 2016;23(2):68–79.
107. Aggarwal R, Naik S. Epidemiology of hepatitis E: current status. J Gastroenterol Hepatol. 2009;24(9):1484–93.

108. Khuroo MS, Hepatitis E. the enterically transmitted non-A, non-B hepatitis. Indian J Gastroenterol. 1991;10(3):96–100.
109. Arankalle VA, Paranjape S, Emerson SU, Purcell RH, Walimbe AM. Phylogenetic analysis of hepatitis E virus isolates from India (1976–1993). J Gen Virol. 1999;80(Pt 7):1691–700.
110. Panda SK, Thakral D, Rehman S. Hepatitis E virus. Rev Med Virol. 2007;17(3):151–80.
111. Ghabrah TM, Stickland GT, Tsarev S, Yarbough P, Farci P, Engle R, et al. Acute viral hepatitis in Saudi Arabia: seroepidemiological analysis, risk factors, clinical manifestations, and evidence for a sixth hepatitis agent. Clin Infect Dis. 1995;21(3):621–7.
112. Dai X, Dong C, Zhou Z, Liang J, Dong M, Yang Y, et al. Hepatitis E virus genotype 4, Nanjing, China, 2001–2011. Emerg Infect Dis. 2013;19(9):1528–30.
113. Delarocque-Astagneau E, Abravanel F, Moshen A, Le Fouler L, Gad RR, El-Daly M, et al. Epidemiological and virological characteristics of symptomatic acute hepatitis E in Greater Cairo, Egypt. Clin Microbiol Infect. 2012;18(10):982–8.
114. Blackard JT, Rouster SD, Nady S, Galal G, Marzuuk N, Rafaat MM, et al. Genotypic characterization of symptomatic hepatitis E virus (HEV) infections in Egypt. J Clin Virol. 2009;46(2):140–4.
115. Pischke S, Heim A, Bremer B, Raupach R, Horn-Wichmann R, Ganzenmueller T, et al. Hepatitis E: an emerging infectious disease in Germany? Z Gastroenterol. 2011;49(9):1255–7.
116. Kamar N, Izopet J, Rostaing L. Hepatitis E virus infection. Curr Opin Gastroenterol. 2013;29(3):271–8.
117. Mansuy JM, Peron JM, Abravanel F, Poirson H, Dubois M, Miedouge M, et al. Hepatitis E in the south west of France in individuals who have never visited an endemic area. J Med Virol. 2004;74(3):419–24.
118. Meng XJ. From barnyard to food table: the omnipresence of hepatitis E virus and risk for zoonotic infection and food safety. Virus Res. 2011;161(1):23–30.
119. Naik SR, Aggarwal R, Salunke PN, Mehrotra NN. A large waterborne viral hepatitis E epidemic in Kanpur, India. Bull World Health Organ. 1992;70(5):597–604.
120. Tandon BN, Gandhi BM, Joshi YK, Irshad M, Gupta H. Hepatitis virus non-A, non-B: the cause of a major public health problem in India. Bull World Health Organ. 1985;63(5):931–4.
121. Teshale EH, Grytdal SP, Howard C, Barry V, Kamili S, Drobeniuc J, et al. Evidence of person-to-person transmission of hepatitis E virus during a large outbreak in Northern Uganda. Clin Infect Dis. 2010;50(7):1006–10.
122. Khuroo MS, Dar MY, Hepatitis E. evidence for person-to-person transmission and inability of low dose immune serum globulin from an Indian source to prevent it. Indian J Gastroenterol. 1992;11(3):113–6.
123. Aggarwal R. Hepatitis E virus and person-to-person transmission. Clin Infect Dis. 2010;51(4):477–8; author reply 8–9.
124. Yugo DM, Meng XJ. Hepatitis E virus: foodborne, waterborne and zoonotic transmission. Int J Environ Res Public Health. 2013;10(10):4507–33.
125. Miyashita K, Kang JH, Saga A, Takahashi K, Shimamura T, Yasumoto A, et al. Three cases of acute or fulminant hepatitis E caused by ingestion of pork meat and entrails in Hokkaido, Japan: zoonotic food-borne transmission of hepatitis E virus and public health concerns. Hepatol Res. 2012;42(9):870–8.
126. Colson P, Borentain P, Queyriaux B, Kaba M, Moal V, Gallian P, et al. Pig liver sausage as a source of hepatitis E virus transmission to humans. J Infect Dis. 2010;202(6):825–34.
127. Garbuglia AR, Alessandrini AI, Pavio N, Tesse S, Grignolo S, Viscoli C, et al. Male patient with acute hepatitis E in Genoa, Italy: figatelli (pork liver sausage) as probable source of the infection. Clin Microbiol Infect. 2015;21(1):e4–6.
128. Shukla P, Chauhan UK, Naik S, Anderson D, Aggarwal R. Hepatitis E virus infection among animals in northern India: an unlikely source of human disease. J Viral Hepat. 2007;14(5):310–7.
129. Arankalle VA, Chobe LP, Joshi MV, Chadha MS, Kundu B, Walimbe AM. Human and swine hepatitis E viruses from Western India belong to different genotypes. J Hepatol. 2002;36(3):417–25.

130. Woo PC, Lau SK, Teng JL, Tsang AK, Joseph M, Wong EY, et al. New hepatitis E virus genotype in camels, the Middle East. Emerg Infect Dis. 2014;20(6):1044–8.
131. Rasche A, Saqib M, Liljander AM, Bornstein S, Zohaib A, Renneker S, et al. Hepatitis E virus infection in dromedaries, North and East Africa, United Arab Emirates, and Pakistan, 1983–2015. Emerg Infect Dis. 2016;22(7):1249–52.
132. Zhuang H, Cao XY, Liu CB, Wang GM. Epidemiology of hepatitis E in China. Gastroenterol Jpn. 1991;26(Suppl 3):135–8.
133. Aye TT, Uchida T, Ma XZ, Iida F, Shikata T, Zhuang H, et al. Complete nucleotide sequence of a hepatitis E virus isolated from the Xinjiang epidemic (1986–1988) of China. Nucleic Acids Res. 1992;20(13):3512.
134. Khuroo MS, Kamili S, Yattoo GN. Hepatitis E virus infection may be transmitted through blood transfusions in an endemic area. J Gastroenterol Hepatol. 2004;19(7):778–84.
135. Matsubayashi K, Nagaoka Y, Sakata H, Sato S, Fukai K, Kato T, et al. Transfusion-transmitted hepatitis E caused by apparently indigenous hepatitis E virus strain in Hokkaido, Japan. Transfusion. 2004;44(6):934–40.
136. Matsubayashi K, Kang JH, Sakata H, Takahashi K, Shindo M, Kato M, et al. A case of transfusion-transmitted hepatitis E caused by blood from a donor infected with hepatitis E virus via zoonotic food-borne route. Transfusion. 2008;48(7):1368–75.
137. Hewitt PE, Ijaz S, Brailsford SR, Brett R, Dicks S, Haywood B, et al. Hepatitis E virus in blood components: a prevalence and transmission study in southeast England. Lancet. 2014;384(9956):1766–73.
138. Fukuda S, Sunaga J, Saito N, Fujimura K, Itoh Y, Sasaki M, et al. Prevalence of antibodies to hepatitis E virus among Japanese blood donors: identification of three blood donors infected with a genotype 3 hepatitis E virus. J Med Virol. 2004;73(4):554–61.
139. Vollmer T, Diekmann J, Johne R, Eberhardt M, Knabbe C, Dreier J. Novel approach for detection of hepatitis E virus infection in German blood donors. J Clin Microbiol. 2012;50(8):2708–13.
140. Holm DK, Moessner BK, Engle RE, Zaaijer HL, Georgsen J, Purcell RH, et al. Declining prevalence of hepatitis E antibodies among Danish blood donors. Transfusion. 2015;55(7):1662–7.
141. Juhl D, Baylis SA, Blumel J, Gorg S, Hennig H. Seroprevalence and incidence of hepatitis E virus infection in German blood donors. Transfusion. 2014;54(1):49–56.
142. Khuroo MS. Association of severity of hepatitis E virus infection in the mother and vertically transmitted infection in the fetus. JK-Practitioner. 2006;13(2):70–4.
143. Bose PD, Das BC, Hazam RK, Kumar A, Medhi S, Kar P. Evidence of extrahepatic replication of hepatitis E virus in human placenta. J Gen Virol. 2014;95(Pt 6):1266–71.
144. Chibber RM, Usmani MA, Al-Sibai MH. Should HEV infected mothers breast feed? Arch Gynecol Obstet. 2004;270(1):15–20.
145. Lee GH, Tan BH, Chi-Yuan Teo E, Lim SG, Dan YY, Wee A, et al. Chronic infection with camelid hepatitis E virus in a liver transplant recipient who regularly consumes camel meat and milk. Gastroenterology. 2016;150(2):355–7.e3.
146. Huang F, Li Y, Yu W, Jing S, Wang J, Long F, et al. Excretion of infectious hepatitis E virus into milk in cows imposes high risks of zoonosis. Hepatology. 2016;64(2):350–9.
147. Ucar E, Cetin M, Kuvandik C, Helvaci MR, Gullu M, Huzmeli C. [Hepatitis E virus seropositivity in hemodialysis patients in Hatay province, Turkey]. Mikrobiyol Bul. 2009;43(2):299–302.
148. Siddiqui AR, Jooma RA, Smego RA Jr. Nosocomial outbreak of hepatitis E infection in Pakistan with possible parenteral transmission. Clin Infect Dis. 2005;40(6):908–9.
149. Ola SO, Odaibo GN, Olaleye OD, Ayoola EA. Hepatitis B and E viral infections among Nigerian healthcare workers. Afr J Med Med Sci. 2012;41(4):387–91.
150. Robson SC, Adams S, Brink N, Woodruff B, Bradley D. Hospital outbreak of hepatitis E. Lancet. 1992;339(8806):1424–5.
151. Pawlotsky JM, Belec L, Gresenguet G, Deforges L, Bouvier M, Duval J, et al. High prevalence of hepatitis B, C, and E markers in young sexually active adults from the Central African Republic. J Med Virol. 1995;46(3):269–72.

152. Keane F, Gompels M, Bendall R, Drayton R, Jennings L, Black J, et al. Hepatitis E virus coinfection in patients with HIV infection. HIV Med. 2012;13(1):83–8.
153. Chauhan A, Jameel S, Dilawari JB, Chawla YK, Kaur U, Ganguly NK. Hepatitis E virus transmission to a volunteer. Lancet. 1993;341(8838):149–50.
154. Khuroo MS, Kamili S. Aetiology and prognostic factors in acute liver failure in India. J Viral Hepat. 2003;10(3):224–31.
155. Hamid SS, Atiq M, Shehzad F, Yasmeen A, Nissa T, Salam A, et al. Hepatitis E virus superinfection in patients with chronic liver disease. Hepatology. 2002;36(2):474–8.
156. Kumar Acharya S, Kumar Sharma P, Singh R, Kumar Mohanty S, Madan K, Kumar Jha J, et al. Hepatitis E virus (HEV) infection in patients with cirrhosis is associated with rapid decompensation and death. J Hepatol. 2007;46(3):387–94.
157. Ramachandran J, Eapen CE, Kang G, Abraham P, Hubert DD, Kurian G, et al. Hepatitis E superinfection produces severe decompensation in patients with chronic liver disease. J Gastroenterol Hepatol. 2004;19(2):134–8.
158. Radha Krishna Y, Saraswat VA, Das K, Himanshu G, Yachha SK, Aggarwal R, et al. Clinical features and predictors of outcome in acute hepatitis A and hepatitis E virus hepatitis on cirrhosis. Liver Int. 2009;29(3):392–8.
159. Khuroo MS. Discovery of hepatitis E: the epidemic non-A, non-B hepatitis 30 years down the memory lane. Virus Res. 2011;161(1):3–14.
160. Izopet J, Kamar N. [Hepatitis E: from zoonotic transmission to chronic infection in immunosuppressed patients]. Med Sci (Paris). 2008;24(12):1023–5.
161. Yamamoto T, Suzuki H, Toyota T, Takahashi M, Okamoto H. Three male patients with sporadic acute hepatitis E in Sendai, Japan, who were domestically infected with hepatitis E virus of genotype III or IV. J Gastroenterol. 2004;39(3):292–8.
162. Khuroo MS, Khuroo MS. Hepatitis E virus. Curr Opin Infect Dis. 2008;21(5):539–43.
163. Kamar N, Selves J, Mansuy JM, Ouezzani L, Peron JM, Guitard J, et al. Hepatitis E virus and chronic hepatitis in organ-transplant recipients. N Engl J Med. 2008;358(8):811–7.
164. Kamar N, Mansuy JM, Cointault O, Selves J, Abravanel F, Danjoux M, et al. Hepatitis E virus-related cirrhosis in kidney- and kidney-pancreas-transplant recipients. Am J Transplant. 2008;8(8):1744–8.
165. Kamar N, Garrouste C, Haagsma EB, Garrigue V, Pischke S, Chauvet C, et al. Factors associated with chronic hepatitis in patients with hepatitis E virus infection who have received solid organ transplants. Gastroenterology. 2011;140(5):1481–9.
166. Dalton HR, Kamar N, van Eijk JJ, McLean BN, Cintas P, Bendall RP, et al. Hepatitis E virus and neurological injury. Nat Rev Neurol. 2016;12(2):77–85.
167. Abid S, Khan AH. Severe hemolysis and renal failure in glucose-6-phosphate dehydrogenase deficient patients with hepatitis E. Am J Gastroenterol. 2002;97(6):1544–7.
168. Au WY, Ngai CW, Chan WM, Leung RY, Chan SC. Hemolysis and methemoglobinemia due to hepatitis E virus infection in patient with G6PD deficiency. Ann Hematol. 2011;90(10):1237–8.
169. Bhagat S, Wadhawan M, Sud R, Arora A. Hepatitis viruses causing pancreatitis and hepatitis: a case series and review of literature. Pancreas. 2008;36(4):424–7.
170. Haffar S, Bazerbachi F, Lake JR. HEV-associated cryoglobulinaemia and extrahepatic manifestations of hepatitis E. Lancet Infect Dis. 2015;15(3):268.
171. Mishra A, Saigal S, Gupta R, Sarin SK. Acute pancreatitis associated with viral hepatitis: a report of six cases with review of literature. Am J Gastroenterol. 1999;94(8):2292–5.
172. Cheung MC, Maguire J, Carey I, Wendon J, Agarwal K. Review of the neurological manifestations of hepatitis E infection. Ann Hepatol. 2012;11(5):618–22.
173. Scharn N, Ganzenmueller T, Wenzel JJ, Dengler R, Heim A, Wegner F. Guillain-Barre syndrome associated with autochthonous infection by hepatitis E virus subgenotype 3c. Infection. 2014;42(1):171–3.
174. Bruffaerts R, Yuki N, Damme PV, Moortele MV, Wautier M, Lagrou K, et al. Acute ataxic neuropathy associated with hepatitis E virus infection. Muscle Nerve. 2015;52(3): 464–5.

175. Wu X, Liu K, Zhang HL. Guillain-Barre syndrome and encephalitis/encephalopathy associated with acute severe hepatitis E infection. Neurol Sci. 2015;36(1):165–6.
176. Cronin S, McNicholas R, Kavanagh E, Reid V, O'Rourke K. Anti-glycolipid GM2-positive Guillain-Barre syndrome due to hepatitis E infection. Ir J Med Sci. 2011;180(1):255–7.
177. Khudyakov Y, Kamili S. Serological diagnostics of hepatitis E virus infection. Virus Res. 2011;161(1):84–92.
178. Zhou H, Jiang CW, Li LP, Zhao CY, Wang YC, Xu YW, et al. [Comparison of the reliability of two ELISA kits for detecting IgM antibody against hepatitis E virus]. Zhonghua Yu Fang Yi Xue Za Zhi. 2008;42(9):667–71.
179. Scobie L, Dalton HR. Hepatitis E: source and route of infection, clinical manifestations and new developments. J Viral Hepat. 2013;20(1):1–11.
180. Lin XL, Ren H, Liang XH. Detection of anti-virus antibody in sera from patients with hepatitis E after ten-years-infection. Endem Dis Bull. 2002;17(3):14–7.
181. Wen GP, Tang ZM, Yang F, Zhang K, Ji WF, Cai W, et al. A valuable antigen detection method for diagnosis of acute hepatitis E. J Clin Microbiol. 2015;53(3):782–8.
182. Chen HY, Lu Y, Howard T, Anderson D, Fong PY, Hu WP, et al. Comparison of a new immunochromatographic test to enzyme-linked immunosorbent assay for rapid detection of immunoglobulin M antibodies to hepatitis E virus in human sera. Clin Diagn Lab Immunol. 2005;12(5):593–8.
183. Brochot E, Choukroun G, Duverlie G. Ribavirin for chronic hepatitis E virus infection. N Engl J Med. 2014;370(25):2446–7.
184. Pas SD, Streefkerk RH, Pronk M, de Man RA, Beersma MF, Osterhaus AD, et al. Diagnostic performance of selected commercial HEV IgM and IgG ELISAs for immunocompromised and immunocompetent patients. J Clin Virol. 2013;58(4):629–34.
185. Zhao ZY, Ruan B, Shao H, Chen ZJ, Liu SL. Detection of hepatitis E virus RNA in sera of patients with hepatitis E by polymerase chain reaction. Hepatobiliary Pancreat Dis Int. 2007;6(1):38–42.
186. Pischke S, Wedemeyer H. Chronic hepatitis E in liver transplant recipients: a significant clinical problem? Minerva Gastroenterol Dietol. 2010;56(2):121–8.
187. Kamar N, Rostaing L, Abravanel F, Garrouste C, Lhomme S, Esposito L, et al. Ribavirin therapy inhibits viral replication on patients with chronic hepatitis E virus infection. Gastroenterology. 2010;139(5):1612–8.
188. Zhang LQ, Zhao FR, Liu ZG, Kong WL, Wang H, Ouyang Y, et al. Simple and rapid detection of swine hepatitis E virus by reverse transcription loop-mediated isothermal amplification. Arch Virol. 2012;157(12):2383–8.
189. Goyal R, Kumar A, Panda SK, Paul SB, Acharya SK. Ribavirin therapy for hepatitis E virus-induced acute on chronic liver failure: a preliminary report. Antivir Ther. 2012;17(6):1091–6.
190. Wang Y, Zhou X, Debing Y, Chen K, Van Der Laan LJ, Neyts J, et al. Calcineurin inhibitors stimulate and mycophenolic acid inhibits replication of hepatitis E virus. Gastroenterology. 2014;146(7):1775–83.
191. Dao Thi VL, Debing Y, Wu X, Rice CM, Neyts J, Moradpour D, et al. Sofosbuvir inhibits hepatitis E virus replication in vitro and results in an additive effect when combined with ribavirin. Gastroenterology. 2016;150(1):82–5.e4.
192. Khuroo MS. Sanitation and sewage disposal in India. http://www.researchgate.net/publication/2694115842014.
193. Khuroo MS. Viral hepatitis in international travellers: risks and prevention. Int J Antimicrob Agents. 2003;21(2):143–52.
194. Kamar N, Legrand-Abravanel F, Izopet J, Rostaing L. Hepatitis E virus: what transplant physicians should know. Am J Transplant. 2012;12(9):2281–7.
195. Zhu FC, Zhang J, Zhang XF, Zhou C, Wang ZZ, Huang SJ, et al. Efficacy and safety of a recombinant hepatitis E vaccine in healthy adults: a large-scale, randomised, double-blind placebo-controlled, phase 3 trial. Lancet. 2010;376(9744):895–902.

196. Zhang J, Shih JW, Xia NS. Long-term efficacy of a hepatitis E vaccine. N Engl J Med. 2015;372(23):2265–6.
197. Azman AS, Luquero FJ, Ciglenecki I. Long-term efficacy of a hepatitis E vaccine. N Engl J Med. 2015;372(23):2265.
198. Hepatitis E vaccine: why wait? Lancet. 2010;376(9744):845.

Clinical Epidemiology of NAFLD

14

Donghee Kim, Osama Siddique, Brandon J. Perumpail, and Aijaz Ahmed

Abstract

Nonalcoholic fatty liver disease (NAFLD) is defined as the presence of hepatic fat accumulation after the exclusion of other causes of hepatic steatosis, including other causes of liver disease, excessive alcohol consumption, and other conditions that may lead to hepatic steatosis. NAFLD encompasses a broad clinical spectrum ranging from nonalcoholic fatty liver to nonalcoholic steatohepatitis (NASH), advanced fibrosis, cirrhosis, and hepatocellular carcinoma. NAFLD is the most common liver disease in the world and NASH may soon become the most common indication for liver transplantation. The ongoing persistence of obesity with increasing rate of diabetes will increase the prevalence of NAFLD, and as this population ages, many will develop cirrhosis and end-stage liver disease. There has been a general increase in the prevalence of NAFLD, with Asia leading the rise, but the United States (U.S.) is following closely behind with prevalence increasing from 15% in 2005 to 25% within 5 years. NAFLD is commonly associated with metabolic comorbidities, including obesity, type II diabetes, dyslipidemia, and metabolic syndrome. Our understanding of the pathophysiology of NAFLD is constantly evolving. Based on NAFLD subtypes, it has the potential to progress into advanced fibrosis, end-stage liver disease and hepatocellular carcinoma. The increasing prevalence of NAFLD with advanced

D. Kim · A. Ahmed (✉)
Division of Gastroenterology and Hepatology, Stanford University School of Medicine, Stanford, CA, USA
e-mail: messmd@chol.com; aijazahmed@stanford.edu

O. Siddique
Department of Medicine, Brown University, Providence, RI, USA
e-mail: osama_siddique@brown.edu

B. J. Perumpail
Department of Medicine, Drexel University College of Medicine, Philadelphia, PA, USA
e-mail: bjp63@drexel.edu

R. J. Wong, R. G. Gish (eds.), *Clinical Epidemiology of Chronic Liver Diseases*,
https://doi.org/10.1007/978-3-319-94355-8_14

fibrosis is concerning because patients appear to experience higher liver-related and non-liver-related mortality than the general population. The increased morbidity and mortality, healthcare costs and declining health related quality of life associated with NAFLD makes it a formidable disease, and one that requires more in-depth analysis.

Keywords
Nonalcoholic fatty liver disease · Hepatic steatosis · Fatty liver · Prevalence · Incidence · Fibrosis · Risk factor · Epidemiology · Outcomes · Nonalcoholic steatohepatitis

14.1 Definition of Nonalcoholic Fatty Liver Disease

Since its first description in 1980 as the "unnamed disease" [1], nonalcoholic fatty liver disease (NAFLD) has become a common cause of chronic liver disease worldwide [2]. It has been studied in depth with a myriad of further investigations being carried out on this soon to be common indication for liver transplantation. NAFLD encompasses a wide histological variety: nonalcoholic fatty liver (NAFL), nonalcoholic steatohepatitis (NASH), fibrosis, NASH cirrhosis and NASH-related hepatocellular carcinoma (HCC) (Table 14.1). NAFLD is characterized by ≥5% of hepatic fat accumulation in the absence of any secondary causes. NAFLD is a diagnosis of exclusion. Therefore, other etiologies leading to similar hepatic histology must be ruled out including excessive alcohol consumption; viral hepatitis; other chronic liver disease such as Wilson's disease,

Table 14.1 Definitions of spectrum of NAFLD

Type	Definition
Nonalcoholic fatty liver disease (NAFLD)	Presence of greater than 5% of hepatic fat accumulation with or without inflammation, hepatocyte ballooning degeneration, and fibrosis. No other causes of secondary hepatic fat accumulation (e.g. alcohol, infections, medications, etc.)
Non alcoholic fatty liver (NAFL)	Presence of hepatic steatosis without hepatocyte ballooning degeneration, or fibrosis. The chances of progression in cirrhosis or hepatocellular carcinoma are minimal
Non alcoholic steatohepatitis (NASH)	Presence of hepatic steatosis with histological manifestation of either lobular inflammation and/or hepatocyte ballooning degeneration, with or without fibrosis
NASH cirrhosis	Presence of cirrhosis with evidence of steatosis or NASH diagnosed via histology
Cryptogenic cirrhosis	Unclear etiology of cirrhosis which is usually enriched with metabolic abnormalities after extensive serological, clinical and pathological assessment has been performed. Progression of NAFLD to cirrhosis may cause difficulty in diagnosing NASH cirrhosis due to reduced hepatic steatosis

hemochromatosis, autoimmune hepatitis, cholestatic liver disease and etc. starvation; lipodystrophy; celiac disease; Cushing's disease; and medications (corticosteroids, methotrexate, diltiazem, oxaliplatin, amiodarone, isoniazid, highly active antiretroviral therapy, etc.). Current guidelines recommend utilizing criteria requiring alcohol exposure of less than 30 g/day for men and less than 20 g/day for women as a component of NAFLD diagnosis [2].

14.2 Incidence and Prevalence of NAFLD

NAFLD has diverse manifestations described in all ethnicities over the world and present in both genders [3]. The variable presentations likely contribute to the underreported new and existing cases of NAFLD as well as the limited studies undertaken to elucidate the exact incidence and prevalence of NAFLD.

14.2.1 Incidence of NAFLD

A study from Japan which followed 3147 patients over 414 days found a 10% annual incidence rate [4]. Another Japanese study evaluated elevated aminotransferase levels, weight gain and insulin resistance development over 5 years to classify patients with NAFLD and their incidence was reported as 31 per 1000 person-year [5]. A retrospective study done in England later demonstrated a much lower incidence of 29 per 100,000 person-years [6]. A recent extensive meta-analysis described a pooled regional incidence of NAFLD in Asia and Israel to be 52 (95% CI: 28–97) per 1000 person-years and 28 (95% CI: 19–41) per 1000 person-years, respectively [3]. Current data on incidence for NAFLD are limited in some regions of the world due to the limited number of studies. Further studies seem warranted to determine the accurate incidence in the general population.

14.2.2 Prevalence of NAFLD

In general, the prevalence of NAFLD has increased over the last 20 years. In addition to the gold standard diagnostic test using a liver biopsy, there are some noninvasive modalities available to diagnose NAFLD. Hepatic ultrasonography, computed tomography, and magnetic resonance imaging are accepted modalities for detecting hepatic fatty infiltration. The difference in sensitivity of diagnostic modalities may account for the discrepancy in prevalence data for NAFLD. Using aminotransferase as a screening laboratory test for liver disease, the prevalence of elevated aminotransferases was 7.9% in the United States (U.S.) general population (1988–1992) with unexplained liver disease in 69% of these subjects [7, 8]. In a recent meta-analysis, hepatic ultrasonography allowed for the reliable and accurate detection of moderate-to-severe fatty liver and is now considered the screening modality of choice [9]. Prevalence of ultrasonographic diagnosis of NAFLD ranged from 17% in India to 46% in the U.S. [7, 10, 11]. Magnetic resonance spectroscopy remains one of the most sensitive and accurate noninvasive tests available with a NAFLD prevalence of 33% reported in the Dallas Heart Study [12, 13]. The Middle East and South America have the highest NAFLD prevalence at 31% and 32%, respectively, with the lowest prevalence in Africa at 13.5% [3]. Recently, Asia has been facing the highest obesity epidemic and thus not surprisingly has been experiencing a rapid rate of increase in the prevalence of NAFLD. Chinese adolescents consuming a "Westernized" diet have a greater than 25% prevalence of NAFLD. Studies from Korea, China, Japan and Taiwan all have reported a prevalence ranging from 11% to 45% [14]. The U.S. has also experienced increasing prevalence. Data from the National Health and Nutrition Examination Survey (NHANES) that used serologic and clinical data to establish liver disease diagnoses showed a doubling of NAFLD prevalence (5.51–11.01%) from 1988 to 2008 [15]. Based on the NHANES-III data collected between 1988 and 1994, the prevalence of ultrasonography-diagnosed NAFLD was 34% [16]. In a major study that used U.S. Medicare claim files to examine the prevalence of chronic liver disease and cirrhosis by underlying etiologies among African Americans, Native Hawaiians, Japanese Americans, Latinos and whites in the Multiethnic Cohort Study (MEC), there were 5783 cases (3575 chronic liver disease and 2208 cirrhosis) between 1999 and 2012. The study showed that in the entire cohort NAFLD was the most common cause of chronic liver disease (52%) and, for the first time, showed that NAFLD was the most common cause of cirrhosis [17]. A meta-regression of studies done globally also displayed an increased prevalence of NAFLD from 15% in 2005 to 25% in 2010 [3]. The discrepancy in the prevalence of NAFLD between studies is most likely due to differences in sample selection, diagnostic modalities, and dietary and lifestyle habits.

14.3 Role of Demographic and Clinical Factors in Predisposition to NAFLD

Based on our current knowledge, it appears that a combination of demographic and clinical factors may play a role in determining the likelihood of NAFLD in a given patient. Therefore, the pathogenesis of NAFLD is a multifactorial and multi-step process.

14.3.1 Impact of Age on NAFLD

Based on the NHANES data from 12 to 19-year-olds (males and females), suspected NAFLD prevalence defined as elevated ALT rose from 3.9% in 1988–1994 to 10.7% in 2007–2010, with increases among all race/ethnic subgroups [18]. These trends were also consistent among adolescents and young adults aged 15–39 years [19]. Although the majority of studies are among people aged 30–70 years, the general trend of increased prevalence is observed with age with NHANES III data showing peak prevalence of NAFLD at age 50–60 in men [20]; with 16.1% at ages 30–40 years, 22.3% at 41–50 years, 29.3% at 51–60 years, and 27.6% at >60 years [21]. In women, prevalence of NAFLD increased with age especially after menopause; with 12.5% at ages 30–40 years, 16.1% at 41–50 years, 21.6% at 51–60 years, and 25.4% at >60 years [21]. A study with octogenarians admitted to a geriatric hospital showed a higher than usual prevalence of 46% [22]. In a cross-sectional analysis of adults prospectively enrolled in the NASH Clinical Research Network studies it was shown that elderly patients had a higher prevalence of NASH compared to the non-elderly (72% versus 56%) and a higher prevalence of advanced fibrosis (44% versus 25%) [23].

14.3.2 Impact of Gender on NAFLD

Generally, gender differences exist in NAFLD. The overall prevalence of NAFLD and NASH has been shown to be higher in men [11]. Among obese adolescents, NAFLD prevalence is also higher in men [18]. However, it has been shown that women are at a reduced risk of NAFLD compared with men during their reproductive period, whereas after menopause women lose the protective effect and have comparable prevalence of NAFLD versus men [24].

14.3.3 Impact of Ethnicity on NAFLD

Ethnicity is another variable affecting the prevalence of NAFLD, with the highest prevalence among Hispanics followed by non-Hispanic whites, and the lowest prevalence in African Americans [11, 12, 25]. The numbers reported are at times double for Hispanics (45–58%) in comparison to African Americans (24–35%), with Latinos of Mexican origin having the highest prevalence in a subgroup analysis of the Latino population [12, 26]. These findings hold true even in studies in the pediatric population [18]. Underlying genetic and lifestyle variations among these ethnicities could further account for the skewed prevalence of NAFLD.

14.3.4 Impact of Genetic Factors on NAFLD

Although obesity, lifestyle variation, and insulin resistance are the most prevalent NAFLD risk factors, NAFLD varies substantially among people with comparable lifestyle factors, environmental impact, and metabolic abnormalities, indicating that other factors contribute to pathogenesis. The familial heritability [27] and interethnic variations in susceptibility [12] suggest that genetic factors may play an important role in determining the phenotypic manifestation and overall risk for NAFLD. NAFLD clusters in families with certain genetic variants on or near

TM6SF2, *PNPLA3*, *NCAN*, and *PPP1R3B* genes that increase the heritability of NAFLD to up to 27% within families [27, 28]. One genetic variant that is associated with NAFLD is a missense mutation [Ile148→Met148 (I148M)] in the palatin-like phospholipase domain-containing 3 gene (*PNPLA3*) [28]. A recent meta-analysis showed that *PNPLA3* exerts a strong influence not only on hepatic fat accumulation (GG homozygous individuals showed a 73% higher hepatic fat content compared with CC homozygous individuals, $p < 1 \times 10^{-9}$) but also on the susceptibility to develop more severe histologic liver damage (GG homozygous individuals had a 3.24-fold greater risk of higher necroinflammatory scores and a 3.2-fold greater risk of developing fibrosis compared with CC homozygous individuals, $p < 1 \times 10^{-9}$, respectively) [29]. These associations were maintained irrespective of the degree of obesity or the presence of diabetes [30–32]. The highest frequency of a single variant in the *PNPLA3* gene (I148M) has been observed in Hispanics followed by non-Hispanic whites, with the lowest frequency seen in African Americans [28]. A minor allele in transmembrane 5 superfamily member 2 (*TM6SF2*) was associated with MRS-measured hepatic triglyceride content from the Dallas Heart Study [33]. In addition, a minor allele of *TM6SF2* was noted to increase the risk for hepatic fibrosis independent of age, obesity, diabetes, and *PNPLA3* genotype [34].

14.3.5 Impact of Obesity and Weight Gain on NAFLD

The prevalence of NAFLD in the obese population ranges from 30% to 37% [7]. Abdominal obesity with higher waist circumference is specifically more strongly correlated with NAFLD [35]. In a recent cohort study of 2017 people during a median 4.4 year follow-up, visceral adiposity was associated with incident NAFLD in a dose-dependent manner, with an adjusted hazard ratio (HR, per one-standard deviation [SD] increase) for incident NAFLD of 1.36 (1.16–1.59) [36]. In addition, this study found significant relationships with subcutaneous adiposity for regressed NAFLD of HR 1.36 (95% CI 1.08–1.72) independent of visceral adiposity [36]. Furthermore, a recent study reported that visceral adiposity increased the risk for NAFLD both with and without significant fibrosis after adjusting for known risk factors [37]. Multivariate analysis showed that the visceral adipose tissue area was independently associated with increased risks of NASH and significant fibrosis [37]. These studies suggest that certain types of abdominal fat are risk factors for NAFLD and more advanced NAFLD-related fibrosis, whereas other types could reduce risk for NAFLD. In recent years, several cohort studies demonstrated an association between body weight change and incident NAFLD [38–41]. Even a modest gain in body weight of 2 kg within the normal range has been shown to increase the risk of developing NAFLD [39]. Obesity has also been noted to be an additive factor causing a twofold increase in steatosis in avid alcohol drinkers [32]. While it is common to have NAFLD in the obese population, it is even more common to have obesity in patients with NAFLD. The pooled prevalence of obesity in NAFLD globally is reported to be 51% [3].

14.3.6 Impact of Diet and Dietary Habits on NAFLD

Some macro- and micro-nutrients contribute more to the epidemic of NAFLD. Fructose is a major player, either from sucrose or high fructose corn syrup found in beverages. Consumption of sugar-containing beverages has increased five-fold in the US since 1950, and drinking two average size servings of these for 6 months ends up mirroring many features of NAFLD [42]. It is hypothesized that sugars promote de novo lipogenesis and trigger inflammatory responses leading to hepatocyte apoptosis via the c-Jun-N-Terminal (JNK) pathway [43]. Multiple studies have also shown a protective effect of higher rates of coffee consumption, including a significant reduction in risk of fibrosis among NASH patients [44]. In a study of the >215,000 participants in the Multiethnic Cohort it was shown that coffee drinking was inversely associated with risk of NAFLD [45]. Compared to not drinking coffee, consumption of 2–3 cups of coffee daily and ≥4 cups daily yielded a reduction in risk for NAFLD-associated chronic liver disease of 15% and 32%, respectively.

14.3.7 Impact of Diabetes on NAFLD

Pre-existing metabolic disorders, especially type 2 diabetes mellitus (T2DM), have a close association with NAFLD, with more than three-quarters of patients with T2DM reportedly having NAFLD [46]. T2DM and insulin resistance promote lipolysis of adipose tissue leading to release of free fatty acids and their deposition in the liver leading to steatosis [43]. T2DM is a significant risk factor for progression of NASH, fibrosis, and cirrhosis and an independent risk factor for mortality in addition to liver-related mortality [47]. Other emerging contributors to NAFLD development include hypothyroidism, hypopituitarism, polycystic ovarian disease and obstructive sleep apnea (Table 14.2) [2].

Table 14.2 Risk factors for NAFLD

Established risk factors:
• Obesity
• Type 2 diabetes mellitus
• Hypertriglyceridemia
• Metabolic syndrome
Risk factors being studied:
• Hypothyroidism
• Hypopituitarism
• Hypogonadism
• Obstructive sleep apnea
• Polycystic ovarian syndrome
• Total parenteral nutrition
• Excess fructose consumption
• Rapid weight loss
• PNPLA3 and TM6SF2 gene

14.4 Natural History of NAFLD

In terms of progression of NAFLD, the cohort of patients falls into two broad categories, NASH and NAFL. They are primarily divided by the likelihood of progression. NAFL represents simple steatosis and steatosis with non-specific inflammatory changes and follows a more indolent course of progression, while NASH may progress more rapidly to end-stage liver disease.

14.4.1 Progression of Histological Damage in NAFLD

NAFL is more readily reversible if lifestyle modifications are implemented in a timely fashion. The benign progression of NAFL and rapid progression of NASH has also been supported by earlier cohort studies from the United Kingdom [48] and Denmark [49]. In one of the earliest histology-based studies, biopsy-proven NAFLD was divided into four types with type 3 (fatty liver and ballooning degeneration) and type 4 (fatty liver, ballooning degeneration, and either Mallory body or fibrosis) representing the modern day definition of NASH [50]. Over follow up periods of 8 years, 21–28% of patients with histological type 3 and type 4 developed cirrhosis compared to only 3% of patients with type 1 (fatty liver alone) and type 2 (fatty liver and lobular inflammation). Liver-related mortality was also increased in types 3 and 4 in comparison to types 1 and 2 (11% vs 2%) [50]. A more recent study using follow-up data from the same cohort reported 18% liver-related mortality in NASH patients compared to 3% in non-NASH patients during 18.5 years [51].

14.4.2 Complications in NAFLD

NAFLD is associated with increased overall mortality, with ranges for the standardized mortality ratio (SMR) of 1.34–2.6 compared to the general population [52]. An early landmark study by Adams et al. documented that patients with NAFLD (n = 435) from Olmsted County, diagnosed histologically or by ultrasonography, demonstrated a significantly higher risk of mortality during 7.6 years of follow-up (SMR 1.34, 95% CI 1.003–1.76) [53]. In this study, liver-related mortality was the third most common cause of death, after malignancy and cardiovascular disease [53]. This is in contrast to the general population where liver-related mortality is the 12th most common cause of death [54]. Previous studies comparing NAFLD to the general population have consistently shown increased mortality in NAFLD. However, these studies did not adjust for metabolic confounders in the setting of NAFLD. Data from NHANES III revealed no significant difference in the overall survival of ultrasonography-diagnosed subjects with NAFLD compared with the non-NAFLD population after adjusting for multiple metabolic factors [16]. These results suggest that NASH and/or fibrosis may be the major driver contributing to significant long-term outcomes [16]. The NAFLD activity score (NAS) has gained popularity for defining NASH, yet histology is still the gold standard. Newer studies are

Table 14.3 Risk factors associated with developing NASH [54]

• Obesity
• Older age
• Non-African American ethnicity
• Type 2 diabetes mellitus
• Hypertension
• High ALT or AST
• Higher AST/ALT ratio
• Low platelet count
• Elevated fasting C-peptide level
• Ultrasound steatosis score

challenging the widespread belief that NAFL has a benign course. Based on histological diagnosis and follow up biopsies of 52 patients, NAFL advanced to NASH in 23% of cases over a period of 3 years [55]. The evolution into NASH can be as high as 44–64% and progression of NAFL into advanced fibrosis was reported in up to 24% of the patients with NAFL [56, 57]. Risk factors causing increasing NASH likelihood include obesity, older age, female sex, non-African American race/ethnicity, T2DM, and hypertension [58] (Table 14.3). The risk for progression of NASH into cirrhosis has been estimated to be between 21% and 26% in 8 years [59]. Although development of cirrhosis further increases the risk of progression to HCC and/or hepatic decompensation, the stages of fibrosis are also an excellent predictor of outcome. A retrospective longitudinal study over 12.6 years showed that increasing fibrosis from stage 1 (HR: 1.88) to stage 4 (HR: 10.49) increased mortality, liver-related events and need for liver transplantation [60]. With fibrosis staging and its progression from one stage to another being an important marker of mortality, recent studies reported that approximately 9–25% of patients developed NASH [61]. NASH cirrhosis has been compared to hepatitis C-related cirrhosis in multiple studies, with the majority of the studies showing decreased or comparable mortality and lower or similar cirrhosis-related complications and/or HCC [52, 61]. However, the cardiovascular mortality was higher in NASH cirrhosis [54]. Increased cardiovascular mortality can be explained by the decreased morbidity when compared to chronic hepatitis C-related cirrhosis. In other words, most patients may outlive their liver disease and thus become more likely to develop fatal complications from cardiovascular disease. As NASH advances to cirrhosis, it loses its characteristic histologic features, including inflammation and steatosis, becoming increasingly recognized as "cryptogenic cirrhosis" which essentially means cirrhosis of unclear etiology. Cryptogenic cirrhosis is referred to as 'burnt out' NASH by experts in the medical literature [7, 62]. Patients with cryptogenic cirrhosis have clinical manifestations commonly observed in patients with NASH such as obesity, dyslipidemia, insulin resistance, T2DM and metabolic syndrome. The incidence of HCC has been increasing in parallel to the rise in NAFLD and its subsets. HCC incidence has grown fourfold from 1973 to 2011 [63]. Advanced fibrosis is an important risk factor for HCC with an 8% 5-year cumulative incidence rate of developing HCC in patients with advanced fibrosis [64]. The annual incidence of NAFLD-related HCC (0.44 per 1000 person-years) is rare at this moment and 15–35 times lower than the incidence of

HCC in chronic hepatitis B [3]. In comparison, the annual incidence rate of NASH-related HCC has been reported as a significant 5.29 cases per 1000 person-years [3]. As the prevalence of NAFLD increases so will the incidence of NASH-related HCC. Younossi et al. described a 9% annual increase of HCC cases related to NAFLD over a period of 6 years from 2004 to 2009 [65]. This highlights the increased need for preventive measures. While previous studies have described progression of advanced fibrosis and cirrhosis as a major link between NAFLD and HCC, the latest studies are describing 35–50% of HCC without cirrhosis [66, 67]. Understanding the underlying pathogenetic pathways remains unclear at best. A few potential mechanisms to explain the link between NAFLD and HCC include hyperinsulinemia or metabolic syndrome, functioning of hepatic progenitor cells activated by hepatocyte damage, activation of CD8+/CD4+ T lymphocytes and natural killer cells causing self-damage, and *PNPLA3*-related pathways [68].

Conclusions

NAFLD remains the most common liver disease globally with increasing prevalence. The current annual medical and societal costs due to NAFLD are estimated at $292 billion in the U.S. [69]. The projected cost of caring for patients is an increase of 18% from year 2000 to 2035 while health-related quality of life of NAFLD patients is described as declining [70, 71]. The population at risk of developing progressive liver disease creates a challenge for the healthcare system in terms of screening for this evolving epidemic of liver disease. Further studies should be conducted to define accurate incidence, current disease burden, and socioeconomic effect of this disease.

Summary Table of Landmark Literature

Study title and authors	Study design	Summary results	Main limitations
Hamaguchi M, et al. The metabolic syndrome as a predictor of nonalcoholic fatty liver disease. Ann Intern Med. 2005;143(10):722–8	A prospective cohort study done over 414 days to investigate the effect of metabolic syndrome on pathogenesis of NAFLD	• Participants with metabolic syndrome had 4–11 times higher risk of future NAFLD	• Abdominal ultrasonography, which is not the gold standard, was used to classify NAFLD
Szczepaniak LS, et al. Magnetic resonance spectroscopy to measure hepatic triglyceride content: prevalence of hepatic steatosis in the general population. Am J Physiol Endocrinol Metab. 2005;288(2):E462–8	Randomized controlled clinical trial to measure hepatic triglyceride content (HTGC) using magnetic resonance spectroscopy	• A value of 5.56% or greater of HTGC defined as abnormal in patients with no risk factors. • Estimated prevalence of NAFLD as 33.6% in the Dallas heart study cohort	• 43% of the study population was obese contributing to the higher prevalence reported in comparison to general population

Study title and authors	Study design	Summary results	Main limitations
Younossi ZM, et al. Changes in the prevalence of the most common causes of chronic liver diseases in the United States from 1988 to 2008. Clin Gastroenterol Hepatol. 2011;9(6):524–30	A retrospective analysis of national health and nutrition examination surveys used to estimate changes in the prevalence and predictors of chronic liver disease (CLD)	• Prevalence of CLD is increasing: 11.78 ± 0.48% (1988–1994), to 14.78 ± 0.58% (2005–2008) ($P < 0.0001$) • Prevalence of NAFLD has increased steadily as well: 5.51 ± 0.31% (1988–1994) to 11.01 ± 0.51% (2005–2008) (P < 0.0001)	• The analysis and results are limited to adults only • There was no histological definition of NAFLD or NASH used to account for prevalence
Younossi ZM, et al. Global epidemiology of nonalcoholic fatty liver disease-meta-analytic assessment of prevalence, incidence, and outcomes. Hepatology. 2016;64(1):73–84	A systematic review and meta-analytic approach to report the incidence, prevalence, disease progression and burden of NAFLD	• Pooled incidence rate from Asia and Israel were 52 and 28 per 1000 person-year respectively • Prevalence of NAFLD in US has increased from 15% to 25% between 2005 and 2010 • Prevalence of NASH is between 1.5% and 6.45% • 9% of NASH patients had advancements in their fibrosis	• High unexplained heterogeneity of included studies • Under representation of under-developed countries and besides two studies all others were from countries with high human development index
Schwimmer JB, et al. Prevalence of fatty liver in children and adolescents. Pediatrics. 2006;118(4):1388–93	A retrospective review to determine the prevalence of pediatric fatty liver as diagnosed by histology in a population-based sample	• Prevalence of fatty liver in pediatric age group 2–19 years old was 9.6% (95% CI: 7.4–11.7) • Prevalence increases with increasing age. Ages 2–4: 0.7 (95% CI: 0–2.0), ages 15–19: 17.3 (95% CI: 13.8–20.8)	• A specific cause of fatty liver disease could not be determined

Study title and authors	Study design	Summary results	Main limitations
Wong VW, et al. Disease progression of non-alcoholic fatty liver disease: a prospective study with paired liver biopsies at 3 years. Gut. 2010;59(7):969–74	Prospective longitudinal hospital based cohort study to investigate disease progression over 36 months of different degrees of NAFLD	• 13 patients with simple steatosis at baseline, three (23%) continued to have simple steatosis at month 36, five (39%) developed borderline NASH and three (23%) developed NASH • Among 17 patients with NASH at baseline, ten (59%) continued to have NASH and six (35%) had borderline NASH at month 36. Only one (6%) patient regressed to simple steatosis	• All patients received lifestyle advice and regular monitoring of metabolic factors. This might have altered the natural history of the disease • Patients with NAFLD in a hospital clinic may have more advanced disease than those in the community • Small sample size precluded more detailed analysis of factors associated with disease progression • Liver biopsy might be limited by sampling bias
Angulo P, et al. Liver fibrosis, but no other histologic features, associated with long-term outcomes of patients with nonalcoholic fatty liver disease. Gastroenterology. 2015;149(2):389–97	A retrospective analysis of 619 patients diagnosed with NAFLD from 1975 through 2005 underwent analysis of their laboratory and biopsies results	• Features associated with death or liver transplantation included fibrosis stage 1 (HR, 1.88; 95% CI, 1.28, 2.77), stage 2 (HR, 2.89; 95% CI, 1.93, 4.33), stage 3 (HR, 3.76; 95% CI, 2.40, 5.89), and stage 4 (HR, 10.9; 95% CI, 6.06, 19.62) compared with stage 0 • Survival free of liver transplantation in patients with non-NASH was significantly lower in those with fibrosis as compared to those without fibrosis ($p < 0.001$)	• Lack of a specific protocol for patient follow-up with regards to endoscopy and imaging procedures in non-cirrhotic patients, and thus it is possible that the number of liver-related events was underestimated • Over-representation of the white population

Study title and authors	Study design	Summary results	Main limitations
Hashimoto E, et al. Hepatocellular carcinoma in patients with nonalcoholic steatohepatitis. J Gastroenterol. 2009;44(Suppl 19):89–95	A large case-control study of NASH patients with and without HCC as well as a prospective cohort study on the natural history of NASH patients with advanced fibrosis who underwent follow-up for HCC at a single tertiary care hospital	• Stage of fibrosis (OR = 4.232; 95% CI, 1.847–9.698; P = 0.001) was an independent predictor of development of HCC • Older age (OR = 1.108; 95% CI, 1.028–1.195; P = 0.008) and low AST levels (OR = 0.956; 95% CI, 0.919–0.995; P = 0.027), were other factors leading to HCC	• As histological diagnosis is a requirement for diagnosis of NASH, the patients diagnosed with this condition consisted of significantly altered liver function test. Findings might be affected by this selection bias
Rafiq N, et al. Long-term follow-up of patients with nonalcoholic fatty liver. Clin Gastroenterol Hepatol. 2009;7(2):234–8	A retrospective analysis of patients with biopsy proven NAFLD and long term follow up (>5 years), to find the long term outcome and specifically liver related mortality in patients with NAFLD	• NASH group had a liver-related mortality of 17.5% in contrast to only 2.7% in the non-NASH group ($P = 0.0048$) • NASH on biopsy ($P = 0.0250$) was an independent predictor of liver related mortality	• A relatively small cohort sample size • There was no histologic or clinical data to assess the development of cirrhosis or other complications during the follow-up period

References

1. Ludwig J, Viggiano TR, McGill DB, Oh BJ. Nonalcoholic steatohepatitis: Mayo Clinic experiences with a hitherto unnamed disease. Mayo Clin Proc. 1980;55(7):434–8.
2. Chalasani N, Younossi Z, Lavine JE, Diehl AM, Brunt EM, Cusi K, et al. The diagnosis and management of non-alcoholic fatty liver disease: practice guideline by the American Gastroenterological Association, American Association for the Study of Liver Diseases, and American College of Gastroenterology. Gastroenterology. 2012;142(7):1592–609.
3. Younossi ZM, Koenig AB, Abdelatif D, Fazel Y, Henry L, Wymer M. Global epidemiology of nonalcoholic fatty liver disease-meta-analytic assessment of prevalence, incidence, and outcomes. Hepatology. 2016;64(1):73–84.
4. Hamaguchi M, Kojima T, Takeda N, Nakagawa T, Taniguchi H, Fujii K, et al. The metabolic syndrome as a predictor of nonalcoholic fatty liver disease. Ann Intern Med. 2005;143(10):722–8.
5. Suzuki A, Angulo P, Lymp J, St Sauver J, Muto A, Okada T, et al. Chronological development of elevated aminotransferases in a nonalcoholic population. Hepatology. 2005;41(1):64–71.
6. Whalley S, Puvanachandra P, Desai A, Kennedy H. Hepatology outpatient service provision in secondary care: a study of liver disease incidence and resource costs. Clin Med (Lond). 2007;7(2):119–24.

7. Vernon G, Baranova A, Younossi ZM. Systematic review: the epidemiology and natural history of non-alcoholic fatty liver disease and non-alcoholic steatohepatitis in adults. Aliment Pharmacol Ther. 2011;34(3):274–85.
8. Clark JM, Brancati FL, Diehl AM. The prevalence and etiology of elevated aminotransferase levels in the United States. Am J Gastroenterol. 2003;98(5):960–7.
9. Hernaez R, Lazo M, Bonekamp S, Kamel I, Brancati FL, Guallar E, et al. Diagnostic accuracy and reliability of ultrasonography for the detection of fatty liver: a meta-analysis. Hepatology. 2011;54(3):1082–90.
10. Amarapurkar D, Kamani P, Patel N, Gupte P, Kumar P, Agal S, et al. Prevalence of non-alcoholic fatty liver disease: population based study. Ann Hepatol. 2007;6(3):161–3.
11. Williams CD, Stengel J, Asike MI, Torres DM, Shaw J, Contreras M, et al. Prevalence of nonalcoholic fatty liver disease and nonalcoholic steatohepatitis among a largely middle-aged population utilizing ultrasound and liver biopsy: a prospective study. Gastroenterology. 2011;140(1):124–31.
12. Browning JD, Szczepaniak LS, Dobbins R, Nuremberg P, Horton JD, Cohen JC, et al. Prevalence of hepatic steatosis in an urban population in the United States: impact of ethnicity. Hepatology. 2004;40(6):1387–95.
13. Szczepaniak LS, Nurenberg P, Leonard D, Browning JD, Reingold JS, Grundy S, et al. Magnetic resonance spectroscopy to measure hepatic triglyceride content: prevalence of hepatic steatosis in the general population. Am J Physiol Endocrinol Metab. 2005;288(2):E462–8.
14. Farrell GC, Wong VW, Chitturi S. NAFLD in Asia—as common and important as in the West. Nat Rev Gastroenterol Hepatol. 2013;10(5):307–18.
15. Younossi ZM, Stepanova M, Afendy M, Fang Y, Younossi Y, Mir H, et al. Changes in the prevalence of the most common causes of chronic liver diseases in the United States from 1988 to 2008. Clin Gastroenterol Hepatol. 2011;9(6):524–30.e1; quiz e60.
16. Kim D, Kim WR, Kim HJ, Therneau TM. Association between noninvasive fibrosis markers and mortality among adults with nonalcoholic fatty liver disease in the United States. Hepatology. 2013;57(4):1357–65.
17. Setiawan VW, Virnig BA, Porcel J, Henderson BE, Le Marchand L, Wilkens LR, et al. Linking data from the Multiethnic Cohort Study to Medicare data: linkage results and application to chronic disease research. Am J Epidemiol. 2015;181(11):917–9.
18. Welsh JA, Karpen S, Vos MB. Increasing prevalence of nonalcoholic fatty liver disease among United States adolescents, 1988–1994 to 2007–2010. J Pediatr. 2013;162(3):496–500.e1.
19. Doycheva I, Watt KD, Rifai G, Abou Mrad R, Lopez R, Zein NN, et al. Increasing burden of chronic liver disease among adolescents and young adults in the USA: a silent epidemic. Dig Dis Sci. 2017;62(5):1373–80.
20. Choi SY, Kim D, Kim HJ, Kang JH, Chung SJ, Park MJ, et al. The relation between non-alcoholic fatty liver disease and the risk of coronary heart disease in Koreans. Am J Gastroenterol. 2009;104(8):1953–60.
21. Lazo M, Hernaez R, Eberhardt MS, Bonekamp S, Kamel I, Guallar E, et al. Prevalence of nonalcoholic fatty liver disease in the United States: the third National Health and Nutrition Examination Survey, 1988–1994. Am J Epidemiol. 2013;178(1):38–45.
22. Kagansky N, Levy S, Keter D, Rimon E, Taiba Z, Fridman Z, et al. Non-alcoholic fatty liver disease—a common and benign finding in octogenarian patients. Liver Int. 2004;24(6):588–94.
23. Noureddin M, Yates KP, Vaughn IA, Neuschwander-Tetri BA, Sanyal AJ, McCullough A, et al. Clinical and histological determinants of nonalcoholic steatohepatitis and advanced fibrosis in elderly patients. Hepatology. 2013;58(5):1644–54.
24. Yang JD, Abdelmalek MF, Pang H, Guy CD, Smith AD, Diehl AM, et al. Gender and menopause impact severity of fibrosis among patients with nonalcoholic steatohepatitis. Hepatology. 2014;59(4):1406–14.
25. Torres DM, Williams CD, Harrison SA. Features, diagnosis, and treatment of nonalcoholic fatty liver disease. Clin Gastroenterol Hepatol. 2012;10(8):837–58.
26. Saab S, Manne V, Nieto J, Schwimmer JB, Chalasani NP. Nonalcoholic fatty liver disease in Latinos. Clin Gastroenterol Hepatol. 2016;14(1):5–12; quiz e9–10.

27. Schwimmer JB, Celedon MA, Lavine JE, Salem R, Campbell N, Schork NJ, et al. Heritability of nonalcoholic fatty liver disease. Gastroenterology. 2009;136(5):1585–92.
28. Romeo S, Kozlitina J, Xing C, Pertsemlidis A, Cox D, Pennacchio LA, et al. Genetic variation in PNPLA3 confers susceptibility to nonalcoholic fatty liver disease. Nat Genet. 2008;40(12):1461–5.
29. Sookoian S, Pirola CJ. Meta-analysis of the influence of I148M variant of patatin-like phospholipase domain containing 3 gene (PNPLA3) on the susceptibility and histological severity of nonalcoholic fatty liver disease. Hepatology. 2011;53(6):1883–94.
30. Rotman Y, Koh C, Zmuda JM, Kleiner DE, Liang TJ, Nash CRN. The association of genetic variability in patatin-like phospholipase domain-containing protein 3 (PNPLA3) with histological severity of nonalcoholic fatty liver disease. Hepatology. 2010;52(3):894–903.
31. Speliotes EK, Butler JL, Palmer CD, Voight BF, Consortium G, Consortium MI, et al. PNPLA3 variants specifically confer increased risk for histologic nonalcoholic fatty liver disease but not metabolic disease. Hepatology. 2010;52(3):904–12.
32. Valenti L, Al-Serri A, Daly AK, Galmozzi E, Rametta R, Dongiovanni P, et al. Homozygosity for the patatin-like phospholipase-3/adiponutrin I148M polymorphism influences liver fibrosis in patients with nonalcoholic fatty liver disease. Hepatology. 2010;51(4):1209–17.
33. Kozlitina J, Smagris E, Stender S, Nordestgaard BG, Zhou HH, Tybjaerg-Hansen A, et al. Exome-wide association study identifies a TM6SF2 variant that confers susceptibility to nonalcoholic fatty liver disease. Nat Genet. 2014;46(4):352–6.
34. Liu YL, Reeves HL, Burt AD, Tiniakos D, McPherson S, Leathart JB, et al. TM6SF2 rs58542926 influences hepatic fibrosis progression in patients with non-alcoholic fatty liver disease. Nat Commun. 2014;5:4309.
35. Farrell GC. The liver and the waistline: fifty years of growth. J Gastroenterol Hepatol. 2009;24(Suppl 3):S105–18.
36. Kim D, Chung GE, Kwak MS, Seo HB, Kang JH, Kim W, et al. Body fat distribution and risk of incident and regressed nonalcoholic fatty liver disease. Clin Gastroenterol Hepatol. 2016;14(1):132–8.e4.
37. Yu SJ, Kim W, Kim D, Yoon JH, Lee K, Kim JH, et al. Visceral obesity predicts significant fibrosis in patients with nonalcoholic fatty liver disease. Medicine (Baltimore). 2015;94(48):e2159.
38. Zelber-Sagi S, Lotan R, Shlomai A, Webb M, Harrari G, Buch A, et al. Predictors for incidence and remission of NAFLD in the general population during a seven-year prospective follow-up. J Hepatol. 2012;56(5):1145–51.
39. Chang Y, Ryu S, Sung E, Woo HY, Cho SI, Yoo SH, et al. Weight gain within the normal weight range predicts ultrasonographically detected fatty liver in healthy Korean men. Gut. 2009;58(10):1419–25.
40. Fan JG, Zhou Q, Wo QH. [Effect of body weight mass and its change on the incidence of nonalcoholic fatty liver disease]. Zhonghua Gan Zang Bing Za Zhi. 2010;18(9):676–9.
41. Kim HK, Park JY, Lee KU, Lee GE, Jeon SH, Kim JH, et al. Effect of body weight and lifestyle changes on long-term course of nonalcoholic fatty liver disease in Koreans. Am J Med Sci. 2009;337(2):98–102.
42. Bray GA, Popkin BM. Calorie-sweetened beverages and fructose: what have we learned 10 years later. Pediatr Obes. 2013;8(4):242–8.
43. Cusi K. Nonalcoholic fatty liver disease in type 2 diabetes mellitus. Curr Opin Endocrinol Diabetes Obes. 2009;16(2):141–9.
44. Molloy JW, Calcagno CJ, Williams CD, Jones FJ, Torres DM, Harrison SA. Association of coffee and caffeine consumption with fatty liver disease, nonalcoholic steatohepatitis, and degree of hepatic fibrosis. Hepatology. 2012;55(2):429–36.
45. Setiawan VW, Porcel J, Wei P, Stram DO, Noureddin N, Lu SC, et al. Coffee drinking and alcoholic and nonalcoholic fatty liver diseases and viral hepatitis in the Multiethnic Cohort. Clin Gastroenterol Hepatol. 2017;15(8):1305–7.
46. Portillo-Sanchez P, Bril F, Maximos M, Lomonaco R, Biernacki D, Orsak B, et al. High prevalence of nonalcoholic fatty liver disease in patients with type 2 diabetes mellitus and normal plasma aminotransferase levels. J Clin Endocrinol Metab. 2015;100(6):2231–8.

47. Stepanova M, Rafiq N, Younossi ZM. Components of metabolic syndrome are independent predictors of mortality in patients with chronic liver disease: a population-based study. Gut. 2010;59(10):1410–5.
48. Teli MR, James OF, Burt AD, Bennett MK, Day CP. The natural history of nonalcoholic fatty liver: a follow-up study. Hepatology. 1995;22(6):1714–9.
49. Dam-Larsen S, Franzmann M, Andersen IB, Christoffersen P, Jensen LB, Sorensen TI, et al. Long term prognosis of fatty liver: risk of chronic liver disease and death. Gut. 2004;53(5):750–5.
50. Matteoni CA, Younossi ZM, Gramlich T, Boparai N, Liu YC, McCullough AJ. Nonalcoholic fatty liver disease: a spectrum of clinical and pathological severity. Gastroenterology. 1999;116(6):1413–9.
51. Rafiq N, Bai C, Fang Y, Srishord M, McCullough A, Gramlich T, et al. Long-term follow-up of patients with nonalcoholic fatty liver. Clin Gastroenterol Hepatol. 2009;7(2):234–8.
52. Kwak M-S, Kim D. Long-term outcomes of nonalcoholic fatty liver disease. Curr Hepatol Rep. 2015;14:69–76.
53. Adams LA, Lymp JF, St Sauver J, Sanderson SO, Lindor KD, Feldstein A, et al. The natural history of nonalcoholic fatty liver disease: a population-based cohort study. Gastroenterology. 2005;129(1):113–21.
54. Heron M. Deaths: leading causes for 2014. Natl Vital Stat Rep. 2016;65(5):1–96.
55. Wong VW, Wong GL, Choi PC, Chan AW, Li MK, Chan HY, et al. Disease progression of non-alcoholic fatty liver disease: a prospective study with paired liver biopsies at 3 years. Gut. 2010;59(7):969–74.
56. Pais R, Charlotte F, Fedchuk L, Bedossa P, Lebray P, Poynard T, et al. A systematic review of follow-up biopsies reveals disease progression in patients with non-alcoholic fatty liver. J Hepatol. 2013;59(3):550–6.
57. McPherson S, Hardy T, Henderson E, Burt AD, Day CP, Anstee QM. Evidence of NAFLD progression from steatosis to fibrosing-steatohepatitis using paired biopsies: implications for prognosis and clinical management. J Hepatol. 2015;62(5):1148–55.
58. Friedman LS. Liver, biliary tract & pancreatic disorders: non-alcoholic fatty liver disease. New York, NY: Academic; 2015. p. 680–1.
59. Ahmed A, Wong RJ, Harrison SA. Nonalcoholic fatty liver disease review: diagnosis, treatment, and outcomes. Clin Gastroenterol Hepatol. 2015;13(12):2062–70.
60. Angulo P, Kleiner DE, Dam-Larsen S, Adams LA, Bjornsson ES, Charatcharoenwitthaya P, et al. Liver fibrosis, but no other histologic features, is associated with long-term outcomes of patients with nonalcoholic fatty liver disease. Gastroenterology. 2015;149(2):389–97.e10.
61. Goh GB, McCullough AJ. Natural history of nonalcoholic fatty liver disease. Dig Dis Sci. 2016;61(5):1226–33.
62. Bugianesi E, Leone N, Vanni E, Marchesini G, Brunello F, Carucci P, et al. Expanding the natural history of nonalcoholic steatohepatitis: from cryptogenic cirrhosis to hepatocellular carcinoma. Gastroenterology. 2002;123(1):134–40.
63. Njei B, Rotman Y, Ditah I, Lim JK. Emerging trends in hepatocellular carcinoma incidence and mortality. Hepatology. 2015;61(1):191–9.
64. Hashimoto E, Yatsuji S, Tobari M, Taniai M, Torii N, Tokushige K, et al. Hepatocellular carcinoma in patients with nonalcoholic steatohepatitis. J Gastroenterol. 2009;44(Suppl 19):89–95.
65. Younossi ZM, Otgonsuren M, Henry L, Venkatesan C, Mishra A, Erario M, et al. Association of nonalcoholic fatty liver disease (NAFLD) with hepatocellular carcinoma (HCC) in the United States from 2004 to 2009. Hepatology. 2015;62(6):1723–30.
66. Mittal S, El-Serag HB, Sada YH, Kanwal F, Duan Z, Temple S, et al. Hepatocellular carcinoma in the absence of cirrhosis in United States veterans is associated with nonalcoholic fatty liver disease. Clin Gastroenterol Hepatol. 2016;14(1):124–31.e1.
67. Rinella ME. Nonalcoholic fatty liver disease: a systematic review. JAMA. 2015; 313(22):2263–73.
68. Wong CR, Nguyen MH, Lim JK. Hepatocellular carcinoma in patients with non-alcoholic fatty liver disease. World J Gastroenterol. 2016;22(37):8294–303.

69. Younossi ZM, Blissett D, Blissett R, Henry L, Stepanova M, Younossi Y, et al. The economic and clinical burden of nonalcoholic fatty liver disease in the United States and Europe. Hepatology. 2016;64(5):1577–86.
70. Martini EM, Garrett N, Lindquist T, Isham GJ. The boomers are coming: a total cost of care model of the impact of population aging on health care costs in the United States by major practice category. Health Serv Res. 2007;42(1 Pt 1):201–18.
71. Younossi ZM, Henry L. Economic and quality-of-life implications of non-alcoholic fatty liver disease. Pharmacoeconomics. 2015;33(12):1245–53.

15 Clinical Epidemiology of Chronic Liver Disease: Hepatocellular Carcinoma

Duminda Suraweera, Peter Konyn, Thomas Vu, and Sammy Saab

Abstract

Hepatocellular carcinoma (HCC) is one of the leading causes of cancer-related deaths in the world. Incidence of HCC is expected to increase in the future with much of this burden concentrated in developing nations, currently accounting for 83% of total HCC deaths. Worldwide rates of HCC vary dramatically by region, reflecting major epidemiologic differences. Incidence is higher in men and the elderly. Chronic hepatitis B and hepatitis C viral infections are the leading causes of HCC with rising rates of obesity, diabetes and nonalcoholic steatohepatitis playing an ever-increasing role in the development and progression of HCC. To develop effective region specific prevention, screening and management strategies will require close examination of the epidemiology of HCC. In this chapter, we aim to explore the global epidemiologic aspects of HCC with a focus on current trends and the risk factors that contribute to these trends.

Keywords

Hepatocellular carcinoma · Hepatitis B virus · Hepatitis C virus · Hepatocellular carcinoma epidemiology

D. Suraweera · T. Vu
Department of Medicine, Olive View-UCLA Medical Center, Sylmar, CA, USA

P. Konyn
Department of Medicine, University of California at Los Angeles, Los Angeles, CA, USA

S. Saab (✉)
Department of Medicine, University of California at Los Angeles, Los Angeles, CA, USA

Pfleger Liver Institute, UCLA Medical Center, Los Angeles, CA, USA
e-mail: SSaab@mednet.ucla.edu

R. J. Wong, R. G. Gish (eds.), *Clinical Epidemiology of Chronic Liver Diseases*,
https://doi.org/10.1007/978-3-319-94355-8_15

15.1 Introduction

Hepatocellular carcinoma (HCC) is one of the leading causes of cancer-related deaths in the world. It is the fifth most common cancer in men, the ninth most common cancer in women and the second most common cause of death in both sexes, accounting for 9% of total deaths from cancer [1, 2]. Incidence of HCC is expected to increase in the future with much of this burden concentrated in developing nations (Fig. 15.1), currently accounting for 83% of total HCC deaths [3]. Based on the World Health Organization's International Agency of Research on Cancer, Africa and East Asia account for approximately 80% of HCC globally [4]. Developed nations are also significantly affected. In the United States the incidence of HCC increased from 4.4/100,000 in 2000 to 6.7/100,000 in 2012 [5]. Chronic viral infections of hepatitis B virus (HBV) and hepatitis C virus (HCV) are well documented risk factors for HCC. These two viruses combined account for 60% of HCC cases worldwide [6]. Furthermore, rising rates of obesity, diabetes and nonalcoholic steatohepatitis play an ever-increasing role in the development and progression of HCC [7, 8]. In this chapter, we aim to explore the global epidemiologic aspects of HCC with a focus on current trends and the risk factors that contribute to these trends (Table).

15.2 Epidemiology by Geography

15.2.1 Africa

Africa has a population of about 1.2 billion people [9]. The true incidence of HCC in Africa is difficult to assess due to incomplete and sometimes inaccurate or biased data [10]. Furthermore, the lack of access to medical care and absence of advanced diagnostic methods contribute to an underestimation of HCC incidence. With the current data available, it is estimated that the incidence of HCC is

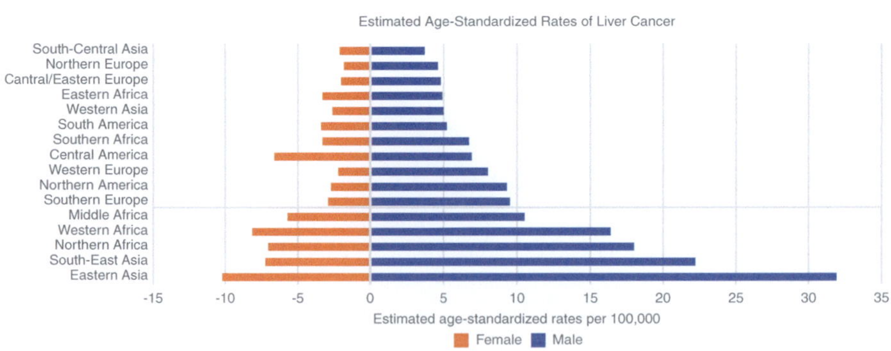

Fig. 15.1 Comparing regional estimates of age standardized rates of liver cancer among men and women [2]

41.2/100,000 in sub-Saharan Africa, 29.7/100,000 in eastern Africa, and 20.9/100,000 in western Africa [11]. HCC is estimated to account for 20% of all malignancies in sub-Saharan Africa [10, 12]. HCC is not uniformly common in African countries with significant regional differences. For example, in Mozambique recorded rates of HCC occur at a higher incidence in eastern areas [10, 13]. Furthermore, differences in HCC rates have been noted between high and low lying geographic areas in Swaziland, between different tribes in Uganda and between urban and rural populations in South Africa [10, 14–16]. These differences highlight the environmental influences that likely play an important role in the epidemiology of HCC in Africa.

Changes in HCC rates in Africa over time are difficult to ascertain due to limited data. In Uganda, the incidence of HCC may have remained unchanged from 1954–1960 to 1993–1997 [10, 17]. However a recent study evaluating HCC incidence in Kampala, Uganda found rates of HCC increasing in the city from 1960–1980 to 1991–2005 [18]. The age-standardized incidence rates of HCC in males remained stable from 6.15/100,000 (95% CI 5.13–7.17) to 5.38/100,000 (95% CI 4.55–6.20) while the incidence in females increased from 2.65/100,000 (95% CI 1.85–3.44) to 4.14/100,000 (95% CI 3.42–4.86) with the male to female ratio decreasing from 2.32 to 1.3. The same study found no indication of increasing prevalence of HBV or HCV. The authors hypothesized that the increasing rates may be due to the large influx of rural populations, who have documented higher exposures to environmental toxins such as aflatoxin. Yet another study in South Africa found a decrease in the rates of HCC by 32% between 1964 and 1994 [19]. The study population were gold miners who often immigrated from neighboring African countries. Interestingly over the same time period there was a significant shift in the labor force with more migrant workers arriving from countries with a lower incidence of HCC, highlighting the complex and dynamic effect of migration in the rates of HCC in African countries.

Chronic HBV is the primary cause of HCC in Africa [20]. It is believed that the vast majority of HBV infections in Africa occur as a result of horizontal transmission, with only a small rate of perinatal infection [21]. The institution of HBV vaccination began in Africa in the 1990s with significant variance in adoption rates in different countries. Overall, the contribution of HCV in the development of HCC is significantly less than that of HBV in Africa [10]. Data from the Republic of the Gambia found that 57% of HCC could be attributed to HBV and 20% attributed to HCV [22]. Furthermore, exposure to environmental toxins like aflatoxin and iron overload also likely contribute to the high incidence of HCC and large geographic variations of HCC rates [23–25].

15.2.2 China

Liver cancer is the second most common cancer in China [26]. Males have an estimated incidence of 40.0/100,000 and females of 15.3/100,000. It is the second leading cause of cancer mortality in males and third in females. The mortality rate in

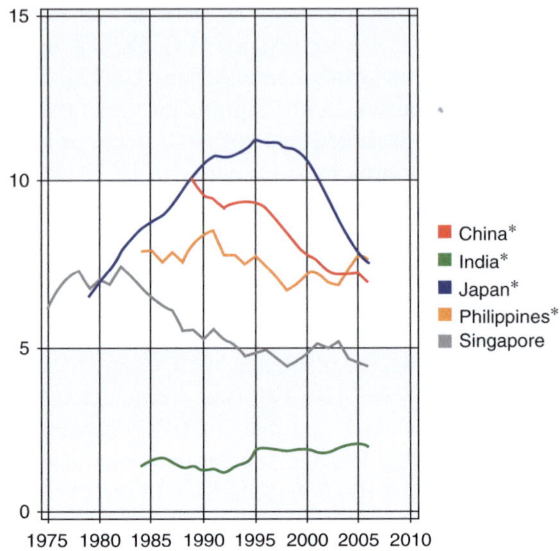

Fig. 15.2 Comparing regional rates of hepatocellular carcinoma to the prevalence of viral hepatitis [2, 26]

males is estimated to be 37.4/100,000 and in females 14.3/100,000. China alone accounts for 50% of all HCC-related deaths worldwide [27].

While trends in disease incidence in China are mixed, there are some signs of decreasing HCC incidence (Fig. 15.2). In Shanghai and Tianjun, there has been a documented decline in HCC incidence rates over the last 30–40 years [28]. In Hong Kong there has been an overall decrease in HCC incidence in all age groups over the past 25 years [29]. This may be partially explained by the decline in HBV infection after the introduction of universal HBV vaccination in Hong Kong in 1988.

Viral hepatitis accounts for the clear majority of HCC in China [30]. According to one systematic assessment of relative risk meta-analyses and large scale observational studies in China, HBV accounts for 63.9% of all cases of HCC, 65.9% among men and 58.4% among women [30]. Hepatitis C virus accounts for 27.7% of all HCC in China, 27.3% in men and 28.6% in women. Other commonly associated risk factors include aflatoxin exposure (25%), alcohol (15.7%) and tobacco use (13.9%).

15.2.3 Europe

HCC accounts for approximately 47,000 deaths per year in Europe [31]. Europe has an overall higher rate of HCC than the United States with significant geographic variation. Southern Europe has the highest incidence of HCC (9.8/100,000) while Northern Europe has the lowest (3.8/100,000). Eastern Europe has an incidence of 4.6/100,000 and Western Europe has a rate of 7.2/100,000.

Blachier et al. conducted a survey of 260 epidemiological studies and found that while the etiology HCC in Europe varies with geographic distribution, HCV is the major risk factor for HCC in Europe, accounting for 60–70% of cases of cirrhosis [32]. Alcohol accounts for 20% and HBV 10–15%. Overall the incidence of chronic HCV in Europe is estimated between 0.13% and 3.26%, compared to HBV at 0.1–0.7%. Many acquired HCV in the 1970s and 1980s prior to the identification of the virus. While the transmission of HCV has been reduced dramatically since then, a high prevalence is still present in injection drug users (IDUs). Prevalence in IDUs ranges from 50% in Cyprus to 83.2% in Italy [33, 34]. However, due to the prolonged progression of the disease, Europe is only seeing the peak of disease burden.

15.2.4 India

Based on recent population-based cancer registries published in 2012, liver cancer is the 7th most common cancer in India among men and the 11th in women [35]. Historical autopsy data revealed the presence of HCC in 0.2–1.9% of cases, with a higher prevalence of HCC in Southeastern states of India [36]. It is estimated that the age adjusted incidence rate of HCC in men ranged from 0.9 to 7.5/100,000 and in women from 0.2 to 2.2/100,000 [35]. The male to female ratio of HCC in India is 4:1.

HCC in India has been increasing (Fig. 15.2). In 1998 there were 10,000 documented cases of HCC, in 2002 13,630 cases and in 2009 25,000 cases; it is predicted that there will be 30,000–50,000 cases by 2016 [35, 37]. Dikshit et al. conducted a landmark population based survey of cancer related mortality in India from 2001 and 2003 using verbal autopsy data from 1.1 million homes across India [38]. The authors used this data along with the United Nations data for deaths in India in 2010 to extrapolate the mortality rates from HCC that occurred in 2010. In men, it is estimated that in 2010, 14,000 deaths might have occurred due to liver cancer with an age standardized mortality rate of 6.5/100,000. In women, it is estimated that approximately 12,000 deaths occurred due to liver cancer with an age standardized mortality rate of 5.1/100,000. Overall there has been a large discrepancy between population-based estimates and documented cases of HCC in India, leading many to believe that there is a considerable underestimation in reporting of HCC [37]. There may, however, be an overestimation of the impact of HBV on development of HCC in India for several reasons. A large portion of HBV cases in India have low HBV DNA, which is associated with lower frequency of HCC. In addition, there may be variances in HBV genotypes and mutations that confer lower risk for HCC. Last, the average life expectancy in India is 68, whereas the incidence of HCC tends to peak in those older than 70 [4].

HBV is the most common cause of HCC in India [39]. In one case-control study involving 213 patients with hepatocellular carcinoma, HBV accounted for 150 cases, 70.42% (OR, 48.02; 95% CI 25.06–91.98). In contrast, HCV accounted for only 26 cases of HCC, 12.21% (OR, 5.45; 95% CI 2.02–14.71). Coinfection with HBV/HCV was found in ten patients (4.69%). Heavy alcohol intake was found in 34, 15.96% (OR, 2.83; 95% CI 1.51–5.28). While the study did not find any synergism between alcohol and HBV, a synergistic effect between HCV and alcohol was found (synergy index, 1.257).

15.2.5 Middle East

The incidence of HCC varies greatly among different regions in the Middle East [40, 41]. Egypt sees the highest incidence of liver cancer with 21.9/100,000 in males and 4.5/100,000 in females [40]. In contrast, Iran has the lowest incidence with 1.4/100,000 in males and 1.9/100,000 in females. In Middle Eastern countries, the prevalence of HCC is high among males and rural residents.

Viral hepatitis is the main etiology of HCC in the Middle East. Depending on the region, HBV or HCV are responsible for most HCC cases. HBV prevalence varies significantly between regions, ranging from 0.8–7% in Iran to 16–20% in Sudan [42–45]. Interestingly, even though HBV is prevalent in the Middle East, the prevalence of HCC is lower than what would be expected when comparing data from Asia. For example, in Iran HBV is the most common etiology of cirrhosis, with up to 35% of the population exposed to the virus and 3% with chronic infection [46]. However HCC is the 16th most prevalent cancer, diverging from higher rates documented in regions with similar prevalence of HBV [4]. This may be due regional variances in HBV genotype and mutations [47, 48]. Overall, HBV is likely the predominant factor in the development of HCC in Jordan, Kuwait, Lebanon, Syria, Iran and Turkey [49]. As with HBV, the prevalence of HCV in the Middle East varies greatly depending on region, ranging from 0.1–0.6% in Lebanon to 22% in Egypt [50]. In one Egyptian case-control study comparing 33 patients with HCC and 35 health patients, HCV was found in 75.8% of patients with HCC and 42.9% in healthy individuals (p = 0.01) [51]. The authors estimated the attributable fraction of HCC to HCV at 64% in the study population and 48% in the general Egyptian population. In addition to Egypt, HCV is likely the most common etiology of HCC in Saudi Arabia [49].

15.2.6 United States

The overall incidence of HCC in the United States is lower than that in the developing world. In 2012, the age adjusted incidence rate for HCC was 6.7/100,000 [5]. The average age of diagnosis of HCC in the United States is 65 years with 95% of patients diagnosed between 2000–2012 older than 45 and 54% diagnosed during age 50–69 years. Males comprise a clear majority of those with HCC at 73%. Males had an incidence rate of 10.8/100,000 and females of 3.2/100,000 in 2012. The racial distribution of HCC is 48% Caucasian, 13% African American, 15% Hispanic and 24% other/Asian [52]. The southern and western regions of the United States have the highest rates of HCC. In 2012, the highest incidence of HCC was in Texas (9.71/100,000), with Hawaii having the second highest (9.68/100,000) [5]. The state with the lowest HCC incidence rate was North Dakota (2.4/100,000).

The incidence of HCC in the United States has been rising. The age-adjusted incidence of HCC has tripled from 1975 to 2005 [53]. Furthermore, data from the National Cancer Institute's Surveillance, Epidemiology and End Results (SEER) Database of the National Cancer institute in the U.S. indicate that the incidence rates of HCC increased by 3.1% per year from 2008 to 2012 [54]. The rate of increase does appear to have slowed, with incidence increasing by 4.5% from 2000 to 2009 but only by 0.7% from 2010 to 2012. This increase in HCC incidence in the United States is likely due to the prevalence of HCV from blood transfusion and injection drug use. The average annual percentage change from 2000 to 2012 was highest in 55–59 year olds at 8.9% [5]. Males have seen a higher rate of increase in incidence with the average annual percentage change from 2000 to 2012 of 3.7% compared to females at 2.7%. Variations in the incidence of HCC in populations in the United States are continuously changing, as well [55]. In 2008, the highest incidence was seen in Asian/Pacific Islanders with an incidence of 11.7/100,000 and the lowest in whites with an incidence of 3.9/100,000 [53]. In 2012, the rates in Hispanics had surpassed that of Asians [5]. Hispanics have seen the fastest sustained rise in HCC age adjusted incidence rates. While the reasons for this are not fully understood, high rates of HCV, alcoholic liver disease, metabolic syndrome and nonalcoholic fatty liver disease (NAFLD) are likely contributing factors [56–60]. The decrease in incidence in Asian/Pacific Islanders is largely thought to be due to the widespread adoption of the HBV vaccine and effective antiviral therapies, as chronic HBV is the predominant cause of HCC in this population [5]. The states that have seen the largest increase in HCC incidence rates are Kansas, Utah, Idaho, Arizona and Georgia.

HCC trends in the United States reflect the changing prevalence of risk factors. The leading risk factor in the United States is HCV with approximately 50–60% of HCC attributed to chronic HCV [27]. Like Europe, the United States is likely only now experiencing the peak of HCV-associated comorbidities. The baby boomer generation (1945–1965), in particular, is heavily affected due to exposure to blood products in the 1970s and potentially higher rates of high risk behavior among this group. This has led to adaptation of HCV screening protocols for this population [61]. Due to the widespread implementation of HBV vaccination programs, HBV only contributes to 10–15% of HCC in the United States [62].

15.3 Risk Factors

15.3.1 Viral Hepatitis

15.3.1.1 Hepatitis B

Much of the worldwide HCC burden is attributed to HBV infection (Fig. 15.3) [63]. HBV is a DNA virus with eight known genotypes. Genotype A is typically found in sub-Saharan Africa, Western Africa and Northern Europe while genotype B is predominantly found in Japan and East Asia. Genotype C can be found in China, Korea, Japan, Southeast Asia and South Pacific Islands. Genotype D has a large distribution

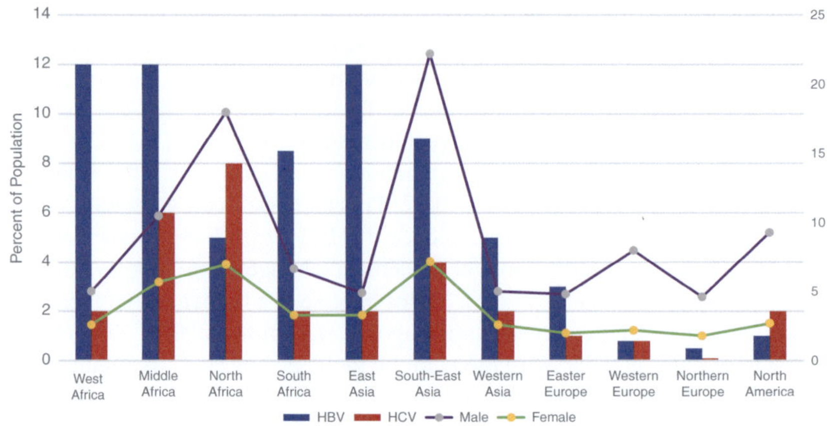

Fig. 15.3 Changing rates of hepatocellular carcinoma in Asia over the last 30 years. *Regional data [2]

including Eastern Europe, the Middle East, North Africa and India. Genotype E is endemic to West Africa, with genotype F and H in Central and South America [64]. In endemic areas, HBV is typically acquired at birth or early childhood. In Asia, the primary modality of transmission is vertical while in Africa horizontal transmission is more common. In the U.S., it is estimated that 850,000 to 2.2 million people are living with chronic HBV [65]. The carcinogenicity of chronic HBV was first established by the Internal Agency for Research on Cancer in 1994 after the analysis of multiple cohort and case-control studies [66]. Unlike many other HCC risk factors, HBV does not require cirrhosis prior to malignant transformation. The likely mechanism of HBV-associated HCC is twofold: one via chronic hepatic injury resulting in hepatocyte regeneration leading to mutations and secondly via direct HBV DNA integration in the host genome resulting in transactivation of oncogenes [67, 68]. Vaccination against HBV has been extremely effective; in fact, HCC was the first malignancy to have rates demonstrably reduced by vaccination. One longitudinal, 20-year follow up study in Taiwan after the introduction of vaccination found that the incidence of HBV decreased significantly among children with the incidence of HBV decreasing in children 6–9 years from 0.51 to 0.15/100,000, in children 10–14 years from 0.6 to 0.19/100,000, and in children 15–19 years from 0.52 to 0.16/100,000 [69].

15.3.1.2 Hepatitis C

The increasing incidence of HCC in the developed world is largely due to chronic HCV infection [7, 70]. HCV is an RNA virus that was first identified in 1989 [71]. There are six major genotypes of HCV. Genotype 1 is the most common worldwide, with genotypes 1a and 1b predominantly found in Europe and the Americas while genotype 1b is found mainly in Asia [72]. Genotype 4 is endemic in Africa. It is estimated that 200 million people are infected with HCV worldwide (Fig. 15.3) [73]. In the U.S., it is estimated that 2.7–3.5 million people have chronic HCV infection [74]. HCV can be acquired at any age via contact with blood and transmission varies depending on country-specific medical and recreational practices. Injection drug use is an important risk factor for HCV. It is estimated that as high as 60–80% of IDUs worldwide have anti-HCV antibodies, a higher incidence of infection than that of human immunodeficiency virus (HIV) in this population [75]. Hepatitis C has a high rate of conversion to chronic progressive infection regardless of the age at which it is acquired. The mechanism of HCV-mediated HCC is likely through the development of liver fibrosis and cirrhosis from chronic inflammation. Malignant transformation is primarily due to viral proteins evoking host responses that lead to apoptosis, reactive oxygen species formation, upregulation of interleukin 1, 2 and tumor necrosis factor α [76]. In contrast to HBV, HCV is unable to integrate directly into the host genome and does not lead to HCC in the absence of cirrhosis. With the advent of direct acting antiviral agents (DAAs), there is now the potential to successfully treat chronic HCV infection with high rates of sustained virologic response (SVR) even in previously difficult to treat populations [77, 78]. A 2013 meta-analysis of 30 studies showed that SVR was associated with a reduced risk of HCC (RR 0.24; 95% CI 0.18–0.31) [79]. HCC developed at a rate of 0.33% per year in patients with SVR compared to 1.67% per year among patients with detectable viral loads.

15.3.2 Toxins

15.3.2.1 Alcohol

Alcoholic cirrhosis is a leading cause of HCC globally [64, 80–82]. Alcohol accounts for around 1.8 million deaths annually, with HCC being a major contributor to alcohol-related mortality [83]. Chronic use of alcohol is associated with a five to tenfold increase in the risk of HCC [84–86]. Daily alcohol use later in life is associated with the development of liver cirrhosis, which is an independent risk factor for HCC [87]. Approximately 8–20% of those who chronically consume alcohol will eventually develop liver cirrhosis, putting them at increased risk for HCC [88]. However, while case studies exist demonstrating development of HCC without cirrhosis, a strong understanding of the carcinogenic effects of alcohol on the liver has yet to be established [81, 89]. A direct, dose-dependent relationship has been identified between alcohol and HCC [84, 90–92]. Alcohol is proposed to affect the development of HCC by way of activating the NF-kB pathway as well as by formation of reactive oxygen species through upregulation of CYP2E1 and metabolic abnormalities caused by increased NADH to NAD+ ratio [93–96]. Among those with alcoholic cirrhosis, the incidence of HCC is 0.2–2.5% per year [85, 97, 98], which is higher than the incidence in alcoholics without cirrhosis (0.01% per year) [85, 86, 99]. Alcohol use has been observed to act synergistically with HCV and HBV infections to increase the risk for HCC [39, 87, 100, 101]. Differences in risk for HCC among those with alcoholic cirrhosis varies based on genetics, and polymorphisms in several genes have been linked to increased risk of HCC in alcoholic cirrhosis, including PNPLA3 rs738409, myeloperoxidase, superoxide dismutase 2, MTHFR,

ALDH2 [102–104]. Other risk factors for progression to HCC in alcoholic liver cirrhosis include diabetes mellitus, male sex, and age [105].

15.3.2.2 Aflatoxin

The aflatoxin class of mycotoxins produced by certain members of the Aspergillus genus is a known hepatic carcinogen, categorized as a Class 1 carcinogen by the International Agency for Research on Cancer [106]. There are four known carcinogenic aflatoxins, which are aflatoxin B1, aflatoxin B2, aflatoxin G1 and aflatoxin G2, with aflatoxin B1 being the strongest carcinogen of the four, and the strongest reported hepatic carcinogen in existence [107]. Exposure to aflatoxins is classically through consumption of food contaminated with Aspergillus molds from unsafe storage methods, or by occupational exposure from those who work with contaminated foods, particularly cereals, oleaginous seeds, cocoa, coffee, grapevine, wine, fruits, spices, and dried fruit [107, 108]. Contamination of food by Aspergillus mold is most common in regions of the world with warm and humid climates which support its growth, such as sub-Saharan Africa, Eastern Asia, and parts of South America [64, 107]. A synergistic relationship in HCC carcinogenesis between aflatoxin B1 and HCC is becoming better established, with recent studies reporting that, while aflatoxin B1 exposure and HBV infection alone had a mean odds ratio of HCC development of 1.9 and 9.5 respectively, a combination of both risk factors had an odds ratio of 63.2 [107]. This is of particular importance, as it is estimated that 4.5–5.5 billion people in the world are at risk of being exposed to aflatoxins, and an estimated 55 million people worldwide currently suffer from exposure to levels of aflatoxins above the safe level of consumption, with many of the regions where aflatoxin exposure is most common having high rates of HBV infection as well [109–111]. The mechanism by which aflatoxin B1 achieves tumorigenesis is most commonly through an arginine to serine mutation at codon 249 of the p53 tumor suppressor gene made possible by a toxic epoxide metabolite of aflatoxin B1 which can bind to DNA [112–114]. Repair of this damage is inhibited in HBV infection due to inhibition of repair enzymes by HBV X protein, the gene for which is often integrated into cellular DNA by HBV virions [115, 116].

15.3.3 Metabolic

15.3.3.1 Nonalcoholic Fatty Liver Disease

Nonalcoholic fatty liver disease (NAFLD) is another important risk factor for HCC to be aware of, especially given the rising rates of obesity, metabolic syndrome, and type 2 diabetes mellitus globally, all of which are risk factors for the development of hepatic steatosis [7, 64, 117–119]. As many as 94% of people with obesity will develop some degree of hepatic steatosis during their lifetime, the severity of which directly correlates with their body mass index (BMI) [64, 120, 121]. With the rising rate of NAFLD, it has become one of the major causes of HCC in developed regions of the world, despite the fact that HCC incidence in NASH-cirrhosis is significantly lower than in HCV-cirrhosis [7, 8, 122, 123]. A U.S.-based population study found that in 2010, 59% of HCC cases could be attributed to NAFLD [124]. A more recent study found that the number of HCC cases associated with NAFLD is increasing by 9% every year [118]. NAFLD and its more severe form nonalcoholic steatohepatitis (NASH), increase the risk for developing liver cirrhosis which puts an individual at increased risk for HCC [120, 125]. However, many non-cirrhotic patients with NAFLD develop HCC, which may be explained by the pro-inflammatory characteristics of obesity, enhanced oxidative stress from increased fatty acid oxidation in hepatocytes, inflammatory and angiogenic influences of insulin resistance often seen alongside NAFLD, and steatosis-induced loss of CD4+ T-lymphocytes in the liver [126–130]. Patients who are obese and suffer from type 2 diabetes mellitus have twice the risk of developing HCC [131, 132]. The yearly cumulative incidence of HCC in patients with cirrhosis is 0.3–4% per year [8, 133–135]. This is particularly significant since as many as 5–7% of people living in the western world currently have NASH, and 2–3% are living with cirrhosis [126, 136, 137].

15.3.3.2 Diabetes

Not only does type 2 diabetes mellitus (DM) increase risk of HCC by increasing risk for NAFLD and cirrhosis, it is also believed to be an independent risk factor for HCC [64, 80, 138–140]. Individuals with type 2 DM (T2DM) have 1.87–4.1 times the risk of developing HCC than non-diabetic persons [101, 127]. The mechanism of tumorigenesis in T2DM-associated HCC involves a complex relationship between cellular proliferation due to hyperinsulinemia and enhanced oxidative stress from the upregulation of inflammatory cytokines [119, 141, 142]. Furthermore, studies have demonstrated that treatment with metformin and statins greatly reduces HCC risk in those with T2DM [143, 144]. T2DM also synergistically increases HCC risk when present alongside heavy consumption of alcohol (>4 drinks per day) and viral hepatitis [101, 145].

15.3.4 Other

Other risk factors for HCC include less common causes of liver cirrhosis such as primary biliary cholangitis, autoimmune hepatitis, alpha-1-antitrypsin deficiency and Wilson's Disease [7]. HIV has also been shown to act synergistically in increasing the severity of HCV infections, further increasing HCC risk [80].

15.3.4.1 Hereditary Hemochromatosis

Hereditary hemochromatosis is an autosomal recessive disorder that results in excess absorption of iron from the gastrointestinal tract, resulting in an iron overload state. It is associated with increased risk for HCC even in non-cirrhotic patients [146]. Yang et al. analyzed the data from the United States National Center for Health Statistics and found that patients with hereditary hemochromatosis had a 23-fold increased risk of developing liver cancer compared to those without the disease (proportionate mortality ratio 22.6; 95% CI 20.6–24.6) [147]. It is believed that iron overload states stimulate hepatic fibrogenesis through the production of oxygen free radicals and cytokines such as tumor growth factor β [148].

15.3.4.2 Tobacco

Data on tobacco as a risk factor for HCC have been mixed. One prospective case control study looking at 210 patients with HCC in Michigan found an increased risk of HCC in those with greater than 20 pack-years compared with cirrhotic patients without HCC (OR 4.9; 95% CI 2.2–10.6) and those with no underlying liver disease (OR 63.7; 95% CI 16.7–144.2) [91]. Another United States-based study using case-control data from the Selected Cancer Study found no increase in risk of primary liver cancer in current smokers, although there was a statistically significant increase in risk of primary liver cancer in former smokers (1.85; 95% CI 1.05–3.25) [149]. A study based in Taiwan involving 12,008 men found that tobacco interacted additively with HCV positivity in the development of HCC, although the synergistic indices were not statistically significant [150]. There is also strong evidence that tobacco use increases mortality in patients with HCC. Jee et al. found that current smoking was associated with an increased risk of mortality among Korean men with HCC (RR 1.4; 95% CI 1.3–1.6) [151].

Conclusion

Hepatocellular carcinoma is a common worldwide malignancy that places a significant burden on global healthcare resources. While the rates of HCC vary greatly by region, the incidence of HCC in general is increasing. The primary driver of HCC is chronic liver disease which may result from a wide variety of etiologies. Of these etiologies, HBV is the leading cause of HCC in the developing world, while HCV is the leading cause in the developed world. Chronic liver disease related to metabolic disorders are increasing in prevalence and likely will play a significant role in HCC development in the future, especially in the developed world. There is an imperative need for further study of the epidemiology of HCC and its risk factors to help guide the prevention, screening and management strategies of tomorrow.

Disclosure The authors of this manuscript have no conflicts of interest to disclose.

Summary Table of Landmark Literature

Study	Study design	Summary results	Main limitations
Wabinga HR et al. British Journal of Cancer. 2000;82(9):1585–92 [17]	Population-based retrospective study in cancer incidence in Kyando country, Uganda	• Incidence of HCC unchanged from 1954 to 1997	• Completeness and quality of registry data available

Study	Study design	Summary results	Main limitations
Ocama et al. British Journal of Cancer. 2009;100(5):799–802 [18]	Population-based retrospective study of liver cancer in Central Uganda	• Incidence of HCC increased in city populations	• Completeness and quality of registry data available
McGlashan et al. British Journal of Cancer. 2003;88(9):1361–9 [19]	Population-based retrospective study of cancer in miners working South Africa	• Incidence of HCC decreased from 1964 to 1994	• Very specific population of miners who were often from varied regions
Kirk et al. Hepatology. 2004;39(1):211–9 [22]	Population-based retrospective study of liver cancer in the Gambia	• HBV accounted for 57% of HCC and HCV for 20%	• Completeness and quality of data available
Chen et al. Annals of Translational Medicine. 2014;2(7):61 [28]	Population-based cross-sectional study of cancer incidence and mortality in China in 2010	• Decrease in incidence of HCC in Shanghai and Tianjun	• Varying representation of different populations and regions in registry data
Yuen et al. Hepatology. 2000;31(2):330–5 [29]	Prospective study of HCC management in Hong Kong from 1995 to 1997	• Screening for HCC in chronic HBV/HCV patients by AFP and/or USG can identify early HCC, resulting in a higher chance of treatment	• Possible lead time bias in early detection group
Fan et al. Asian Pacific Journal of Cancer Prevention. 2013;14(12):7251–6 [30]	Systemic assessment of several population-based studies on risk factors of HCC in China	• HBV accounts for 63.9% of HCC, HCV for 27.7%	• Some risk factors were not assessed, i.e. diabetes/obesity • Possible interaction on liver cancer mortality not assessed
Blachier et al. Journal of Hepatology. 2013;58(3):593–608 [32]	Systemic assessment of several population-based studies on risk factors of HCC in Europe	• HCV is major risk factor of HCC in Europe	• Quality of studies included in analysis

Study	Study design	Summary results	Main limitations
Dikshit et al. Lancet. 2012;379(9828):1807–16 [38]	Population-based retrospective study in cancer mortality in India	• Age standardized HCC mortality in India in 2010 was 6.5/100,000 in men and 5.1/100,000 in women	• Study accuracy dependent on accuracy of verbal autopsy
Kumar et al. Hepatology. 2007;22(7):1104–11 [39].	Case-control study in risk factor analysis of HCC in India	• HBV accounts for 70.42% of HCC, HCV for 12.21%	• Small number of cases studied for certain conclusions
Hassan et al. Journal of Clinical Gastroenterology. 2001;33(2):123–6 [51]	Case-control study in role of HCV in HCC in Egypt	• HCV found in 75.8% of HCC patients and 42.9% of healthy individuals	• Most patients were from low socioeconomic status that likely resulted in a higher prevalence of HCV
White et al. Gastroenterology. 2016 [Epub ahead of print] [5]	Population-based retrospective study in incidence of HCC in U.S. from 2000 to 2012	• Incidence of HCC has increased but rate of increase has decreased from 2010 to 2012	• Cancer registry used did not provide data on risk factors to determine etiology or clinical data needed to determine stage of HCC
Ryerson et al. Cancer. 2016;122(9):1312–37 [54]	Population-based retrospective study in incidence of HCC from 1975 to 2012 in U.S.	• Incidence of HCC increased by 3.1% per year from 2008 to 2012	• Local level variations in data quality • Incomplete geographic or population reporting
Younossi et al. BMC Gastroenterology. 2016;16:45 [61]	Prospective multi-center study evaluating HCV screening protocol and linkage to care	• Screening leads to high linkage to care	• Study populations was based on referrals indicating access to insurance coverage thus biased to excluding uninsured

References

1. Ferlay J, Soerjomataram I, Dikshit R, Eser S, Mathers C, Rebelo M, et al. Cancer incidence and mortality worldwide: sources, methods and major patterns in GLOBOCAN 2012. Int J Cancer. 2015;136(5):E359–86.
2. Ferlay J, Soerjomataram I, Ervik M, Dikshit R, Eser S, Mathers C, et al. GLOBOCAN 2012 v1.0, Cancer Incidence and Mortality Worldwide: IARC CancerBase no. 11 [Internet]. Lyon: International Agency for Research on Cancer; 2013. http://globocan.iarc.fr. Accessed 11 Jan 2017.

3. Venook AP, Papandreou C, Furuse J, de Guevara LL. The incidence and epidemiology of hepatocellular carcinoma: a global and regional perspective. Oncologist. 2010;15(Suppl 4):5–13.
4. International Agency for Research on Cancer (IARC-WHO). http://Ci5.iarc.fr. Accessed 11 Jan 2017.
5. White DL, Thrift AP, Kanwal F, Davila J, El-Serag HB. Incidence of hepatocellular carcinoma in all 50 United States, from 2000 through 2012. Gastroenterology. 2017;152(4):812–820.e5.
6. de Martel C, Maucort-Boulch D, Plummer M, Franceschi S. World-wide relative contribution of hepatitis B and C viruses in hepatocellular carcinoma. Hepatology (Baltimore, MD). 2015;62(4):1190–200.
7. Dhanasekaran R, Limaye A, Cabrera R. Hepatocellular carcinoma: current trends in worldwide epidemiology, risk factors, diagnosis, and therapeutics. Hepat Med. 2012;4:19–37.
8. White DL, Kanwal F, El-Serag HB. Association between nonalcoholic fatty liver disease and risk for hepatocellular cancer, based on systematic review. Clin Gastroenterol Hepatol. 2012;10(12):1342–59.e2.
9. United Nations DoEaSA, Population Division. World population prospects: the 2015 revision, methodology of the United Nations population estimates and projections (ESA/P/WP.242); 2015.
10. Kew MC. Epidemiology of hepatocellular carcinoma in sub-Saharan Africa. Ann Hepatol. 2013;12(2):173–82.
11. Parkin D, Ferlay J, Hamdi-Cherif M, Thomas J, Wabinga H, Whelan S. Cancer in Africa: epidemiology and prevention. IARC Sci Publ. 2003;153:1–414.
12. Steiner PE. Comparison of liver cancer and cirrhosis in nine areas in trans-Saharan Africa. Acta Unio Int Contra Cancrum. 1961;17:798–825.
13. Prates MD, Torres FO. A cancer survey in Lourenco Marques, Portuguese East Africa. J Natl Cancer Inst. 1965;35(5):729–57.
14. Peers FG, Gilman GA, Linsell CA. Dietary aflatoxins and human liver cancer. A study in Swaziland. Int J Cancer. 1976;17(2):167–76.
15. Alpert ME, Hutt MS, Davidson CS. Primary hepatoma in Uganda. A prospective clinical and epidemiologic study of forty-six patients. Am J Med. 1969;46(5):794–802.
16. Kew MC, Fujita Y, Takahashi H, Coppins A, Wands JR. Comparison between polyclonal and first and second generation monoclonal radioimmunoassays in the detection of hepatitis B surface antigen in patients with hepatocellular carcinoma. Hepatology (Baltimore, MD). 1986;6(4):636–9.
17. Wabinga HR, Parkin DM, Wabwire-Mangen F, Nambooze S. Trends in cancer incidence in Kyadondo County, Uganda, 1960–1997. Br J Cancer. 2000;82(9):1585–92.
18. Ocama P, Nambooze S, Opio CK, Shiels MS, Wabinga HR, Kirk GD. Trends in the incidence of primary liver cancer in Central Uganda, 1960–1980 and 1991–2005. Br J Cancer. 2009;100(5):799–802.
19. McGlashan ND, Harington JS, Chelkowska E. Changes in the geographical and temporal patterns of cancer incidence among black gold miners working in South Africa, 1964–1996. Br J Cancer. 2003;88(9):1361–9.
20. Kew MC. Clinical, pathologic, and etiologic heterogeneity in hepatocellular carcinoma: evidence from southern Africa. Hepatology (Baltimore, MD). 1981;1(4):366–9.
21. Kew MC. Progress towards the comprehensive control of hepatitis B in Africa: a view from South Africa. Gut. 1996;38(Suppl 2):S31–6.
22. Kirk GD, Lesi OA, Mendy M, Akano AO, Sam O, Goedert JJ, et al. The Gambia liver cancer study: infection with hepatitis B and C and the risk of hepatocellular carcinoma in West Africa. Hepatology (Baltimore, MD). 2004;39(1):211–9.
23. Tognarelli J, Ladep NG, Crossey MM, Okeke E, Duguru M, Banwat E, et al. Reasons why West Africa continues to be a hotbed for hepatocellular carcinoma. Niger Med J. 2015;56(4):231–5.
24. Gordeuk VR. African iron overload. Semin Hematol. 2002;39(4):263–9.

25. Gong YY, Egal S, Hounsa A, Turner PC, Hall AJ, Cardwell KF, et al. Determinants of aflatoxin exposure in young children from Benin and Togo, West Africa: the critical role of weaning. Int J Epidemiol. 2003;32(4):556–62.
26. Tanaka M, Katayama F, Kato H, Tanaka H, Wang J, Qiao YL, et al. Hepatitis B and C virus infection and hepatocellular carcinoma in China: a review of epidemiology and control measures. J Epidemiol. 2011;21(6):401–16.
27. El-Serag HB. Epidemiology of viral hepatitis and hepatocellular carcinoma. Gastroenterology. 2012;142(6):1264–73.e1.
28. Chen W, Zheng R, Zhang S, Zhao P, Zeng H, Zou X. Report of cancer incidence and mortality in China, 2010. Ann Transl Med. 2014;2(7):61.
29. Yuen MF, Cheng CC, Lauder IJ, Lam SK, Ooi CG, Lai CL. Early detection of hepatocellular carcinoma increases the chance of treatment: Hong Kong experience. Hepatology (Baltimore, MD). 2000;31(2):330–5.
30. Fan JH, Wang JB, Jiang Y, Xiang W, Liang H, Wei WQ, et al. Attributable causes of liver cancer mortality and incidence in China. Asian Pac J Cancer Prev. 2013;14(12):7251–6.
31. Ferlay J, Parkin DM, Steliarova-Foucher E. Estimates of cancer incidence and mortality in Europe in 2008. Eur J Cancer (Oxford, England). 2010;46(4):765–81.
32. Blachier M, Leleu H, Peck-Radosavljevic M, Valla DC, Roudot-Thoraval F. The burden of liver disease in Europe: a review of available epidemiological data. J Hepatol. 2013;58(3):593–608.
33. Demetriou VL, van de Vijver DA, Hezka J, Kostrikis LG, Kostrikis LG. Hepatitis C infection among intravenous drug users attending therapy programs in Cyprus. J Med Virol. 2010;82(2):263–70.
34. Camoni L, Regine V, Salfa MC, Nicoletti G, Canuzzi P, Magliocchetti N, et al. Continued high prevalence of HIV, HBV and HCV among injecting and noninjecting drug users in Italy. Ann Ist Super Sanita. 2010;46(1):59–65.
35. National Cancer Registry Program. http://ncrpindia.org/.
36. Dhir V, Mohandas KM. Epidemiology of digestive tract cancers in India. III. Liver. Indian J Gastroenterol. 1998;17(3):100–3.
37. Acharya SK. Epidemiology of hepatocellular carcinoma in India. J Clin Exp Hepatol. 2014;4(Suppl 3):S27–33.
38. Dikshit R, Gupta PC, Ramasundarahettige C, Gajalakshmi V, Aleksandrowicz L, Badwe R, et al. Cancer mortality in India: a nationally representative survey. Lancet (London, England). 2012;379(9828):1807–16.
39. Kumar M, Kumar R, Hissar SS, Saraswat MK, Sharma BC, Sakhuja P, et al. Risk factors analysis for hepatocellular carcinoma in patients with and without cirrhosis: a case-control study of 213 hepatocellular carcinoma patients from India. J Gastroenterol Hepatol. 2007;22(7):1104–11.
40. Salim EI, Moore MA, Al-Lawati JA, Al-Sayyad J, Bazawir A, Bener A, et al. Cancer epidemiology and control in the Arab world—past, present and future. Asian Pac J Cancer Prev. 2009;10(1):3–16.
41. Lehman EM, Soliman AS, Ismail K, Hablas A, Seifeldin IA, Ramadan M, et al. Patterns of hepatocellular carcinoma incidence in Egypt from a population-based cancer registry. Hepatol Res. 2008;38(5):465–73.
42. Pourshams A, Malekzadeh R, Monavvari A, Akbari MR, Mohamadkhani A, Yarahmadi S, et al. Prevalence and etiology of persistently elevated alanine aminotransferase levels in healthy Iranian blood donors. J Gastroenterol Hepatol. 2005;20(2):229–33.
43. Jahani MR, Motevalian SA, Mahmoodi M. Hepatitis B carriers in large vehicle drivers of Iran. Vaccine. 2003;21(17–18):1948–51.
44. Uzunalimoglu O, Yurdaydin C, Cetinkaya H, Bozkaya H, Sahin T, Colakoglu S, et al. Risk factors for hepatocellular carcinoma in Turkey. Dig Dis Sci. 2001;46(5):1022–8.
45. Qirbi N, Hall AJ. Epidemiology of hepatitis B virus infection in the Middle East. East Mediterr Health J. 2001;7(6):1034–45.

46. Merat S, Rezvan H, Nouraie M, Jamali A, Assari S, Abolghasemi H, et al. The prevalence of hepatitis B surface antigen and anti-hepatitis B core antibody in Iran: a population-based study. Arch Iran Med. 2009;12(3):225–31.
47. Poustchi H, Mohamadkhani A, Bowden S, Montazeri G, Ayres A, Revill P, et al. Clinical significance of precore and core promoter mutations in genotype D hepatitis B-related chronic liver disease. J Viral Hepat. 2008;15(10):753–60.
48. Amini-Bavil-Olyaee S, Sarrami-Forooshani R, Adeli A, Sabahi F, Abachi M, Azizi M, et al. Complete genomic sequence and phylogenetic relatedness of hepatitis B virus isolates from Iran. J Med Virol. 2005;76(3):318–26.
49. Poustchi H, Sepanlou S, Esmaili S, Mehrabi N, Ansarymoghadam A. Hepatocellular carcinoma in the world and the middle East. Middle East J Dig Dis. 2010;2(1):31–41.
50. Ezzat S, Abdel-Hamid M, Eissa SA, Mokhtar N, Labib NA, El-Ghorory L, et al. Associations of pesticides, HCV, HBV, and hepatocellular carcinoma in Egypt. Int J Hyg Environ Health. 2005;208(5):329–39.
51. Hassan MM, Zaghloul AS, El-Serag HB, Soliman O, Patt YZ, Chappell CL, et al. The role of hepatitis C in hepatocellular carcinoma: a case control study among Egyptian patients. J Clin Gastroenterol. 2001;33(2):123–6.
52. El-Serag HB, Rudolph KL. Hepatocellular carcinoma: epidemiology and molecular carcinogenesis. Gastroenterology. 2007;132(7):2557–76.
53. Altekruse SF, McGlynn KA, Reichman ME. Hepatocellular carcinoma incidence, mortality, and survival trends in the United States from 1975 to 2005. J Clin Oncol. 2009;27(9):1485–91.
54. Ryerson AB, Eheman CR, Altekruse SF, Ward JW, Jemal A, Sherman RL, et al. Annual report to the nation on the status of cancer, 1975–2012, featuring the increasing incidence of liver cancer. Cancer. 2016;122(9):1312–37.
55. McPherson S, Anstee QM. Changing epidemiology of chronic liver disease among ethnic groups in the United States. Hepatology (Baltimore, MD). 2016;64(6):1843–6.
56. Armstrong GL, Wasley A, Simard EP, McQuillan GM, Kuhnert WL, Alter MJ. The prevalence of hepatitis C virus infection in the United States, 1999 through 2002. Ann Intern Med. 2006;144(10):705–14.
57. Setiawan VW, Wei PC, Hernandez BY, Lu SC, Monroe KR, Le Marchand L, et al. Disparity in liver cancer incidence and chronic liver disease mortality by nativity in Hispanics: the Multiethnic Cohort. Cancer. 2016;122(9):1444–52.
58. Browning JD, Szczepaniak LS, Dobbins R, Nuremberg P, Horton JD, Cohen JC, et al. Prevalence of hepatic steatosis in an urban population in the United States: impact of ethnicity. Hepatology (Baltimore, MD). 2004;40(6):1387–95.
59. Kallwitz ER, Daviglus ML, Allison MA, Emory KT, Zhao L, Kuniholm MH, et al. Prevalence of suspected nonalcoholic fatty liver disease in Hispanic/Latino individuals differs by heritage. Clin Gastroenterol Hepatol. 2015;13(3):569–76.
60. Mittal S, Sada YH, El-Serag HB, Kanwal F, Duan Z, Temple S, et al. Temporal trends of nonalcoholic fatty liver disease-related hepatocellular carcinoma in the veteran affairs population. Clin Gastroenterol Hepatol. 2015;13(3):594–601.e1.
61. Younossi ZM, LaLuna LL, Santoro JJ, Mendes F, Araya V, Ravendhran N, et al. Implementation of baby boomer hepatitis C screening and linking to care in gastroenterology practices: a multi-center pilot study. BMC Gastroenterol. 2016;16:45.
62. Mittal S, El-Serag HB. Epidemiology of hepatocellular carcinoma: consider the population. J Clin Gastroenterol. 2013;47(Suppl):S2–6.
63. Parkin DM. The global health burden of infection-associated cancers in the year 2002. Int J Cancer. 2006;118(12):3030–44.
64. Lafaro KJ, Demirjian AN, Pawlik TM. Epidemiology of hepatocellular carcinoma. Surg Oncol Clin N Am. 2015;24(1):1–17.
65. Kowdley KV, Wang CC, Welch S, Roberts H, Brosgart CL. Prevalence of chronic hepatitis B among foreign-born persons living in the United States by country of origin. Hepatology (Baltimore, MD). 2012;56(2):422–33.
66. Hepatitis viruses. IARC Monogr Eval Carcinog Risks Hum. 1994;59:1–255.

67. But DY, Lai CL, Yuen MF. Natural history of hepatitis-related hepatocellular carcinoma. World J Gastroenterol. 2008;14(11):1652–6.
68. Feitelson MA. Hepatitis B virus in hepatocarcinogenesis. J Cell Physiol. 1999;181(2):188–202.
69. Chang MH, You SL, Chen CJ, Liu CJ, Lee CM, Lin SM, et al. Decreased incidence of hepatocellular carcinoma in hepatitis B vaccines: a 20-year follow-up study. J Natl Cancer Inst. 2009;101(19):1348–55.
70. Gower E, Estes C, Blach S, Razavi-Shearer K, Razavi H. Global epidemiology and genotype distribution of the hepatitis C virus infection. J Hepatol. 2014;61(1 Suppl):S45–57.
71. Choo QL, Kuo G, Weiner AJ, Overby LR, Bradley DW, Houghton M. Isolation of a cDNA clone derived from a blood-borne non-A, non-B viral hepatitis genome. Science (New York, NY). 1989;244(4902):359–62.
72. Zaltron S, Spinetti A, Biasi L, Baiguera C, Castelli F. Chronic HCV infection: epidemiological and clinical relevance. BMC Infect Dis. 2012;12(Suppl 2):S2.
73. Yoshizawa H. Hepatocellular carcinoma associated with hepatitis C virus infection in Japan: projection to other countries in the foreseeable future. Oncology. 2002;62(Suppl 1):8–17.
74. Edlin BR, Eckhardt BJ, Shu MA, Holmberg SD, Swan T. Toward a more accurate estimate of the prevalence of hepatitis C in the United States. Hepatology (Baltimore, MD). 2015;62(5):1353–63.
75. Nelson PK, Mathers BM, Cowie B, Hagan H, Des Jarlais D, Horyniak D, et al. Global epidemiology of hepatitis B and hepatitis C in people who inject drugs: results of systematic reviews. Lancet (London, England). 2011;378(9791):571–83.
76. Tsai WL, Chung RT. Viral hepatocarcinogenesis. Oncogene. 2010;29(16):2309–24.
77. Suraweera D, Saab EG, Tong MJ, Saab S. Timing of hepatitis C antiviral therapy in liver transplant recipients with direct-acting agents. Exp Clin Transplant. 2016;14(3):243–51.
78. Suraweera D, Weeratunga AN, Saab S. Spotlight on grazoprevir-elbasvir once-daily combination and its potential in the treatment of hepatitis C. Drug Des Devel Ther. 2016;10:2119–27.
79. Morgan RL, Baack B, Smith BD, Yartel A, Pitasi M, Falck-Ytter Y. Eradication of hepatitis C virus infection and the development of hepatocellular carcinoma: a meta-analysis of observational studies. Ann Intern Med. 2013;158(5 Pt 1):329–37.
80. Gomaa AI, Khan SA, Toledano MB, Waked I, Taylor-Robinson SD. Hepatocellular carcinoma: epidemiology, risk factors and pathogenesis. World J Gastroenterol. 2008;14(27):4300–8.
81. Fattovich G, Stroffolini T, Zagni I, Donato F. Hepatocellular carcinoma in cirrhosis: incidence and risk factors. Gastroenterology. 2004;127(5 Suppl 1):S35–50.
82. Stickel F. Alcoholic cirrhosis and hepatocellular carcinoma. Adv Exp Med Biol. 2015;815:113–30.
83. Ezzati M, Lopez AD, Rodgers A, Vander Hoorn S, Murray CJ. Selected major risk factors and global and regional burden of disease. Lancet (London, England). 2002;360(9343):1347–60.
84. Donato F, Tagger A, Gelatti U, Parrinello G, Boffetta P, Albertini A, et al. Alcohol and hepatocellular carcinoma: the effect of lifetime intake and hepatitis virus infections in men and women. Am J Epidemiol. 2002;155(4):323–31.
85. Adami HO, Hsing AW, McLaughlin JK, Trichopoulos D, Hacker D, Ekbom A, et al. Alcoholism and liver cirrhosis in the etiology of primary liver cancer. Int J Cancer. 1992;51(6):898–902.
86. Kuper H, Ye W, Broome U, Romelsjo A, Mucci LA, Ekbom A, et al. The risk of liver and bile duct cancer in patients with chronic viral hepatitis, alcoholism, or cirrhosis. Hepatology (Baltimore, MD). 2001;34(4 Pt 1):714–8.
87. Corrao G, Arico S. Independent and combined action of hepatitis C virus infection and alcohol consumption on the risk of symptomatic liver cirrhosis. Hepatology (Baltimore, MD). 1998;27(4):914–9.
88. Altamirano J, Bataller R. Alcoholic liver disease: pathogenesis and new targets for therapy. Nat Rev Gastroenterol Hepatol. 2011;8(9):491–501.
89. El-Serag HB. Hepatocellular carcinoma: an epidemiologic view. J Clin Gastroenterol. 2002;35(5 Suppl 2):S72–8.

90. Bagnardi V, Rota M, Botteri E, Tramacere I, Islami F, Fedirko V, et al. Alcohol consumption and site-specific cancer risk: a comprehensive dose-response meta-analysis. Br J Cancer. 2015;112(3):580–93.
91. Marrero JA, Fontana RJ, Fu S, Conjeevaram HS, Su GL, Lok AS. Alcohol, tobacco and obesity are synergistic risk factors for hepatocellular carcinoma. J Hepatol. 2005;42(2):218–24.
92. Corrao G, Bagnardi V, Zambon A, La Vecchia C. A meta-analysis of alcohol consumption and the risk of 15 diseases. Prev Med. 2004;38(5):613–9.
93. Tsuchishima M, George J, Shiroeda H, Arisawa T, Takegami T, Tsutsumi M. Chronic ingestion of ethanol induces hepatocellular carcinoma in mice without additional hepatic insult. Dig Dis Sci. 2013;58(7):1923–33.
94. Wang F, Yang JL, Yu KK, Xu M, Xu YZ, Chen L, et al. Activation of the NF-kappaB pathway as a mechanism of alcohol enhanced progression and metastasis of human hepatocellular carcinoma. Mol Cancer. 2015;14:10.
95. Zhu H, Jia Z, Misra H, Li YR. Oxidative stress and redox signaling mechanisms of alcoholic liver disease: updated experimental and clinical evidence. J Dig Dis. 2012;13(3):133–42.
96. McKillop IH, Schrum LW. Role of alcohol in liver carcinogenesis. Semin Liver Dis. 2009;29(2):222–32.
97. Mancebo A, Gonzalez-Dieguez ML, Cadahia V, Varela M, Perez R, Navascues CA, et al. Annual incidence of hepatocellular carcinoma among patients with alcoholic cirrhosis and identification of risk groups. Clin Gastroenterol Hepatol. 2013;11(1):95–101.
98. Uetake S, Yamauchi M, Itoh S, Kawashima O, Takeda K, Ohata M. Analysis of risk factors for hepatocellular carcinoma in patients with HBs antigen- and anti-HCV antibody-negative alcoholic cirrhosis: clinical significance of prior hepatitis B virus infection. Alcohol Clin Exp Res. 2003;27(8 Suppl):47s–51s.
99. Sorensen HT, Friis S, Olsen JH, Thulstrup AM, Mellemkjaer L, Linet M, et al. Risk of liver and other types of cancer in patients with cirrhosis: a nationwide cohort study in Denmark. Hepatology (Baltimore, MD). 1998;28(4):921–5.
100. Hassan MM, Hwang LY, Hatten CJ, Swaim M, Li D, Abbruzzese JL, et al. Risk factors for hepatocellular carcinoma: synergism of alcohol with viral hepatitis and diabetes mellitus. Hepatology (Baltimore, MD). 2002;36(5):1206–13.
101. Yuan JM, Govindarajan S, Arakawa K, Yu MC. Synergism of alcohol, diabetes, and viral hepatitis on the risk of hepatocellular carcinoma in blacks and whites in the U.S. Cancer. 2004;101(5):1009–17.
102. Trepo E, Guyot E, Ganne-Carrie N, Degre D, Gustot T, Franchimont D, et al. PNPLA3 (rs738409 C>G) is a common risk variant associated with hepatocellular carcinoma in alcoholic cirrhosis. Hepatology (Baltimore, MD). 2012;55(4):1307–8.
103. Nahon P, Sutton A, Rufat P, Ziol M, Akouche H, Laguillier C, et al. Myeloperoxidase and superoxide dismutase 2 polymorphisms comodulate the risk of hepatocellular carcinoma and death in alcoholic cirrhosis. Hepatology (Baltimore, MD). 2009;50(5):1484–93.
104. Fabris C, Toniutto P, Falleti E, Fontanini E, Cussigh A, Bitetto D, et al. MTHFR C677T polymorphism and risk of HCC in patients with liver cirrhosis: role of male gender and alcohol consumption. Alcohol Clin Exp Res. 2009;33(1):102–7.
105. Kikuchi M, Horie Y, Ebinuma H, Taniki N, Nakamoto N, Kanai T. Alcoholic liver cirrhosis and significant risk factors for the development of alcohol-related hepatocellular carcinoma—Japan, 2012. Nihon Arukoru Yakubutsu Igakkai Zasshi. 2015;50(5):222–34.
106. Group IW. Aflatoxins. IARC Monogr Eval Carcinog Risks Hum. 2002;82:171–300.
107. Kew MC. Aflatoxins as a cause of hepatocellular carcinoma. J Gastrointestin Liver Dis. 2013;22(3):305–10.
108. Viegas S, Veiga L, Malta-Vacas J, Sabino R, Figueredo P, Almeida A, et al. Occupational exposure to aflatoxin (AFB(1)) in poultry production. J Toxicol Environ Health A. 2012;75(22–23):1330–40.
109. Williams JH, Phillips TD, Jolly PE, Stiles JK, Jolly CM, Aggarwal D. Human aflatoxicosis in developing countries: a review of toxicology, exposure, potential health consequences, and interventions. Am J Clin Nutr. 2004;80(5):1106–22.

110. Strosnider H, Azziz-Baumgartner E, Banziger M, Bhat RV, Breiman R, Brune MN, et al. Workgroup report: public health strategies for reducing aflatoxin exposure in developing countries. Environ Health Perspect. 2006;114(12):1898–903.
111. Liu Y, Wu F. Global burden of aflatoxin-induced hepatocellular carcinoma: a risk assessment. Environ Health Perspect. 2010;118(6):818–24.
112. Hsu IC, Metcalf RA, Sun T, Welsh JA, Wang NJ, Harris CC. Mutational hotspot in the p53 gene in human hepatocellular carcinomas. Nature. 1991;350(6317):427–8.
113. Bressac B, Kew M, Wands J, Ozturk M. Selective G to T mutations of p53 gene in hepatocellular carcinoma from southern Africa. Nature. 1991;350(6317):429–31.
114. Moudgil V, Redhu D, Dhanda S, Singh J. A review of molecular mechanisms in the development of hepatocellular carcinoma by aflatoxin and hepatitis B and C viruses. J Environ Pathol Toxicol Oncol. 2013;32(2):165–75.
115. Kew MC. Hepatitis B virus x protein in the pathogenesis of hepatitis B virus-induced hepatocellular carcinoma. J Gastroenterol Hepatol. 2011;26(Suppl 1):144–52.
116. Ahn JY, Jung EY, Kwun HJ, Lee CW, Sung YC, Jang KL. Dual effects of hepatitis B virus X protein on the regulation of cell-cycle control depending on the status of cellular p53. J Gen Virol. 2002;83(Pt 11):2765–72.
117. Goh GB, Chang PE, Tan CK. Changing epidemiology of hepatocellular carcinoma in Asia. Best Pract Res Clin Gastroenterol. 2015;29(6):919–28.
118. Younossi ZM, Otgonsuren M, Henry L, Venkatesan C, Mishra A, Erario M, et al. Association of nonalcoholic fatty liver disease (NAFLD) with hepatocellular carcinoma (HCC) in the United States from 2004 to 2009. Hepatology (Baltimore, MD). 2015;62(6):1723–30.
119. Reeves HL, Zaki MY, Day CP. Hepatocellular carcinoma in obesity, type 2 diabetes, and NAFLD. Dig Dis Sci. 2016;61(5):1234–45.
120. Neuschwander-Tetri BA, Caldwell SH. Nonalcoholic steatohepatitis: summary of an AASLD single topic conference. Hepatology (Baltimore, MD). 2003;37(5):1202–19.
121. Argo CK, Caldwell SH. Epidemiology and natural history of non-alcoholic steatohepatitis. Clin Liver Dis. 2009;13(4):511–31.
122. Pocha C, Kolly P, Dufour JF. Nonalcoholic fatty liver disease-related hepatocellular carcinoma: a problem of growing magnitude. Semin Liver Dis. 2015;35(3):304–17.
123. Streba LA, Vere CC, Rogoveanu I, Streba CT. Nonalcoholic fatty liver disease, metabolic risk factors, and hepatocellular carcinoma: an open question. World J Gastroenterol. 2015;21(14):4103–10.
124. Sanyal A, Poklepovic A, Moyneur E, Barghout V. Population-based risk factors and resource utilization for HCC: US perspective. Curr Med Res Opin. 2010;26(9):2183–91.
125. Margini C, Dufour JF. The story of HCC in NAFLD: from epidemiology, across pathogenesis, to prevention and treatment. Liver Int. 2016;36(3):317–24.
126. Torres DM, Harrison SA. Nonalcoholic steatohepatitis and noncirrhotic hepatocellular carcinoma: fertile soil. Semin Liver Dis. 2012;32(1):30–8.
127. Noureddin M, Rinella ME. Nonalcoholic fatty liver disease, diabetes, obesity, and hepatocellular carcinoma. Clin Liver Dis. 2015;19(2):361–79.
128. Perumpail RB, Wong RJ, Ahmed A, Harrison SA. Hepatocellular carcinoma in the setting of non-cirrhotic nonalcoholic fatty liver disease and the metabolic syndrome: US experience. Dig Dis Sci. 2015;60(10):3142–8.
129. Piscaglia F, Svegliati-Baroni G, Barchetti A, Pecorelli A, Marinelli S, Tiribelli C, et al. Clinical patterns of hepatocellular carcinoma in nonalcoholic fatty liver disease: a multicenter prospective study. Hepatology (Baltimore, MD). 2016;63(3):827–38.
130. Ma C, Kesarwala AH, Eggert T, Medina-Echeverz J, Kleiner DE, Jin P, et al. NAFLD causes selective CD4(+) T lymphocyte loss and promotes hepatocarcinogenesis. Nature. 2016;531(7593):253–7.
131. Calle EE, Rodriguez C, Walker-Thurmond K, Thun MJ. Overweight, obesity, and mortality from cancer in a prospectively studied cohort of U.S. adults. N Engl J Med. 2003;348(17):1625–38.

132. Mori S, Yamasaki T, Sakaida I, Takami T, Sakaguchi E, Kimura T, et al. Hepatocellular carcinoma with nonalcoholic steatohepatitis. J Gastroenterol. 2004;39(4):391–6.
133. Ascha MS, Hanouneh IA, Lopez R, Tamimi TA, Feldstein AF, Zein NN. The incidence and risk factors of hepatocellular carcinoma in patients with nonalcoholic steatohepatitis. Hepatology (Baltimore, MD). 2010;51(6):1972–8.
134. Ratziu V, Bonyhay L, Di Martino V, Charlotte F, Cavallaro L, Sayegh-Tainturier MH, et al. Survival, liver failure, and hepatocellular carcinoma in obesity-related cryptogenic cirrhosis. Hepatology (Baltimore, MD). 2002;35(6):1485–93.
135. Yatsuji S, Hashimoto E, Tobari M, Taniai M, Tokushige K, Shiratori K. Clinical features and outcomes of cirrhosis due to non-alcoholic steatohepatitis compared with cirrhosis caused by chronic hepatitis C. J Gastroenterol Hepatol. 2009;24(2):248–54.
136. Hashimoto E, Yatsuji S, Tobari M, Taniai M, Torii N, Tokushige K, et al. Hepatocellular carcinoma in patients with nonalcoholic steatohepatitis. J Gastroenterol. 2009;44(Suppl 19):89–95.
137. Lazo M, Clark JM. The epidemiology of nonalcoholic fatty liver disease: a global perspective. Semin Liver Dis. 2008;28(4):339–50.
138. Wideroff L, Gridley G, Mellemkjaer L, Chow WH, Linet M, Keehn S, et al. Cancer incidence in a population-based cohort of patients hospitalized with diabetes mellitus in Denmark. J Natl Cancer Inst. 1997;89(18):1360–5.
139. Li CI, Chen HJ, Lai HC, Liu CS, Lin WY, Li TC, et al. Hyperglycemia and chronic liver diseases on risk of hepatocellular carcinoma in Chinese patients with type 2 diabetes—National Cohort of Taiwan Diabetes Study. Int J Cancer. 2015;136(11):2668–79.
140. Adami HO, Chow WH, Nyren O, Berne C, Linet MS, Ekbom A, et al. Excess risk of primary liver cancer in patients with diabetes mellitus. J Natl Cancer Inst. 1996;88(20):1472–7.
141. Chettouh H, Lequoy M, Fartoux L, Vigouroux C, Desbois-Mouthon C. Hyperinsulinaemia and insulin signalling in the pathogenesis and the clinical course of hepatocellular carcinoma. Liver Int. 2015;35(10):2203–17.
142. Capone F, Guerriero E, Colonna G, Maio P, Mangia A, Marfella R, et al. The cytokinome profile in patients with hepatocellular carcinoma and type 2 diabetes. PLoS One. 2015;10(7):e0134594.
143. Chen HH, Lin MC, Muo CH, Yeh SY, Sung FC, Kao CH. Combination therapy of metformin and statin may decrease hepatocellular carcinoma among diabetic patients in Asia. Medicine. 2015;94(24):e1013.
144. Donadon V, Balbi M, Mas MD, Casarin P, Zanette G. Metformin and reduced risk of hepatocellular carcinoma in diabetic patients with chronic liver disease. Liver Int. 2010;30(5):750–8.
145. El-Serag HB, Tran T, Everhart JE. Diabetes increases the risk of chronic liver disease and hepatocellular carcinoma. Gastroenterology. 2004;126(2):460–8.
146. Elmberg M, Hultcrantz R, Ekbom A, Brandt L, Olsson S, Olsson R, et al. Cancer risk in patients with hereditary hemochromatosis and in their first-degree relatives. Gastroenterology. 2003;125(6):1733–41.
147. Yang Q, McDonnell SM, Khoury MJ, Cono J, Parrish RG. Hemochromatosis-associated mortality in the United States from 1979 to 1992: an analysis of multiple-cause mortality data. Ann Intern Med. 1998;129(11):946–53.
148. Lata J. Chronic liver diseases as liver tumor precursors. Dig Dis (Basel, Switzerland). 2010;28(4–5):596–9.
149. Zhu K, Moriarty C, Caplan LS, Levine RS. Cigarette smoking and primary liver cancer: a population-based case-control study in US men. Cancer Causes Control. 2007;18(3):315–21.
150. Sun CA, Wu DM, Lin CC, Lu SN, You SL, Wang LY, et al. Incidence and cofactors of hepatitis C virus-related hepatocellular carcinoma: a prospective study of 12,008 men in Taiwan. Am J Epidemiol. 2003;157(8):674–82.
151. Jee SH, Ohrr H, Sull JW, Samet JM. Cigarette smoking, alcohol drinking, hepatitis B, and risk for hepatocellular carcinoma in Korea. J Natl Cancer Inst. 2004;96(24):1851–6.

Autoimmune Hepatitis and Immune-Mediated Cholestatic Liver Diseases

16

Albert J. Czaja

Abstract

Autoimmune hepatitis, primary biliary cholangitis, and primary sclerosing cholangitis are immune-mediated chronic liver diseases of uncertain cause that have a global distribution and highly variable occurrence. The goals of this review are to describe the epidemiological studies that have identified the populations at risk, estimated the incidence and prevalence of each disease, suggested environmental and genetic bases for their occurrence, and indicated trends that should direct the allocation of healthcare resources and investigational efforts. Population-based epidemiological studies have described patterns of susceptibility for each liver disease that reflect predilections for certain age groups, gender, geographical regions, and ethnic background. Familial studies and genetic analyses have implicated a genetic predisposition for each disease, and population-based studies have suggested associations with triggering agents, including pollutants, xenobiotics, viruses, bacteria, and the intestinal microbiome. Variations in prevalence between ethnic groups within regions or between countries may reflect differences in early diagnosis, management, and outcome, and the increasing incidence of these diseases in certain regions and ethnic groups may help identify pivotal etiological factors that might be modified. Population-based epidemiological studies are lacking in China, India, and developing countries, and they are needed to complete the global perspective of these diseases and their consequences. In conclusion, autoimmune hepatitis and the immune-mediated cholangiopathies are rare, but they constitute a global healthcare burden that is increasing in certain geographical regions and ethnic groups. Populations at risk and susceptibility factors must continue to be characterized, and interventions must be tailored to meet individual and regional needs.

A. J. Czaja
Division of Gastroenterology and Hepatology, Mayo Clinic College of Medicine and Science, Rochester, MN, USA
e-mail: czaja.albert@mayo.edu

R. J. Wong, R. G. Gish (eds.), *Clinical Epidemiology of Chronic Liver Diseases*,
https://doi.org/10.1007/978-3-319-94355-8_16

Keywords
Autoimmune hepatitis · Primary biliary cholangitis · Primary sclerosing cholangitis · Epidemiology

16.1 Introduction

Population-based epidemiological studies are essential for understanding the genetic susceptibilities and the possible antigenic triggers of autoimmune liver disease [1, 2]. They are also necessary to correctly allocate resources for improving the early diagnosis and management of this disease category [3]. Autoimmune liver disease encompasses acute and chronic forms of liver injury that are defined by cell- and antibody-mediated immune responses that lack a definable etiological agent [4]. They may have variable clinical phenotypes and severity, but they all tend to be persistent, progressive, and variably responsive to current therapies. Autoimmune hepatitis is the prototypic autoimmune liver disease, and primary biliary cholangitis (PBC) and primary sclerosing cholangitis (PSC) complete the disease category. Variant phenotypes also exist in which the features of autoimmune hepatitis can be intermixed with those of PBC or PSC [5–7]. The lack of codified diagnostic criteria for these variant or overlap syndromes and uncertainty about their pathogenic basis have limited the performance of epidemiological studies that clarify their disease burden.

Autoimmune liver disease is a consequence of misdirected and dysregulated immune responses against self-antigens in a genetically susceptible individual [4]. The triggering antigens may reflect molecular mimicry between environmental or infectious agents and normal proteins within the liver [8]. Chronic or repeated exposures to these extrinsic agents may break immune tolerance of these normal self-proteins, and liver-infiltrating, antigen-sensitized, cytotoxic T lymphocytes may initiate and sustain hepatic injury [4, 9, 10]. The class II molecules of the major histocompatibility complex (MHC) can contribute to the presentation of antigens, sensitization of T helper lymphocytes, and differentiation of the activated immune cells along cytokine-mediated pathways that result in cellular- and antibody-dependent immune responses [11–16]. Genetic factors outside the MHC, including polymorphisms of genes that influence the production of various cytokines and immune modulators, may also affect the propensity for tissue damage and its severity [17, 18]. Epigenetic factors that influence the transcriptional activity of regulatory genes without altering the sequence of deoxyribonucleic acid (DNA) can unbalance homeostatic mechanisms that maintain immune tolerance of self-antigens, alter susceptibility for immune-mediated disease, and create an inheritable trait that has transgenerational consequences [19–21].

Autoimmune liver disease has a global distribution, and its occurrence varies between ethnic groups within the same geographical region, in different age groups, and in different countries [1, 22]. The diversity of individual susceptibilities for autoimmune liver disease may reflect genetic and epigenetic differences and variations in the nature and duration of exposure to environmental and microbial antigens within a specific age range or geographical location [21, 23]. Region-specific environmental antigens may derive from water and food sources, industrial pollutants, or toxic waste sites [24], and the microbial antigens may be indigenous infectious agents [25] or region-specific microflora within the intestinal microbiome that are affected by factors such as diet, sanitation, socioeconomic status, and antibiotic exposure [26–32]. Epigenetic alterations in gene activity can be induced by these environmental factors [33, 34], and they can influence the risk for immune-mediated disease in individuals and their progeny in different geographical regions and ethnicities [35]. Population-based epidemiological studies are key mechanisms by which to identify these antigenic sources and develop management strategies that impact on disease occurrence.

Autoimmune liver disease constitutes only a fraction of patients with chronic liver disease, but it affects most individuals during productive phases of life [3]. Accordingly, its indirect costs due to years of productive life lost may far exceed its direct costs for medical care [3]. Furthermore, the recognition of differences in liver-related mortality among different ethnic groups in the same geographical region can direct efforts to understand and improve outcomes [36]. Hispanics in the United States have an overall liver-related mortality that is 49% higher than in non-Hispanic whites (13.7 cases per 100,000 persons versus 9.2 cases per 100,000 persons) and 82% higher than in African Americans (13.7 cases per 100,000 persons versus 7.5 cases per 100,000 persons) [37]. The proper allocation of medical resources, the formulation of healthcare policies, and the direction of future investigation in the autoimmune liver diseases require epidemiological studies that define the burden of each disease type in the general population and in different ethnic groups within that population.

The goals of this review are to describe the epidemiology of autoimmune hepatitis, PBC and PSC and to indicate how continued strengthening of this knowledge base can clarify pathogenic mechanisms, identify at risk subgroups, and direct the allocation of healthcare resources and future investigational efforts.

16.2 Epidemiology of Autoimmune Hepatitis

Population-based studies that have estimated the incidence and prevalence of autoimmune hepatitis have been performed in Alaska [38], Australia [39], Denmark [40], southern Israel [41], the Netherlands [42], New Zealand [43], Norway [44], Singapore [45], Spain [46, 47], and Sweden [48]. Population-based studies within the United States have been performed mainly in the pediatric population [49] (Table 16.1). These assessments have indicated the rarity of autoimmune hepatitis (defined as an annual incidence less than 50 cases per 100,000 persons [50]) and the regional variability of its occurrence [38–42, 45]. Countries with healthcare systems that provide universal access, systematic data accumulation, and prescribed follow-up examinations (Sweden, Netherlands, Denmark, Norway, and New Zealand) have

Table 16.1 Incidence and prevalence of autoimmune hepatitis in different regions (lowest to highest annual incidence)

Geographical region	Annual incidence per 100,000 persons	Prevalence per 100,000 persons
Canada (children) [52, 53] (2000–2009)	0.23	2.4, non-First Nations children 9.9, First Nations children
United States (children) [49] (1986–2011)	0.4	3.0
Singapore [45]	Not reported	4.0 (similar in Chinese, Malaysian, and Indian subgroups)
Australia (Capital Territory) [39]	Not reported	8.0
Israel (southern) [41]	0.67	11.0
Spain (Sagunto/Valencia) [46, 47]	0.83–1.07 (women, 1.37–1.96; men, −0.12 to 0.26) (increasing incidence in women)	11.61 (women, 19.17; men, 3.66)
Sweden [48]	0.85	10.7
Netherlands [42]	1.1 (increasing incidence over 10 years)	18.3
Denmark [40] (1994–2012)	1.68 (rising incidence from 1.37 to 2.33)	23.9 (women, 34.6; men, 13.0)
Norway (Oslo) [44]	1.9	16.9
New Zealand (Canterbury Region) [43] (2001–2007)	2.0 (1.7, age-standardized) (stable incidence over 6 years)	24.5 (18.9, age-standardized)
Alaska (native population) [38]	Not reported	42.9

Numbers in brackets are references

performed the strongest population-based evaluations [51]. They have also been able to describe changes in occurrence, phenotype, and mortality, albeit mainly in homogeneous white populations.

16.2.1 Annual Incidence of Autoimmune Hepatitis

The annual incidence of autoimmune hepatitis in adults ranges from 0.67 cases per 100,000 persons in southern Israel [41] to 2.0 cases per 100,000 persons in the Canterbury Region of New Zealand (95% confidence interval [CI]: 0.8–3.3 per 100,000) (Table 16.1). The annual incidence of autoimmune hepatitis in Canadian children was 0.23 cases per 100,000 persons between 2000 and 2009 [52], and it was 0.4 cases per 100,000 persons in children residing in the United States (Utah) between 1986 and 2011 [49].

Two studies evaluating temporal trends have suggested that the incidence of autoimmune hepatitis has been increasing in the adult populations of Spain [46, 47] and Denmark [40] over 10–18 years, whereas a third study in New Zealand has suggested a stable incidence over a 6 year period from 2001 to 2007 [43]. Temporal trends may reflect changes in the methods of case-recognition, but they may also indicate a true increase in disease occurrence that warrants additional scrutiny. The wide range in incidence may reflect variations in the type and frequency of antigenic exposures, differences in genetic predispositions, or the effects of gender-specific (possibly hormonal) modifiers of the immune response [1, 4].

16.2.2 Prevalence of Autoimmune Hepatitis

The prevalence of autoimmune hepatitis in adults ranges from 4.0 cases per 100,000 persons in Singapore (with a similar prevalence in the Chinese, Malaysian and Indian subpopulations) [45] to 42.9 cases per 100,000 persons in Alaskan natives [38] (Table 16.1). The prevalence of autoimmune hepatitis in Alaskan natives is 1.7-fold greater than the highest reported prevalence of autoimmune hepatitis elsewhere [38]. In children, the prevalence of autoimmune hepatitis is 3.0 cases per 100,000 persons in Utah [49] and 2.4 cases per 100,000 persons in the non-native children of British Columbia, Canada [49, 53]. In contrast, the prevalence of autoimmune hepatitis in the First Nations (Aboriginal) children of British Columbia (9.9 cases per 100,000 persons) is nearly fourfold greater than that of the non-native children within this same geographical region (2.4 cases per 100,000 persons) [53].

The differences in prevalence between children and adults from different geographical regions and between children within the same geographical region suggest that predispositions for autoimmune hepatitis may be associated with age-related antigenic exposures and hereditary or culturally-specific factors. Other differences in prevalence among populations with autoimmune hepatitis have less apparent associations. Whereas the prevalence of autoimmune hepatitis is similar in Sweden and Spain (10.7–11.6 cases per 100,000 persons) [46–48], it is higher in Norway, the Netherlands, and Denmark (16.9–23.9 case per 100,000 persons) despite similarly predominant white adult populations, geographical proximity, and availability of tertiary medical care [40, 42, 44] (Table 16.1).

16.2.3 Variations of Phenotype in Different Geographical Regions and Ethnic Groups

The phenotype of autoimmune hepatitis can vary between different ethnic groups and geographical regions [1]. Autoimmune hepatitis is characterized by its inflammatory nature, and codified diagnostic criteria and scoring systems have been refined to exclude prominent cholestatic features [54–56]. In Alaskan natives [38], Somalians [57], and individuals from the Middle East [58] who have autoimmune hepatitis, clinical, laboratory, and histological changes of cholestasis are common (57–67%) (Table 16.2).

In the United Kingdom, 50% of children with autoimmune hepatitis have cholangiographic changes that suggest an autoimmune sclerosing cholangitis [59],

Table 16.2 Regional and ethnic differences in phenotypic manifestations of autoimmune hepatitis

Variable feature	Manifestations	Regional or ethnic differences
Age	Children and adults in same geographical region have different frequencies of AIH [40, 43, 49, 52] Adults in different countries have different ages of disease onset [40, 42] Peak age shift to elderly adults [40, 43]	Highest prevalence in adults [40, 42, 43, 49, 52] Peak age (New Zealand), 60 years [43] Peak age (Denmark), 70 years [40] Median age (Netherlands), 43–48 years [42]
Gender	Female predilection varies in different countries [38, 40, 41, 44, 45, 47]	Young Somalian men affected [57] Unusual high female frequency in Alaskan natives and southern Israelis (91–95%) [38, 41] F:M ratio (Singapore), 11:1 [45] F:M ratio (USA, Europe), 2.6–5.2:1 [40, 44, 47, 63]
Cholestasis	Clinical, laboratory or histological findings of cholestasis [38, 57, 58]	Present in 57–67% of Alaskan natives, Somalians, Middle Easterners [38, 57, 58] Unusual in white North American and European adults [54, 55]
Autoimmune sclerosing cholangitis	Focal strictures and dilations by cholangiography in otherwise classical AIH [59]	Present in 50% of British children with AIH [59] Present in 21% of Utah children with AIH [49] Rare in North American and European adults (1–10%) unless CUC present (44%) [60–62]
Antibodies	Variable frequencies of serological markers of AIH in children and adults between countries [52, 67, 70, 71, 73]	Anti-LKM1 occur mainly in children [66] • 13% of Canadian children with AIH [52] • 38% of British children with AIH [59, 67] • 1% in American adults [68, 69] Alaskan natives versus American adults • Anti-dsDNA, 48% versus 23–34% [70, 71] • ANCA, 38% versus 96% [70, 72] • Anti-Ro, 11% versus 40% [70, 73, 74] Japanese versus American adults • Anti-Ro, 62% versus 38% [73]

AIH autoimmune hepatitis, *ANCA* anti-neutrophil cytoplasmic antibodies, *anti-dsDNA* antibodies to double-stranded deoxyribonucleic acid, *anti-LKM1* antibodies to liver kidney microsome type 1, *anti-Ro* antibodies to ribonucleoprotein, *CUC* chronic ulcerative colitis, *F:M ratio* female-to-male ratio, *USA* United States of America

Numbers in brackets are references

whereas in the United States (Utah), only 21% of children with autoimmune hepatitis have features of autoimmune sclerosing cholangitis [49] (Table 16.2). The overall incidence of autoimmune sclerosing cholangitis in Utah is 0.1 cases per 100,000 persons, and the prevalence is 0.6 cases per 100,000 persons [49]. Cholangiographic changes of sclerosing cholangitis (focal biliary strictures and dilations) are even less frequent (2–10%) in white North American and European adults with autoimmune hepatitis [60, 61] unless they have concurrent chronic ulcerative colitis [62].

Autoimmune hepatitis has had a female propensity in all countries with the possible exception of Somalia where the disease appears to affect young males [57] (Table 16.2). Among Alaskan natives, 91% of patients with autoimmune hepatitis are women [38], and in southern Israel, 95% of patients are women [41]. The female-to-male ratio in Singapore is 11:1 [45]. In contrast, women constitute 72–78% of patients with autoimmune hepatitis in Denmark [40], Sweden [48], the Netherlands [42], and the United States [63], and the prevalence of autoimmune hepatitis in northern Europe is only 2.6–5.2 times greater in women than in men [40, 44, 46, 47]. Women may also have a predilection to have concurrent immune diseases more commonly than men in white North American and European populations [64, 65].

Autoimmune hepatitis affects all ages, but its prevalence is higher in adults than children [40, 42–44, 49, 52] (Table 16.2). Furthermore, the age of onset in adults may be shifting from the young and middle-aged populations to the elderly. In New Zealand, the peak age at presentation was in the sixth decade, and 72% of patients presented after the age of 40 years [43]. In Denmark, the peak incidence of autoimmune hepatitis in both genders was at the age of 70 years [40]. In contrast, the peak incidence of autoimmune hepatitis in the Netherlands was in the middle age range. The median age at presentation was 48 years in Dutch women and 43 years in Dutch men [42].

The serological manifestations of autoimmune hepatitis can also vary between age ranges, ethnic groups, and countries [1] (Table 16.2). Antibodies to liver kidney microsome type 1 (anti-LKM1) occur mainly in children with autoimmune hepatitis [66]. They are detected in 13–38% of children with autoimmune hepatitis in the United Kingdom [59, 67] and in Canada [52], but they are present in only 1% of North American adults with autoimmune hepatitis [68, 69]. In Alaskan natives with autoimmune hepatitis, there is a higher frequency of antibodies to double stranded deoxyribonucleic acid (anti-dsDNA) (48% versus 23–34% depending on the assay) than in white North American patients [70, 71], and the frequencies of anti-neutrophil cytoplasmic antibodies (ANCA) (38% versus 96%) [70, 72] and antibodies to ribonucleoprotein (anti-Ro) are lower (11% versus 40%) [70, 73, 74]. In contrast, antibodies to Ro are detected more commonly in Japanese patients with autoimmune hepatitis than in North American patients (62% versus 38%, $P < 0.0001$) [73].

Plasma cells that stain for immunoglobulin G4 (IgG4) and number more than 5 per high power field are present in the liver tissue of 3–35% of patients with autoimmune hepatitis [75–77]. These patients have been classified as having IgG4-associated autoimmune hepatitis, and they commonly, but not invariably, have increased serum levels of IgG4 [76–78]. The frequency of IgG4-associated autoimmune hepatitis varies with the stringency of the diagnostic criteria. Application of the most stringent criteria (definite autoimmune hepatitis by international criteria, ≥10 IgG4-staining plasma cells/high power field, and serum IgG4 level ≥135 mg/dL) has recognized the variant form in only 3.3% of patients with autoimmune hepatitis [76, 78].

IgG4-associated autoimmune hepatitis may represent a variant clinical phenotype of autoimmune hepatitis that is within a spectrum of IgG4-related diseases that includes autoimmune pancreatitis and IgG4-associated cholangitis [79]. Liver injury is recognized in 60–70% of patients with autoimmune pancreatitis, and the associated IgG4-hepatopathy is characterized by IgG4-staining plasma cells near the portal vein, portal inflammation, portal sclerosis, bile duct damage, lobular hepatitis, and cholestasis [76, 78]. The features of IgG4-associated autoimmune hepatitis have typical histological findings of autoimmune hepatitis except for the prominent infiltration of IgG4-staining plasma cells [76].

IgG4-associated autoimmune hepatitis has been described mainly in Japan and China, and all experiences have emphasized responsiveness to conventional glucocorticoid therapy [75–77, 80]. The *de novo* occurrence of IgG4-associated autoimmune hepatitis after liver transplantation [80], the absence of relapse after drug withdrawal [77], the development of autoimmune pancreatitis 2 years after diagnosis in one patient [81], and the occurrence of IgG4-associated cholangitis 5 years later in another patient [76] are clinical vignettes that emphasize the uncertain nature and consequences of this variant [76].

Patients with IgG4-associated autoimmune hepatitis have higher serum immunoglobulin E (IgE) levels than patients with classical autoimmune hepatitis, and this finding suggests that the IgG4-associated autoimmune hepatitis may be triggered by antigens that generate an allergic response [76]. Both IgG4 and IgE are immune responses that have been recognized in allergic reactions [82, 83], and they are mediated by IL-10-secreting regulatory T cells which are abundant in autoimmune pancreatitis and IgG4-associated cholangitis [84]. The IgG4-staining histological phenotype of autoimmune hepatitis may reflect an allergic reaction to environmental antigens in a genetically-predisposed individual. Epidemiological studies are required to clarify the global distribution of IgG4-associated autoimmune hepatitis and the antigenic exposures associated with this variant form of autoimmune hepatitis.

16.2.4 Variations in Liver-Related Mortality in Different Geographical Regions and Ethnic Groups

Mortality rates can vary between ethnic groups and geographical regions, and these differences may reflect variable access to medical care, promptness of diagnosis and treatment, frequency of cirrhosis at presentation, type of treatment administered, diligence of follow-up, frequency of co-morbidities (concurrent diseases, alcohol intake), and socioeconomic status [1]. Regional- and ethnic-specific differences in the intrinsic behavior of the liver disease cannot be excluded, but they are more difficult to discover beneath an overlay of cultural, economic, and healthcare disparity [1]. Furthermore, the liver-related death burden may be underestimated in population studies that apply only one diagnostic category of the International Classification of Diseases (ICD). Liver-specific descriptors, such as hepatic encephalopathy, hepatorenal syndrome, and liver malignancy, must also be included in all outcome analyses [85].

Liver-related mortality can vary in different ethnic groups within the same geographical region [1]. Liver failure is more common at presentation in African-Americans with autoimmune hepatitis than in white American adults (38% versus 9%) [86] (Table 16.3). African-Americans with autoimmune hepatitis are younger at diagnosis than white Americans; they have cirrhosis more frequently (57–85% versus 38%); they require liver transplantation more often (51% versus 23%); and their overall mortality is significantly higher (24% versus 6%), especially in black

Table 16.3 Regional and ethnic differences in outcomes of autoimmune hepatitis

Outcomes	Findings	Regional or ethnic differences
Liver-related mortality	Different between ethnic groups in same region [86] Different between geographical regions [40, 41, 45, 95–97]	African-American versus white American adults • Liver failure at presentation, 38% versus 9% [86] • Mortality, 24% versus 6% [86] • Highest mortality in black males [86] Regional differences in mortality • 10 years, 7–10.3% in Europe, Israel, USA [40, 41, 95, 96] • 5 years, 29% in Singapore [45] • <3 years (mean, 15.7 ± 17 months), 25% in India [97]
Cirrhosis	Different in ethnic groups in same region [86] Different between geographical regions [40, 41, 45, 95–97] Differences may reflect disease severity, genetic predisposition, or socioeconomic status [86]	African-Americans versus white Americans • Younger at presentation [86] • Cirrhosis at presentation, 57–85% versus 38% [86, 87] Regional differences in cirrhosis at presentation • 42% in Singapore [45] • 76% in India [97] • 12–29% in Europe, Israel, USA [40–42, 96] Mortality hazard (1st year), 3.25 (95% CI: 2.25–4.7) [40]
Liver transplantation	Differences may reflect disease severity, delayed diagnosis, or limited access to medical care [86, 92]	African-Americans versus white Americans • Liver transplantation indicated, 51% versus 23% [86] • Access to transplantation may be less [92, 94]

(continued)

Table 16.3 (continued)

Outcomes	Findings	Regional or ethnic differences
Hepatocellular carcinoma	Differences may reflect limited access to treatment in ethnic groups of same or different region [89–94] Referral bias in tertiary medical centers may over-estimate occurrence [100]	African-Americans versus white Americans • Higher mortality with localized HCC [88, 89] • Lower frequency of liver transplantation [94] Regional differences in occurrence • 0.8 cases per 1000 person-years in Denmark [40] • 0.7% 10 year cumulative risk in Denmark [40] • 1% frequency (median, 6 years) in Netherlands [42] • 1 case per 965 person-years in USA [99] • 10.9 cases per 1000 person-years in UK [100] Male predominant except in UK [40, 42, 98, 100] Develops in cirrhosis only except in UK [40, 98, 100]

CI confidence interval, *HCC* hepatocellular carcinoma, *UK* United Kingdom, *USA* United States of America
Numbers in brackets are references

males [86, 87]. African-Americans also have a higher mortality associated with small, non-metastatic hepatocellular carcinoma [88, 89]. These findings may reflect a more aggressive autoimmune hepatitis, possibly because of different antigenic triggers or genetic predispositions in the black population, or they could reflect cultural or socioeconomic differences between the white and black populations that prevent early diagnosis and limit access to medical interventions, especially liver transplantation [90–94].

Liver-related mortality can also vary in different geographical regions. Autoimmune hepatitis has a 10-year all-cause mortality of 26.4% in Denmark (95% CI: 23.7–29.1%), but only 38.6% of the known causes of death are liver-related [40] (Table 16.3). The estimated 10-year liver-related mortality in Denmark is 10.2% and similar to the 10-year liver-related mortality of 9% in the United Kingdom [95], 10.3% in southern Israel [41], and 7% in North America [96]. In each of these non-Asian countries, the mortality estimates are lower than the 5-year liver-related mortality of 29% in Singapore [45] and the overall mortality of 25% in India during a mean observation period of only 15.7 ± 17 months [97].

The presence of cirrhosis at presentation in 42% of the patients in Singapore [45] and 76% of the patients in India [97] may explain the differences in mortality (Table 16.3). Cirrhosis at presentation occurs in only 12–29% of patients with autoimmune hepatitis in Denmark [40], southern Israel [41], the Netherlands [42], and the United States [96], and it has a greater mortality hazard during the first year after diagnosis than the absence of cirrhosis (mortality hazard of cirrhosis, 3.25; 95% CI: 2.25–4.70) [40].

Hepatocellular carcinoma has an incidence of 0.8 cases per 1000 person-years (95% CI: 0.3–1.5) in Denmark, especially in men with cirrhosis, and the 10-year cumulative risk of hepatocellular carcinoma has been 0.7% (95% CI: 0.3–1.5) [40] (Table 16.3). These findings are similar to those in the Netherlands where the frequency of hepatocellular carcinoma has been 1% during a median observation interval of 6 years [42]. In the United States, hepatocellular carcinoma has developed only in patients with longstanding cirrhosis (≥5 years duration) [98]; it has been male predominant [98]; and its incidence has been 1 per 965 person-years [99]. In the United Kingdom, hepatocellular carcinoma has occurred at a rate of 10.9 cases per 1000 patient-years or 1.1% per year [100]. It has affected 3.4% of patients without cirrhosis, and it has developed equally in men and women (6.4% versus 6.1%) [100]. The study in the United Kingdom was performed in a tertiary medical center, and it may have reflected referral bias associated with more advanced and severe autoimmune hepatitis than encountered elsewhere.

16.2.5 Variations of Genetic Predisposition in Different Geographical Regions and Ethnic Groups

Autoimmune hepatitis has a complex genetic predisposition that can vary in children and adults within the same geographical region and between adults in different regions [11]. Autoimmune hepatitis does not have a causative gene, but a constellation of normal genes within and outside the MHC may favor immune reactivity. Familial occurrence is rare (0.2% in Brazil [101] and 0.3% in the Netherlands [42]), but monozygotic (not dizygotic) twins have been affected [42]. Furthermore, 42% of first-degree relatives in the Netherlands have had other autoimmune diseases (rheumatoid arthritis, type 1 diabetes, and autoimmune thyroid disease) [42]. The antibodies associated with autoimmune hepatitis have been uncommon in first degree relatives of juvenile patients in Britain, but the frequency of the human leukocyte antigen (HLA) DRB1*0301, which has been associated with autoimmunity, has been similar in both populations [102]. These findings suggest a familial propensity for immune reactivity.

16.2.5.1 Genetic Susceptibilities Within the MHC

Genes within the MHC encode the antigen-binding groove of the class II MHC molecules, and they can affect the presentation of antigens and the nature of the autoreactive response [11]. *DRB1*0301* and *DRB1*0401* are the principal susceptibility alleles in white North American and European adults with autoimmune hepatitis [103, 104] (Table 16.4). Each allele encodes a six amino acid sequence (leucine-leucine-glutamic acid-glutamine-lysine-arginine) at positions DRβ67–72 of the antigen binding groove, and this sequence has been associated with the occurrence of autoimmune hepatitis in these adult populations [103, 105].

Table 16.4 Ethnic differences in genetic factors for autoimmune hepatitis

Genetic factors	Principal associations in ethnic groups with autoimmune hepatitis	Clinical associations
Alleles inside MHC	White North American and European adults • *DRB1*0301* and *DRB1*0401* [103, 104] Japanese, Chinese, Mexicans, South Koreans • *DRB1*0404* and *DRB1*0405* [106–110] Argentina, Brazil, Venezuela, Peru • *DRB1*1301* (children) [111–115] • *DRB1*0405* (adults) [23] • *DRB1*1301*, *DRB1*0405*, *DQB1*02*, *DQB1*0603* (meta-analysis) [116] North American and European children • *DQB1*0201* [122, 123] • Linked with *DRB1*07*, *DRB1*03* [123]	*DRB1*03 and DRB1*04 alleles* • Encode similar amino acid sequences in class II MHC molecules [11, 103, 105] • May present similar triggering antigens [4] *DRB1*1301* • Encodes different amino acid sequence than *DRB1*03* and *DRB1*04* alleles in class II MHC molecules [11, 117] • Affects mainly children [23, 111] • Associated with HAV infection [25] • May favor viral triggers [4] *DQB1*0201*, *DRB1*07* and *DRB1*03* • Associated with anti-LKM1 [122, 123] • Affects mainly children [122, 123] • May favor CYP2D6 or homologous viral epitopes [128, 129]
Variants outside MHC	North American adults • *CTLA-4* [131, 135] • *TNFRSF (Fas)* [137] • *TNFA* [138, 139] European and Chinese adults • *Vitamin D receptor* (*VDR*) [140, 141] European adults • *SH2B3* [104] • *CARD10* [104] Japanese adults • *TNFRSF (Fas)* [136] • *STAT4* [142] South American children and adults • *TGF-β1* [18]	Controversial pathogenic significance [134] Statistical associations in small cohorts [132] Not disease-specific [17, 130–132] Uncertain functional differences between variants of same gene [4] Variable presence in ethnic groups [131, 133] No direct comparisons between ethnicities [1] Constellations may be more important than any single variant [4, 11]

CARD10 caspase recruitment domain family member 10 gene, *CTLA-4* cytotoxic T lymphocyte antigen-4 gene, *MHC* major histocompatibility complex, *SH2B3* Scr homology 2 adaptor protein 3 gene, *STAT4* signal transducer and activator of transcription 4 gene, *TGF-β1* transforming growth factor-beta 1 gene, *TNFA* tumor necrosis factor-α gene, *TNFRSF* tumor necrosis factor receptor super-family (Fas) gene
Numbers in brackets are references

*DRB1*0404* and *DRB1*0405* are the principal susceptibility alleles in Japan [106, 107], mainland China [108], and Mexico [109], and *DRB1*0405* and *DQB1*0401* are the main susceptibility alleles in South Korea [110] (Table 16.4). The *DRB1*0404* and *DRB1*0405* alleles differ from the *DRB1*0301* and *DRB1*0401* alleles by encoding an arginine for lysine at the DRβ71 position. This substitution of a similarly structured and charged amino acid for lysine would not greatly alter antigen selection and presentation by the class II MHC molecules. Accordingly, the autoimmune hepatitis associated with the alleles, *DRB1*0301*, *DRB1*0401*, *DRB1*0404* and *DRB1*0405*, could be triggered in different geographical regions and ethnic groups by antigens with homologous epitopes [4].

In contrast, *DRB1*1301* is the principal susceptibility allele in Argentina [23, 111], Brazil [112, 113], Venezuela [114], and Peru [115], and *DRB1*0405*, *DQB1*02*, and *DQB1*0603* have also been implicated by meta-analysis [116] (Table 16.4). Children with autoimmune hepatitis in Argentina have mainly *DRB1*1301* [111], whereas adults with autoimmune hepatitis in Argentina have mainly *DRB1*0405* [23]. *DRB1*1301* encodes a different amino acid sequence (isoleucine-leucine-glutamic acid-aspartic acid-glutamic acid-arginine) between positions DRβ67–72 than the *DRB1*03* and *DRB1*04* alleles, and this sequence would change the steric and electrostatic properties of the antigen binding groove of the class II MHC molecules [117].

The substitution of the negatively charged aspartic acid and glutamic acid at positions DRβ70 and 71 within the antigen binding groove suggest that the autoimmune hepatitis in South American children with *DRB1*1301* is triggered by antigens different than those encountered in South American, North American, and European adults who have mainly *DRB1*03* and *DRB1*04* alleles. The association of protracted hepatitis A virus infection in patients with *DRB1*1301* [25] has supported speculation that the hepatitis A virus is a cause of autoimmune hepatitis, especially in areas like South America that are endemic for the virus [118–121]. This hypothesis might also extend elsewhere to other infectious agents that are more common in children than adults.

*DQB1*0201* has been proposed as the principal susceptibility allele of autoimmune hepatitis that is characterized by the presence of anti-LKM1 [122, 123] (Table 16.4). This allele is in strong linkage disequilibrium with *DRB1*07* and *DRB1*03* [123], and HLA DRB1*07 has been associated with this type of autoimmune hepatitis in Brazil [112, 113, 124, 125], Britain [126], and Germany [127]. The cytochrome P450 2D6 (CYP2D6) is the target antigen of anti-LKM1, and it has homologies with peptide sequences in the hepatitis C virus, cytomegalovirus, and herpes simplex type 1 virus [128, 129]. The autoimmune hepatitis characterized by anti-LKM1 in European children may be a reflection of exposures to indigenous infectious or environmental agents that mimic CYP2D6. Susceptibility might be enhanced by alleles of the MHC that favor presentation of these antigens.

16.2.5.2 Genetic Susceptibilities Outside the MHC

Genetic polymorphisms outside the MHC are not antigen-directed, and they may modify the immune response and modulate the mechanisms of tissue damage and repair in a fashion that is not disease-specific [17, 130–132]. They are frequently present in non-hepatic immune-mediated diseases, and they are commonly absent in the same immune-mediated disease but in different ethnic groups [131, 133]. Accordingly, their presence is not essential for disease occurrence, and their true role in autoimmune hepatitis has been unclear and controversial [134].

Polymorphisms of the *cytotoxic T lymphocyte antigen-4 gene* (*CTLA-4*) [131, 135], *Fas* gene (*tumor necrosis factor receptor super-family [TNFRSF] gene*) [136, 137], *tumor necrosis factor-α* (*TNFA*2*) *gene* [138, 139], *vitamin D receptor* (*VDR*) *gene* [140, 141], *signal transducer and activator of transcription 4* (*STAT4*) *gene* [142], *transforming growth factor-beta 1 (TGF-β1) gene* [18], the *Scr homology 2 adaptor protein 3 (SH2B3) gene* [104], and the *caspase recruitment domain family member 10* (*CARD10*) *gene* [104] have been implicated as genetic factors in autoimmune hepatitis (Table 16.4). Each has been described in region- and ethnic-specific cohorts; each has been implicated by statistical association of varying strength; and none has an established role in the occurrence or manifestations of autoimmune hepatitis. A constellation of polymorphisms may be a more critical determinant of the phenotype and behavior of autoimmune hepatitis in different populations than a single prime variant.

16.2.5.3 Genetic Associations with Clinical Course

The alleles within the MHC have been associated with differences in the phenotype and behavior of autoimmune hepatitis in patients of the same or different ethnicity [11]. *DRB1*0301* has been associated with an earlier age of onset, more severe disease, higher frequency of treatment failure, and greater requirement for liver transplantation than patients with *DRB1*0401* in white North American and European adults [16, 64, 105, 143]. In contrast, patients with *DRB1*0401* are more commonly women, have concurrent immune diseases more frequently, respond better to immunosuppressive therapy, and are older at disease onset than patients with *DRB1*0301* [16, 64, 105]. Elderly patients (aged ≥60 years) have *DRB1*0401* more often than young adults (aged ≤30 years), and they respond better to immunosuppressive therapy despite having a greater frequency of cirrhosis at presentation [144, 145].

*DRB1*0301* is rare in the Japanese population, and *DRB1*0405* is the principal susceptibility allele for autoimmune hepatitis [106, 146, 147]. Japanese patients with autoimmune hepatitis are typically women with late onset disease, few or no symptoms, mild disease severity, responsiveness to treatment, and favorable long-term prognosis [148–150]. In this ethnic group, the common association of *DRB1*0405* with autoimmune hepatitis and the almost complete absence of *DRB1*0301* in the general population may have shaped a disease phenotype that is similar to that of women in western countries who also have *DRB1*04* alleles. Genome wide association studies (GWAS) in diverse geographical regions and ethnic groups may be able to identify other genetic factors that influence outcome and help individualize management strategies.

16.2.6 Possible Epigenetic Changes Affecting Predisposition and Outcome

Micro-ribonucleic acids (miRNAs) are regulatory molecules that exert an epigenetic effect on the transcriptional activity of genes by binding with the messenger RNA (mRNA) produced by the gene and marking it for degradation by an RNA-induced silencing complex (RISC) [151, 152]. This gene silencing effect can repress the activity of protein-encoding genes, and it may alter the expressions of pro- and anti-inflammatory genes in autoimmune liver disease [21]. Serum levels of the miRNAs miR-21 and miR-122 have fluctuated with the serum ALT concentrations in Japanese patients with autoimmune hepatitis, and the circulating level of miR-21 has correlated with the histological grade of inflammation [153].

miRNAs have organ but not disease specificity, and their association with inflammatory activity in autoimmune hepatitis suggests that they may affect susceptibility and outcome. The expression of miRNAs is influenced by genetic factors, and the genes expressing the miRNAs themselves can be affected by epigenetic mechanisms that may be cued from the environment [154, 155]. Epidemiological studies are required to determine if differences in clinical phenotype and outcome in diverse populations can be ascribed to variations in the expression of miRNAs as a result of genetic variation or environmental cues.

Vitamin D deficiency occurs in 51–92% of patients with non-cholestatic chronic liver disease [156–158] and 81% of Turkish patients with autoimmune hepatitis [159]. Low serum levels of 25-hydroxyvitamin D3 may result from impaired liver hydroxylation of the skin-derived vitamin D3 [156, 157] or impaired synthesis, absorption, or consumption of vitamin D3 [160]. Variations in sun exposure, seasonal climate, diet, and contact with toxins that alter the metabolic activity of P450 cytochromes can promote vitamin D deficiency and perturb the immunomodulatory actions of vitamin D [161].

Vitamin D has diverse immunomodulatory effects on the innate and adaptive immune systems [162–164], and the vitamin D receptor (VDR) is expressed on multiple cell types [165, 166]. Furthermore, the hydroxylating enzyme (25-hydroxyvitamin D-1α hydroxylase) that converts inactive 25-hydroxyvitamin D3 to the active 1,25-dihydroxyvitamin D3 is not restricted to the kidney. The expression of 25-hydroxyvitamin D-1α hydroxylase can be induced in diverse cell types, and the hydroxylating enzyme can activate vitamin D outside the kidney [167, 168].

The activated 1,25-dihydroxyvitamin D3 can in turn interact with the vitamin D response element (VDRE) in regulatory genes, and it can modulate the immune response by exerting an epigenetic effect on the transcriptional activity of the targeted gene [169]. Genetic factors can affect the structure and avidity of the VDR, and differences in vitamin D availability and metabolism may also affect susceptibility to autoimmune hepatitis and its clinical phenotype in diverse populations [140, 141]. Population-based epidemiological studies will be pivotal in determining the impact of vitamin D deficiency and epigenetic changes on the distribution and consequences of autoimmune hepatitis.

16.3 Epidemiology of Primary Biliary Cholangitis

Primary biliary cholangitis is a progressive chronic liver disease in which the biliary epithelial cells rather than the hepatocytes are the primary targets of the immune response [170]. Clinical, laboratory, and histological changes (bile duct injury, destruction or loss) define a cholestatic phenotype that typifies PBC and distinguishes it from autoimmune hepatitis [171]. Importantly, the classical cholestatic components can be absent at presentation [172] or intermixed with features of autoimmune hepatitis (overlap syndrome) [6]. Furthermore, many patients may be asymptomatic and escape early detection [173, 174]. For these reasons, population-based epidemiological studies of PBC can be influenced greatly by the level of clinical expertise within the community being scrutinized [175].

16.3.1 Annual Incidence of Primary Biliary Cholangitis

The annual incidence of PBC has ranged from 0 to <1 case per 100,000 persons in Brunei, Darussalem [176] and Estonia [177] to 3.2 cases per 100,000 persons in Newcastle, United Kingdom [178, 179] (Table 16.5). Olmsted County, Minnesota (2.7 cases per 100,000 persons) [180], Calgary, Canada (3.03 cases per 100,000 persons) [181], and Newcastle, United Kingdom (3.2 cases per 100,000 persons) [178, 179] have reported an annual incidence of PBC that is almost twofold greater than the annual incidence of PBC in Denmark (1.14 cases per 100,000 persons) [182], Sweden (1.4 cases per 100,000 persons) [173], Norway (1.6 cases per 100,000 persons) [44], Italy (1.67 cases per 100,000 persons) [182], and Spain (1.72 cases per 100,000 persons) [183]. Furthermore, the annual incidence of PBC in Olmsted

Table 16.5 Incidence and prevalence of primary biliary cholangitis in different regions (lowest to highest annual incidence)

Geographical region	Annual incidence per 100,000 persons	Prevalence per 100,000 persons
Australia (Victoria) [194, 198]	Not reported	1.9–5.1 (Australian-born, 3.72; Italian-born, 19.9; Greek-born, 20.8; British-born, 14.1)
Brunei, Darussalem [176, 306]	0–1	2.6 (Malaysian, 2.3; Chinese, 4.1)
Estonia [177]	0.23	2.69
Japan [175, 195]	Not reported	2.7–5.4
China (southern) [196]	Not reported	4.92 (15.6 in women aged >40 years)
Israel (southern) [197]	Not reported	5.5
Denmark [182]	1.14	11.5
Sweden [173]	1.4	12.8
Norway (Oslo) [44]	1.6	14.6
Italy (Lombardia) [182]	1.67	16 (increasing prevalence)
Spain (Sabadell) [183]	1.72	19.5
United States (Olmsted County, Minnesota) [180]	2.7 (women, 4.5; men, 0.7) (stable for 20 years)	40.2 (women, 65.4; men, 12.1)
Canada (Calgary) [181]	3.03 (women, 4.84; men, 1.04) (stable from 1996 to 2003)	22.7 (increased from 10 over 6 years)
United Kingdom (Newcastle) [178, 179, 199]	3.2 (increased from 2.3 over 7 years)	25.1 (increased from 14.9 over 7 years)

Numbers in brackets are references

County, Calgary, and Newcastle is almost 14-fold greater than the annual incidence of PBC in Estonia (0.23 cases per 100,000 persons) [177]. Importantly, each region with the highest annual incidence of PBC (Olmsted County, Minnesota, Calgary, Canada, and Newcastle, United Kingdom) has an academic medical center with a long-standing interest and expertise in PBC.

The annual incidence of PBC has been stable for 7 years in Calgary, Canada [181] and for 20 years in Olmsted County, Minnesota [180], but it has increased in Newcastle, United Kingdom (2.3–3.2 cases per 100,000 persons over 7 years) [178, 179] (Table 16.5). In adults aged ≥20 years in Newcastle, the annual incidence has increased from 3.1 to 4.3 cases per 100,000 persons, and in women aged ≥40 years, it has increased from 9.1 to 10 cases per 100,000 women [179]. These trends have not been statistically significant, but they have been consistent in each analyzed subgroup. Since the three regions with the highest annual incidence of PBC have academic medical centers with similar interest and expertise in PBC, the increasing annual incidence of PBC in one area is unlikely to reflect a difference in case detection. Continued separation of the Newcastle region from the other two regions would suggest a newly introduced environmental factor for PBC or a changing population by age, gender or genetic composition.

The annual incidence of PBC in women has been 4.5 cases per 100,000 persons in Olmsted County, Minnesota [180] and 4.84 cases per 100,000 persons in Calgary, Canada [181]. The annual incidence of PBC in women has been 4.6- to 6.4-fold greater than in men residing in these same regions (Table 16.5). The female-to-male ratio of patients with PBC has been 2.3:1 in Lombardia, Italy [182], 4.2:1 in Denmark [182], and 9–10:1 in most other studies [50, 175, 184]. The bases for the female predisposition for PBC and the variable sex ratios in different regions are unclear [170]. Recent studies have suggested that the composition of the intestinal microbiome can influence the immune response in PBC [185–188]. The intestinal microflora may also contribute to gender bias by influencing serum sex hormone levels and altering the antigenic stimuli that modulate the immune response [32, 189, 190].

The annual incidence of PBC is highly dependent on age, and in Calgary, the highest incidence is among individuals aged 60–79 years (annual incidence, 6.3 cases per 100,000 persons) [181]. Primary biliary cholangitis does not affect children, and the absence of childhood PBC also distinguishes it from autoimmune hepatitis and PSC [59, 67, 191–193]. The bases for protection against PBC in children are unknown, and this uncertainty must generate speculation about the pathogenic role of post-pubescent female hormones, infections, environmental factors, and age-related changes in the intestinal microbiome [32, 170].

16.3.2 Prevalence of Primary Biliary Cholangitis

The prevalence of PBC ranges from 1.9 cases per 100,000 persons in Victoria, Australia [194] to 40.2 cases per 100,000 persons in Olmsted County, Minnesota [180]. Asian countries (Japan [195] and China [196]) and southern Israel [197] have a prevalence of PBC that is one third the prevalence of PBC in Europe and one fifth the prevalence in North America (Table 16.5). In contrast, Australia, whose population is descended mainly from European settlers, has a lower prevalence of PBC than Europe, North America, Asia and southern Israel [194, 198]. Prevalence has been 5.4-fold higher in women than men in the United States (65.4 cases per 100,000 women versus 12.1 cases per 100,000 men) [180], and it has been 15-fold higher in patients aged 60–79 years than in patients aged 20–39 years in Canada (57.3 cases per 100,000 persons versus 3.8 cases per 100,000 persons) [181].

Australian-born women aged ≥24 years have a prevalence of 5.1 cases per 100,000 persons (95% CI: 3.75–6.79) [194], but this estimate is still lower than that reported in Europe [44, 173, 178, 179, 182, 183], North America [180, 181], and Japan [195] (Table 16.5). Australian-born individuals also have a lower prevalence of PBC (3.72 cases per 100,000 persons) compared to individuals who have migrated to Australia from Britain (14.1 cases per 100,000 persons), Italy (19.9 cases per 1000,000 persons), and Greece (20.8 cases per 100,000 persons) [198]. Genetic factors are unlikely to be the basis for protection from PBC since most Australians are descended from British and European settlers [194] whose native populations have had a higher prevalence of PBC than native Victorians [179, 198]. These findings have justified speculation that individuals in Australia are protected from PBC because they lack an environmental factor encountered elsewhere [194, 198].

The prevalence of PBC has increased by more than twofold over a 6 year period in Calgary, Canada (from 10 to 22.7 cases per 100,000 persons) and by 1.7-fold over a 7 year period in Newcastle, United Kingdom [178, 179, 199] (Table 16.5). The prevalence may also have increased in Lombardia, Italy [182]. An increasing prevalence of PBC in certain regions suggests that the disease is being recognized at earlier asymptomatic stages and individuals with the disease are living longer [179]. Whereas greater recognition of the disease can be a consequence of improved case-detection, improved survival may relate to changes in the behavior, management or cause of the disease.

16.3.3 Variations in Liver-Related Mortality in Different Geographical Regions

The number of liver transplants performed in patients with PBC has been decreasing [3, 200], and this finding suggests that earlier detection and improved management have had an impact on prevalence. This possibility has not been established (or excluded) by comparisons of mortality between regions with rising and stable prevalence of PBC. The annual mortality of PBC in Calgary, Canada has been 3.4%; the standardized mortality ratio (SMR) has been 2.1 (95% CI: 1.2–3.4); the frequency of liver transplantation over 5.8 years (range, 10 days–10.9 years) has been 4.4%; and the 5- and 10-year survivals have been 83% and 73%, respectively [181]. The 5- and 10-year survivals of women with PBC in Calgary are 87% and 80%, respectively, compared to those of men (64% and 0%, respectively). Calgary has had a greater increase in prevalence of PBC than Newcastle, England and Lombardia, Italy. Survival has also been better in this region.

The SMR for PBC has been 2.85 (95% CI: 2.54–3.19) in Newcastle, United Kingdom [179], and the 5- and 10-year survivals have been 70% and 61%, respectively, in Lombardia Italy [182]. Women with PBC in Lombardia have had 5- and 10-year survivals of 77% and 67%, respectively, compared to those of men (55% and 47%, respectively). In contrast, the estimated 10-year survival of PBC in Olmsted County, Minnesota, which has had a stable prevalence of PBC for 20 years, is 59% [180]. Countering the suggestion that increased survival is a basis for increasing prevalence of PBC in certain communities is the lack of statistically valid comparisons of survival between the regions of interest.

The marked predilection of women for PBC [50, 175, 177, 180, 182], the lower occurrence but higher mortality of men than women with the disease [181, 182], the relative protection of native-born Australians from PBC [194, 198], and the sparing of children [170] are epidemiological observations that lack an explanation, and these findings should direct future investigations.

16.3.4 Environmental Factors and the Occurrence of Primary Biliary Cholangitis

Environmental agents and conditions have been implicated as risk factors for PBC, and they may help explain the clustering of cases in certain areas within the same geographical region [201, 202].

16.3.4.1 Tobacco Smoking

Tobacco smoking has been strongly implicated as an environmental risk factor for PBC (Table 16.6). Regular smoking and a history of previous smoking have been more frequent in patients with PBC than control populations [203–209], and patients with PBC have had a higher frequency of persistent passive exposure to tobacco smoke [209, 210]. Furthermore, smoking history and the amount of tobacco consumed have been associated with advanced hepatic fibrosis [211, 212]. Smoking intensity, defined by the number of pack-years, has been higher in patients with advanced hepatic fibrosis (stages 3 and 4) than in patients without these histological findings, and the likelihood of advanced hepatic fibrosis at presentation has increased by 5% (95% CI: 1.3–8.7%) for each increase in pack-year exposure [212]. Smoking has also been more frequent in other immune-mediated diseases, including rheumatoid arthritis (RA), systemic lupus erythematosus (SLE), multiple sclerosis (MS), and Graves' disease [213]. These observations have supported concerns that tobacco smoke has deleterious effects on the immune system.

Smokers in general have increased plasma levels of the pro-inflammatory cytokines, interleukin (IL)-1, IL-6, IL-8, and interferon-gamma (IFN-γ) [214–216]. The anti-inflammatory cytokine, IL-10, is also increased, but plasma IFN-γ (not IL-10) levels are higher in female smokers than male smokers [208, 217]. The predominance of IFN-γ in women in conjunction with other pro-inflammatory cytokines favor a type 1 cytokine pathway of lymphocyte differentiation and proliferation in

Table 16.6 Environmental risk factors for primary biliary cholangitis

Risk factor	Possible mechanism(s)	Evidence
Cigarette smoking	Releases polycyclic aromatic hydrocarbons (including benzene) and ROS [216, 222, 223] Pro-inflammatory cytokines increased [215] Protective dendritic cell functions less [220] Risk of infection increased [220] Xenobiotic transformation of mitochondrial antigen into neo-antigen [216, 224]	History of smoking associated with PBC [205] Regular smoking more common in PBC [209] More lifetime exposure to second hand smoke [209] Associated with advanced fibrosis [211, 212] Dose-dependent effect on fibrosis risk [212] Linked to RA, SLE, MS, Graves' disease [213]
Toxic waste exposure	Possible exposures to benzene, trichloroethylene, and other aromatic and halogenated hydrocarbons [227] Toxic liver injury may trigger autoreactive immune response [227]	Increased frequency of PBC on liver transplant list in zip code areas in or adjacent to Superfund toxic waste sites in New York [227]
Water source	Soft water, low fluoride levels found [226] Uncertain pathogenic effects [216]	PBC >10-fold more common in areas of Sheffield, England receiving water from one reservoir [184]
Nail polish Hair dye	May alter or complex with self-proteins changing structure to induce immune response (xenobiotic effect) [228]	Controlled interview-based study showed increased association with PBC [205]
HRT	Uncertain pathogenic effect [233] Improves liver tests in PBC [234]	HRT use more frequent in PBC [205] May be prescribed more commonly [205]
Urban living	Presumed exposure to industrial pollution, infectious agents, toxic waste [230]	Associated with higher prevalence than in rural community [230]
Seasonality	May relate to seasonal infections, pollutants, exercises, diets, sunlight/UV exposure [235]	Peak diagnosis of PBC in northeast England during month of June [235]

HRT hormonal replacement therapy, *MS* multiple sclerosis, *PBC* primary biliary cholangitis, *RA* rheumatoid arthritis, *ROS* reactive oxygen species, *SLE* systemic lupus erythematosus, *UV* ultraviolet
Numbers in brackets are references

PBC [218]. Predominance of the type 1 cytokine pathway can in turn promote hepatic fibrosis [219]. Tobacco smoking can also suppress the secretion of cytokines, IL-12 and IL-23, by dendritic cells and weaken the immune response to bacterial lipopolysaccharide [220]. A compromised immune defense could favor the occurrence of infections that might also trigger PBC [220]. Chronic expression of IFN-γ in a mouse model can produce an autoimmune cholangitis with female predominance that mimics human PBC [221].

Numerous other cytotoxic agents are also inhaled during tobacco smoking, including nicotine, polycyclic aromatic hydrocarbons (benzene), and reactive oxygen species (ROS) [222, 223]. Chemical transformation of benzene through halogenation can have a xenobiotic effect, and it may contribute to the development of PBC by altering mitochondrial antigens and inducing an autoreactive response [224]. ROS may also contribute by altering mitochondrial function, inducing apoptosis, provoking nitrosative stress, and stimulating hepatic fibrosis [225].

16.3.4.2 Water Sources, Toxic Waste Sites, Nail Polish, and Hormonal Replacement Therapy

The unusual occurrence of PBC in certain areas within a geographical region has supported the concept that a toxic agent might predispose to the disease by exerting a xenobiotic effect [24, 224, 226, 227]. Xenobiotics are foreign substances (chemicals, drugs, and pollutants) that are not naturally produced or consumed. Their introduction into the system is usually fortuitous and unsuspected, and they can have deleterious consequences. The mitochondrial component, pyruvate dehydrogenase complex-E2 (PDC-E2), can be altered *in vitro* by a xenobiotic [224, 228], and this molecular alteration could create a neo-antigen that enhances or extends an autoreactive response [229]. Modification of the PDC-E2 peptide with 2-octynoic acid induces a greater reactivity against PBC sera than against control sera, and the use of 2-octynoic acid in perfumes, lipstick, and food colorings ensures ample opportunity for environmental exposure to this xenobiotic [224].

Epidemiological studies have supported the concept of a xenobiotic effect in PBC (Table 16.6). A single water source in Sheffield, England has supplied an area in which the prevalence of PBC has been >10-fold higher than the prevalence of PBC in areas supplied by other water sources [226]. Neighborhoods in close proximity to a toxic waste site have had more patients with PBC awaiting liver transplantation than other neighborhoods of New York [227], and case-control studies have indicated a statistical association between the occurrence of PBC and yearly exposures to nail polish ($P < 0.0001$) and hair dye ($P = 0.04$) [205]. The higher prevalence of PBC in urban communities (14.4 cases per 100,000 persons) than in rural communities (3.7 cases per 100,000 persons) supports speculation that PBC-causing xenobiotics are more plentiful in the urban environment [230].

Drugs may also exert a xenobiotic effect or cause drug-induced liver injury which may in turn promote a pro-inflammatory immune response [231]. A case-control study by questionnaire has demonstrated a statistically higher frequency of hormonal replacement therapy (HRT) in patients with PBC than in unaffected women [205] (Table 16.6). The pathogenic significance of this finding remains speculative since HRT is frequently prescribed in PBC as part of a management strategy to prevent or improve osteoporosis [232]. Estrogen receptors are present in the biliary epithelial cells of patients with PBC (in contrast to normal liver), but they disappear in advanced stages and their role in disease progression is unclear [233]. Furthermore, estradiol therapy has actually improved liver tests in PBC [234].

16.3.4.3 Seasonal Variation

The diagnosis of PBC has a seasonality that may influence its detection at early stages and its prognosis (Table 16.6). The symptoms of PBC have been recognized most commonly in the Spring and early Summer in northeast England [230, 235], and the peak month for diagnosing PBC in this region has been June [235]. Furthermore, the distribution of patients with survivals >10 years has had a similar seasonality that has not been evident in the distribution of patients with survivals <5 years [235]. These findings have suggested that the summer occurrence of symptoms may have contributed to an early diagnosis of PBC that in turn favored an improved survival.

The seasonality of the diagnosis of PBC in northeast England could not be attributed to changes in the number of patients attending medical clinics or admitted to hospital, and a transient seasonal factor with a short lag time between exposure and effect has been suspected [235, 236]. Infections [237–241] and air pollutants whose occurrence can vary with weather conditions [242, 243] have been prime considerations, but other seasonal factors (activities, dietary adjustments, and exposure to sunlight and ultraviolet radiation) cannot be overlooked. Similar epidemiological studies have not been performed in other countries to assess the regional specificity of the observations.

16.3.5 Infectious Agents and the Occurrence of Primary Biliary Cholangitis

Infectious agents may trigger an immune-mediated disease by sensitizing immune cells to peptide sequences within the pathogen that resemble those within the host (molecular mimicry) [9, 244]. They may also cause tissue damage, create or expose neo-antigens within the host, and promote a pro-inflammatory immune response that breaks self-tolerance [4]. Some infectious agents may metabolize xenobiotics, and these metabolic products may then alter the immunogenicity of normal host proteins (xenobiotic effect) [238]. An infectious etiology has long been considered in PBC [245–247], and this speculation has been supported by several epidemiological studies. *Escherichia coli* has been the most commonly implicated organism, and it induces the expression of antibodies to PDC-E2 and histological changes of cholangitis in a mouse model [244]. Multiple other pathogens have also been proposed [247], but only *Novoshingobium aromaticivorans* [238, 241, 248, 249] and β-retrovirus [250–254] have been well studied.

16.3.5.1 *Escherichia coli* and Urinary Tract Infections

Escherichia coli and PDC-E2 have structural similarities, and these homologies between the pathogen and the host (molecular mimicry) may generate a promiscuous immune response that breaks self-tolerance of PDC-E2 and triggers PBC [9, 244, 255, 256] (Table 16.7). In the United Kingdom, the frequency of urinary tract infection (UTI) has been higher in women with PBC (19%) than in women with

Table 16.7 Infectious agents and the occurrence of primary biliary cholangitis

Infectious agent	Laboratory evidence	Clinical evidence
Escherichia coli	Structural homologies with PDC-E2 [9] Induces antibodies to PDC-E2 and cholangitis in mouse model [244]	UTIs more common in PBC [257, 258] Most UTIs caused by *E. coli* [257] Multiple UTIs are risk factors [259] Association exists across regions [209, 210]
Novoshingobium aromaticivorans	Metabolizes xenobiotics [238] Two homologies with PDC-E2 [241] PBC sera reactive against bacteria [238] Infected mice develop cholangitis [244]	PBC sera react to bacterial proteins [240] Reactivity consistent with AMA [240] FDRs may also react (1.2%) [240] Bacteria in 25% PBC fecal specimens [240]
Human β-retrovirus	Viral sequences in diseased livers [251] Exogenous virus signature [251] Retroviral antibodies in serum [250] Retroviral sequences in genome [253] Virus-like particles in biliary cells [237]	Better after anti-retroviral therapy [254] Retroviral infection not in all PBC [252] Retrovirus not disease-specific [262]
Less robust candidates • Epstein-Barr virus • *Mycobacterium gordonae* • *Helicobacter pylori* • *Chlamydia pneumoniae* • *Mycoplasma pneumoniae*	Increased EBV DNA in PBMC, liver tissue, and saliva of PBC patients [263] PBC sera react against *M. gordonae* [264] *M. gordonae* and AMA cross-react [264] *H. pylori* in PBC liver tissue [265] *C. pneumoniae* antigen and RNA in PBC liver tissue [266] PDC subunits on mycoplasma [267] Reactivity to mycoplasma in PBC [267]	No epidemiological studies or treatment trials [247]

AMA antimitochondrial antibodies, *EBV DNA* Epstein-Barr virus deoxyribonucleic acid, *FDRs* first degree relatives, *PBC* primary biliary cholangitis, *PBMC* peripheral blood mononuclear cells, *PDC-E2* pyruvate dehydrogenase complex E2 subunits, *RNA* ribonucleic acid, *UTIs* urinary tract infections
Numbers in brackets are references

other chronic liver (7%) or non-liver (8%) diseases, and most UTIs have been caused by *Escherichia coli* [257, 258]. Furthermore, most women with PBC have had multiple, often asymptomatic UTIs that have disappeared and re-appeared spontaneously in patterns unaffected by antibiotic therapy [259].

Similar associations between UTIs and PBC have been recognized in the United States [205, 209, 216] and France [210] (Table 16.7). Multiple UTIs have been common in women with PBC (>1 episode per year in the United States [209] to >5 episodes per lifetime in France [210]), and the infections have occurred mainly before the diagnosis of PBC [260]. The highest adjusted odds ratio (OR) for the occurrence of PBC (OR: 2.60 [1.02–6.63]) has been in British women aged

<55 years who have had pyelonephritis 5 years prior to the diagnosis of PBC [260]. Animal studies have supported the epidemiological findings by demonstrating the development of autoimmune cholangitis and antimitochondrial antibodies (AMA) in genetically susceptible mice after infection with *Escherichia coli* [244].

16.3.5.2 *Novoshingobium aromaticivorans*

Novoshingobium aromaticivorans is an alphaproteobacterium. Alphaproteobacteria are ubiquitous, gram-negative, non-spore-forming, rod-shaped, aerobic organisms that are found mainly in soil sediments [239]. *Novoshingobium aromaticivorans* degrades aromatic compounds which may then act as xenobiotics, and it also activates environmental estrogens [238, 241] (Table 16.7). Two lipoylated proteins within *Novoshingobium aromaticivorans* have homology with PDC-E2, and sera from patients with PBC have uniformly reacted against these bacterial proteins in titers 100- to 1000-fold higher than against *Escherichia coli* [238]. Furthermore, genetically-modified mice infected with *Novoshingobium aromaticivorans* have developed biliary changes, albeit less severe than in mice infected with *Escherichia coli* [244].

In Iceland, the sera of patients with PBC have reacted against the proteins of *Novoshingobium aromaticivorans* in a fashion consistent with their AMA status, and the one of 85 first-degree relatives (1.2%) who had AMA also had reactivity to the proteins of *Novoshingobium aromaticivorans* [239, 240] (Table 16.7). *Novoshingobium aromaticivorans* has been isolated in 25% of fecal specimens from patients with PBC, but it has also been recovered with similar frequency in healthy individuals from the same household (26%) and healthy individuals from different households (27%) [238].

There have been no epidemiological studies within the same geographical region or between regions to define the distribution or clustering of PBC that is associated with *Novoshingobium aromaticivorans*. Furthermore, there have been no studies that suggest routes of bacterial transmission, identify genetic, ethnic or age-related predispositions, characterize the clinical phenotype, or determine differences in outcome. Causal relationships are difficult to establish by demonstrating molecular mimicries in the laboratory, coincident colonization of comparable frequency in patients and healthy individuals, and compatible but nonspecific biliary changes in genetically-modified animal models.

16.3.5.3 Human β-Retrovirus

Human β-retrovirus emerged as an etiological consideration in PBC when explorative studies in the livers of patients with PBC failed to demonstrate bacterial infection [254]. Subsequent studies using subtractive hybridization techniques found viral sequences in the diseased livers that were consistent with an exogenous virus that had nucleotide similarities with a β-retrovirus associated with breast cancer in mice [251] (Table 16.7). Later studies in PBC demonstrated retroviral antibodies in serum samples [250], virus-like particles in biliary epithelial cells [237], and retroviral sequences in the genome of biliary epithelium [253]. Biochemical responses to a treatment combination of reverse transcriptase inhibitor and protease inhibitor in patients with PBC provided a proof of principle that retrovirus might cause PBC [254, 261].

Subsequent studies have challenged the role of β-retrovirus in PBC. Immunological and molecular evidence of retroviral infection has been absent in one study [252], and retrovirus has been detected in liver diseases other than PBC in another study [262] (Table 16.7). Furthermore, the frequency of retroviral detection has been higher in other liver diseases than in PBC (27% versus 12%) [262]. There have been no epidemiological studies demonstrating the incidence, prevalence, distribution and consequences of human β-retroviral infection in PBC, and the pathogenic relationship between this viral agent and PBC remains uncertain.

16.3.5.4 Other Infectious Candidates

Epstein-Barr virus (EBV) [263], *Mycobacterium gordonae* [264], *Helicobacter pylori* [265], *Chlamydia pneumoniae* [266], and *Mycoplasma pneumoniae* [267] have all been proposed as causative agents of PBC, but none has been validated or aggressively pursued [247] (Table 16.7). Infection may be a consequence of chronic liver disease rather than its cause. Furthermore, the burden of infection with one or more organisms may be the critical factor triggering the disease rather than any individual agent [268].

16.3.6 Variations in Genetic Predisposition in Different Geographical Regions and Ethnic Groups

Epidemiological studies have implicated genetic factors in the occurrence of PBC [269–271], and these observations have been supported by genome-wide association studies in North American, European, and Japanese cohorts [272–275]. PBC has occurred in 5 of 8 monozygotic twin sets within families that have had at least one index case of PBC, and it has not occurred in 8 dizygotic twin sets selected by the same criteria [270] (Table 16.8). The concordance rate of 0.63 among individuals that have genetic identity and shared environmental background (monozygotic twins) contrasts with the absence of disease in individuals that lack genetic identity but have shared environmental background (dizygotic twins). The findings strongly implicate genetic factors in the occurrence of PBC, and they are supported by other studies of familial occurrence.

PBC has clustered in families, including 5 of 8 sisters of Palestinian origin [202], and familial occurrence has been documented in 0.72% of first degree relatives in Newcastle, England [276]; 1% in Brazil [277]; 1.3% in London, England [278]; 5.1–5.8% in different regions of Japan [269, 279]; 6.4% in New York, New York [280]; and 9.9% in Crete, Greece [271] (Table 16.8). First degree family members may also manifest autoantibodies, hypergammaglobulinemia, and extrahepatic autoimmune diseases that suggest a genetic propensity for immune reactivity. AMA have been demonstrated in 13% of first degree relatives in Olmsted County, Minnesota [281] and 18.8% in Larissa, Greece [282]. Immune mediated diseases of

Table 16.8 Genetic associations with primary biliary cholangitis

Sources	Principal associations	Clinical implications
Twin studies	PBC in 5 of 8 MZ twin sets [270] PBC in 0 of 8 DZ twin sets [270] High concordance with genetic identity (0.63) [270]	Genetic identity a risk factor [270] Shared environment less critical [270]
Familial occurrence	PBC in 5 of 8 Palestinian sisters [202] PBC in 0.72–10% of FDR [271, 276] AMA in 13–19% of FDR [281, 282] Autoimmune diseases in 4–14% of FDR [277, 283] PBC in 1.2% of offspring [276]	Hereditary propensity for PBC [280] Low penetrance of genotype [276]
HLA associations	*DRB1*08-DQB1*0402* haplotype [285] Extends weakly to *DPB1*0301* in British [285] Extends weakly to *DPB1*0501* in Japanese [285] DRB1, DQA1, DQB1 loci by GWAS [275, 287, 288]	Contributory not causative [275] Weak association [285]
Non-HLA associations	Located on chromosomes 6p21.3 and 2q [275] *IL-12A, IL-12RB2* are major factors [289] *CTLA-4* implicated [17, 130]	Lack disease specificity [275] Modulate immune reactivity [290]

AMA antimitochondrial antibodies, *CTLA-4* cytotoxic T lymphocyte antigen-4 gene, *DZ* dizygotic, *FDR* first degree relatives, *HLA* human leukocyte antigen, *IL* interleukin, *MZ* monozygotic, *PBC* primary biliary cholangitis
Numbers in brackets are references

a non-liver nature have also been present in 4% of first degree relatives in Brazil [277] and 14% of first degree relatives in Newcastle, England [283].

These findings are consistent with a hereditary propensity for the development of PBC, but they do not indicate a disease-related genotype of strong penetrance (Table 16.8). Only 1.2% of the offspring of PBC patients develop PBC [276], and the frequency of first degree relatives developing PBC is only 0.7% in the absence of AMA [284]. First degree relatives have a greater frequency of developing PBC if they express AMA (24%), but only if the serum alkaline phosphatase level is also increased [284]. The occurrence of PBC may be favored by hereditary factors, but other infectious, toxic or environmental agents may be necessary to trigger the disease. The variations in the occurrence of PBC, its laboratory manifestations, and other immune-mediated diseases in first degree relatives from different geographical regions and ethnic groups support these considerations.

PBC has been associated with the *DRB1*08-DQB1*0402* haplotype, and this haplotype extends weakly to include *DPB1*0301* in British patients and *DPB1*0501* in Japanese patients [285] (Table 16.8). Polymorphisms of genes that can affect the immune response in PBC are located on chromosomes 6p21.3 and 2q [286], and a polymorphism of the *cytotoxic T lymphocyte antigen-4* (*CTLA-4*) *gene* has been implicated in PBC [17, 130]. Genome wide association studies have demonstrated genetic associations in PBC within and outside the MHC, and at least 27 risk loci unrelated to the human leukocyte antigen (HLA) have been associated with PBC [275, 287, 288]. The HLA variants that have been described in PBC by GWAS are at DRB1, DQA1 and DQB1 loci, and the non-HLA loci have been mainly genes that affect the production of IL-12 and the family of cytokines that modulate immune reactivity [275]. Variants of *IL-12A* and *IL-12RB2* have had strong associations with PBC [289], and they encode subunits on $CD4^+$ T lymphocytes that induce molecular signaling pathways that promote the immune response [275, 290]. These loci have not been disease-specific, have been shared in other immune-mediated diseases, and can vary in different ethnic groups. They probably constitute a genetic background that favors immune reactivity after exposure to one or more environmental or infectious agents.

16.3.7 Possible Epigenetic Changes Affecting Predisposition and Outcome

Epigenetic changes that affect the expression of the chemokine receptor CXCR3 may influence the migration of activated T lymphocytes and natural killer (NK) cells to sites of liver injury in PBC [291], and the miRNAs miR-451a and miR-642a-3p may silence immune regulatory genes and contribute to disease severity [292]. Demethylation of the DNA molecule enwrapped with histones within the nucleosomes of chromatin can enhance the accessibility of transcription factors to DNA binding sites, increase the activity of ribonucleic acid polymerase (RNAP), and promote the transcriptional activity of immunomodulatory genes [21, 293, 294]. In PBC, the CXCR3 gene promoter in the X chromosome of $CD4^+$ T lymphocytes is demethylated [291], and this epigenetic change may affect the migration of liver-infiltrating inflammatory cells and the severity of PBC [295]. Similarly, the over-expression of miR-451a and miR-642a-3p in exosomes isolated from the plasma of patients with PBC may silence anti-inflammatory genes and increase disease severity as described in patients with rheumatoid arthritis [296]. Epigenetic changes are under-evaluated factors in the autoimmune liver diseases, and they may be affected by environmental cues, inherited as stable traits, and help shape susceptibility and phenotypic diversity.

16.4 Epidemiology of Primary Sclerosing Cholangitis

The epidemiology of PSC has been difficult to study because its diagnosis has been dependent on evolving criteria and techniques [297–303]. Older studies may not have applied the same diagnostic tools or had the same interpretative expertise as more recent studies [61], and the same diagnostic methods may not have been applied uniformly in all centers in the same study or in different studies. Furthermore, certain aspects of the disease, such as small duct PSC [304], PSC unrelated to inflammatory bowel disease [305], PSC in children [192] and asymptomatic PSC [303], may have been overlooked in some medical centers. Consequently, variations in the incidence and prevalence of PSC between studies in different regions may reflect differences in diagnostic methods and case identification rather than actual regional differences in the occurrence of the disease. These interpretive difficulties may be more pronounced in population-based studies of PSC than in population-based studies of autoimmune hepatitis and PBC [306].

16.4.1 Annual Incidence of Primary Sclerosing Cholangitis

The annual incidence of PSC has ranged from 0 cases per 100,000 persons among Alaskan natives [38, 307] to 1.3 cases per 100,000 persons in Norway [44] (Table 16.9). The most recent studies in Sweden (1992–2005) [305] and the Netherlands (2008–2011) [308] indicate a more than twofold difference in the annual incidence of PSC between the countries (1.22 cases per 100,000 persons in Sweden versus 0.5 cases per 100,000 cases in the Netherlands). Swedish men have a threefold higher incidence of PSC than Dutch men (1.78 cases per 100,000 persons versus 0.6 cases per 100,000 persons), whereas Swedish women have a 1.7-fold higher incidence of PSC than Dutch women (0.69 cases per 100,000 persons versus 0.4 cases per 100,000 persons) [305, 308].

The United Kingdom [309, 310], the Netherlands [308]), the United States [311, 312] and Canada [313] have annual incidences of PSC that are less than 1 case per 100,000 persons (0.41–0.91 cases per 100,000 persons in the United Kingdom, 0.5 cases per 100,000 persons in the Netherlands, 0.41–0.9 cases per 100,000 persons in the United States, and 0.92 cases per 100,000 persons in Canada) (Table 16.9). Spain is an exception among the European countries as the annual incidence of PSC was only 0.07 cases per 100,000 persons in a questionnaire study performed between 1984 and 1988 [314]. Small duct PSC has an incidence of 0.15 cases per 100,000 persons in Calgary, Canada, whereas the overall incidence of PSC in this region is more than sixfold greater at 0.92 cases per 100,000 persons [313].

In contrast to the European and North American experiences, the Scandinavian countries (Sweden, Norway) have an annual incidence of PSC that is greater than 1 case per 100,000 persons (1.22 cases per 100,000 persons in Sweden and 1.31 cases per 100,000 persons in Norway), and the incidences are similar to each other despite differences in the time intervals of each study [44, 305] (Table 16.9). In all studies, PSC has been more common in men than women, and in the few pediatric studies, children have been less commonly affected than adults. The annual incidence of PSC among children in the United States (Utah) is 0.2 cases per 100,000 persons [49], and this incidence is lower than the annual incidence of 0.9 cases per 100,000 persons among adults in the United States (Olmsted County, Minnesota) [311]. The annual incidence of PSC in Canadian children is 0.23 cases per 100,000 persons, and it is also lower than the annual incidence of PSC in Canadian adults (1.11 cases per 100,000 persons) [313]. The similar incidence of PSC in the children of Utah and Canada suggests that possible differences in ethnicity or cultural background were inconsequential.

Table 16.9 Incidence and prevalence of primary sclerosing cholangitis in different regions (lowest to highest annual incidence)

Geographical region	Annual incidence Per 100,000 persons	Prevalence Per 100,000 persons
Alaska (Natives) [38, 307] (1984–2000)	0	Not reported
Spain [314] (1984–1988)	0.07 Increased from 0.02 to 0.07 over 5 years	0.22 (December 31, 1988) Increased from 0.08 to 0.22 over 5 years
United States (Utah) [49] (1986–2011)	0.2 (children)	1.5 (children)
United Kingdom [309, 310] (1991–2001 and 1984–2003)	0.41–0.91 No significant increase over 10 years	3.85 (2001)–12.7 (July 1, 2003) United Kingdom versus South Wales
Netherlands [308] (2008–2011)	0.5 (men, 0.6; women, 0.4) 0.25, female adolescents 0.93, men aged 40–49 years	6.0 (January 1, 2008) Increasing prevalence (possible greater frequency of IBD)
United States [311, 312] (1991–2000 and 2000–2006)	0.41–0.9 (men, 0.45–1.25; women, 0.37–0.54) No increase in men or women	4.03 (men, 4.92; women, 3.19) to 13.6 (men, 20.9; women, 6.3) California versus Minnesota
Canada (Calgary) [313] (2000–2005)	0.92 (adults, 1.11; children, 0.23) Small duct PSC, 0.15	Not reported
Japan [367] (2007)	Not reported	0.95 (2007)
Sweden [305] (1992–2005)	1.22 (men, 1.78; women, 0.69) Increased overall AAPC, 3.06 Increased AAPC for women: • IBD-associated PSC, 7.01 • Large duct PSC, 6.32 Increased AAPC for men: • Non-IBD related, 9.69 • Small duct PSC, 17.88	16.2 (December 31, 2005) (men, 23.7; women, 8.9)
Norway [44, 315] (1986–1995)	0.7–1.31	5.6–8.5 (December 31, 1995)

AAPC average annual percentage change, *IBD* inflammatory bowel disease, *PSC* primary sclerosing cholangitis
Numbers in brackets are references

A meta-analysis restricted to eight population-based studies [44, 305, 309–311, 313–315] has estimated the overall annual incidence of PSC as 1.0 case per 100,000 persons [316]. The incidence of PSC was considered to be similar in North America and Europe, and the incidence ratio for males versus females was 1.7 (range, 1.34–2.07). The median age at diagnosis was 41 years (range, 35–47 years), and the frequency of concurrent inflammatory bowel disease was 67%. Importantly, the average annual percentage change (AAPC) in the incidence of PSC had increased in four studies, ranging from 3.06% to 27.2% [316]. A population-based study in

Sweden has indicated that the AAPC for large duct PSC has increased by 6.32% in women and that the AAPC for small duct PSC has increased by 17.88% in men [305] (Table 16.9).

The disparities between studies may reflect differences in the time intervals of each study, the methods that were applied for detection of PSC, and the level of expertise and interest in PSC among the participating institutions. Alternatively, the disparities may reflect true differences in susceptibility to the disease. Predispositions for PSC may be influenced by genetic factors [15, 132, 317–326], exposure to environmental agents [327–329], alterations in the intestinal microbiome [330–332], and the presence of inflammatory bowel disease, especially ulcerative colitis [333, 334]. These predisposing factors may vary among age groups, races, and regions within a country or between countries [321].

Inflammatory bowel disease (IBD), mainly ulcerative colitis, has been present in 67–80% of patients with PSC in Europe and North America [311, 316, 335], and men with PSC have had IBD more commonly than women with PSC in the United States (73% versus women 52%) [312]. Since 2.4–7.5% of patients with IBD have PSC [303, 336, 337], an increasing frequency of IBD in a population may impact on the annual incidence of PSC in that region. The annual incidence of ulcerative colitis has increased from 22.1 cases per 100,000 persons in Finland to 27.4 cases per 100,000 persons from 2001 to 2007 [338]. The annual incidence of ulcerative colitis is also higher in Finnish men than women (27.8 cases per 100,000 persons versus 21.9 cases per 100,000 persons). An increasing frequency of men with ulcerative colitis may explain in part an increasing annual incidence of PSC in some regions. An increase in the annual incidence of IBD has also been reported in Denmark [339] and suggested in the Netherlands [308].

16.4.2 Prevalence of Primary Sclerosing Cholangitis

The prevalence of PSC has been as low as 0.22 cases per 100,000 persons in Spain [314] to as high as 16.2 cases per 100,000 persons in Sweden [305] (Table 16.9). Sweden (16.2 cases per 100,000 persons) [305], Olmsted County, Minnesota in the United States (13.6 persons per 100,000 persons) [311], and Norway (8.5 cases per 100,000 persons) [44] have had the highest prevalence of the disease, and these regions have also had tertiary medical centers with long-standing expertise and interest in PSC. Men have had a 2.7-fold greater prevalence of PSC than women in Sweden [305] and a 3.3-fold greater prevalence in Olmsted County, Minnesota [311].

Prevalence in a geographic region has not closely reflected the incidence of the disease in that region (Table 16.9). Countries with similar annual incidences of PSC (United Kingdom [309] and the Netherlands [308], and Sweden [305] and Norway [44]) have had 1.9–2.3-fold differences in prevalence. A striking increase in the prevalence of PSC in Spain from 0.08 cases per 100,000 persons to 0.22 cases per 100,000 persons over a 5 year period may have reflected improved case detection [314], but a more recent population-based study in the Netherlands using current diagnostic criteria and methods has also suggested that the prevalence of PSC is increasing [308]. A factor that may account for this apparent increase in prevalence is improved survival through early diagnosis and the availability of liver transplantation.

16.4.3 Variations in Clinical Phenotype

16.4.3.1 Variant ("Overlap") Syndromes

PSC may have clinical features that resemble autoimmune hepatitis or PBC [340], and the mixed manifestations may be present concurrently [341, 342] or emerge later [343–346]. Features reminiscent of autoimmune hepatitis are present in 4–54% of patients with PSC [347, 348], and cholangiographic features of PSC are present in 2–10% of patients with autoimmune hepatitis [60, 61]. The frequency that findings of PSC and PBC coexist is estimated at 0.76% based on the presence of a mixed syndrome in two of 261 patients with autoimmune liver disease [346]. The diagnostic criteria for the variant ("overlap") syndromes of PSC have not been codified, and treatment recommendations are based on weak clinical evidence [6, 7, 301, 349]. Immunosuppressive therapy (prednisone or prednisolone with azathioprine) in combination with ursodeoxycholic acid has been recommended by the European Association for the Study of the Liver (EASL) [350] and the American Association for the Study of Liver Diseases (AASLD) [301]. The epidemiology of the variant syndromes of PSC is unknown.

16.4.3.2 IgG4-Associated Cholangitis

IgG4-associated cholangitis has cholangiographic features that are indistinguishable from those of PSC [351, 352]. The inflammatory lesions usually involve the extrahepatic, hilar, and perihilar bile ducts by cholangiography [352], but histological examination of the liver can indicate small bile duct damage in 26% [353]. The histological manifestations of small bile duct injury are most common (80%) in patients with intrahepatic strictures [353], and the histological spectrum includes portal inflammation, >10 IgG4-staining plasma cells, and distinctive portal-based fibro-inflammatory micro-nodules composed of fibroblasts, plasma cells, lymphocytes, and eosinophils [354, 355].

IgG4-associated cholangitis is within the spectrum of IgG4-related diseases that have been characterized as fibro-inflammatory processes with a dense lymphoplasmacytic infiltrate enriched with IgG4-staining plasma cells, storiform fibrosis, and obliterative phlebitis [355, 356]. The IgG4-related diseases have affected the colon, salivary glands, periorbital tissues, kidneys, lungs, thyroid, prostate, skin, and pericardium in addition to the pancreas, liver, and biliary tract [356]. The diagnostic criteria of the Japan Biliary Association for IgG4-associated cholangitis include coexistence of IgG4-related disease outside the biliary tract [357]. The other criteria are characteristic cholangiographic changes, elevated serum IgG4 level, and typical histopathological findings.

Autoimmune pancreatitis occurs in 19–92% of patients with IgG4-associated cholangitis, depending in part on the presence or absence of jaundice [351, 358], and the lungs, kidneys, colon, mesentery, retroperitoneum, and salivary glands may also be involved [359]. A lymphoplasmacytic infiltrate that contains >50 IgG4-staining plasma cells/high power field may involve the colon in patients with IgG4-associated cholangitis and mimic ulcerative colitis [359–361]. IgG4-related colitis should be differentiated from the ulcerative colitis more frequently associated with PSC.

Serum IgG4 levels are increased in 74–90% of patients with IgG4-associated cholangitis (versus 9–15% in patients with PSC) [358, 359, 362], and a ratio of serum IgG4/IgG1 >0.24 has been proposed as a feature distinguishing IgG4-associated cholangitis from PSC [359]. IgG4-associated cholangitis must be distinguished from PSC and cholangiocarcinoma [363], and its characteristic responsiveness to glucocorticoid therapy can be a distinguishing feature and another criterion for its diagnosis [357]. The epidemiology of the IgG4-related diseases is unknown, albeit the early reports of this disease have been mainly from Japan.

16.4.4 Variations in Outcomes of Primary Sclerosing Cholangitis in Different Age Groups

The estimated median survival from diagnosis to liver transplantation or death from PSC was 21.2 years in a population-based study from the Netherlands, and the duration of transplant-free survival was 20.6 years [308]. Small duct PSC was associated with a better survival than large duct PSC, and the main causes of death were cholangiocarcinoma (32%), liver failure (18%), complications of liver transplantation (9%), and colorectal carcinoma (8%) [308].

The median transplant-free survival for pediatric patients with PSC has been 12.7 years, and overall survival has been shorter than in an age- and gender-matched population [364]. Small duct PSC may be more common in children than adults (36% versus 6–11%), but the shorter transplant-free survival for children than adults suggests differences in the stage of PSC at diagnosis or the aggressiveness of the liver disease [365]. The 5-year survival with the native liver in children has been 80%, and the 10-year survival after liver transplantation has been 89%. Unlike PSC in adults, the PSC in children has not been complicated by cholangiocarcinoma [364, 365].

Survival in adults has been better in studies based on population-based cohorts that are not weighted by disease severity compared to studies from tertiary medical centers where referrals for advanced disease are likely (median survival, 21.3 years in population-based cohorts versus 13.2 years in cohorts from tertiary referral centers) [308]. These observations may also apply to the pediatric experiences which are mainly derived from referral institutions [59, 192, 364, 365]. Variations in the prevalence of PSC among countries with a similar incidence of the disease may reflect differences in the severity and stage of the disease at presentation which may in turn vary with the nature of the medical centers participating in the study.

16.4.5 Variations in the Occurrence of PSC in Different Geographic Regions and Ethnic Groups

Population-based epidemiological studies of PSC have been sparse in developing countries and different ethnic groups. PSC has been described in Japan [366, 367], India [368], and Singapore [369], and the major phenotypic difference between the PSC of Asia and western countries has been a lower frequency of concurrent IBD in Asia. PSC has been associated with IBD in only 20% of patients in Singapore [369], 37% in Japan [366], and 50% in India [368]. A questionnaire-based epidemiological study in Japan in 2007 (which excluded sclerosing cholangitis associated with immunoglobulin-4) estimated the prevalence of PSC as 0.95 cases per 100,000 persons [367]. This prevalence was at least fourfold lower than in western countries (Table 16.9). The basis for this disparity remains uncertain, albeit a lower frequency of IBD in these countries may have contributed.

Disparities in the occurrence of PSC have also been recognized in certain regions within the same country, and ethnic diversity may have been a contributing factor. The prevalence of PSC has been 3.3-fold greater in a region of the United Kingdom (South Wales) [310] than in the entire country [309], and the annual incidence (0.41 versus 0.91 cases per 100,000 persons) and overall prevalence (4.03 versus 13.6 cases per 100,000 persons) of PSC have varied in different regions of the United States (northern California [312] versus Olmsted County, Minnesota [311]).

Non-Hispanic whites in northern California (Oakland) account for 80% of the cases of IBD [312, 370]. African Americans account for 16% of cases, and Asians account for 9% [312, 370]. These ethnic variations in the occurrence of IBD may explain in part the regional differences in the occurrence of PSC. Importantly, the occurrence of IBD may not closely correlate with the occurrence of PSC as each disease has genetic factors that are independent of each other [319, 320]. Well-designed, population-based epidemiological studies are required to understand the regional differences within the same country.

16.4.6 External and Internal Environmental Factors in Primary Sclerosing Cholangitis

The major external environmental risk factor that has been implicated in PSC has been non-smoking (Table 16.10). Four case control studies have indicated that patients with PSC are more commonly non-smokers than healthy control subjects (66–70% versus 39–47%) [327–329, 371]. Furthermore, the odds ratio for PSC in current smokers compared to never-smokers is reduced (odds ratio, 0.13–0.21). The decreased odds for PSC in current and former smokers has been independent of the presence or absence of IBD, and a systemic protective effect of smoking on the occurrence of PSC has been proposed [327, 371]. Tonsillectomy has also been associated with a decreased risk of PSC [329], whereas the protective effect of appendectomy that had been proposed for ulcerative colitis [372] has not been recognized in PSC [328, 329, 371].

Investigational scrutiny has also focused on the intestinal microbiome as a reservoir of microbial antigens, metabolic products, and activated immune cells that could affect susceptibility to IBD and PSC [32] (Table 16.10). Biliary epithelial cells in PSC express toll-like receptors (TLR4 and TLR9) that can respond to bacterial-derived lipopolysaccharide and produce pro-inflammatory cytokines [331, 373]; atypical perinuclear anti-neutrophil cytoplasmic antibodies (pANCA) are directed against β-tubulin which cross-reacts with an intestinal bacterial antigen (FtsZ) [330]; and commensal bacteria in a murine model of PSC are protective against the disease [332]. Preliminary translational studies have supported the potential pathogenic role of the intestinal microbiome by demonstrating clinical and laboratory improvement in patients with PSC after antibiotic therapy [374]. The internal environment may be more important than the external environment in modulating the occurrence of this disease and affecting its distribution among different ethnic groups and countries [375].

16.4.7 Genetic Factors in the Occurrence of Primary Sclerosing Cholangitis

The disparities in the occurrence of PSC between age-groups, different ethnicities, and various countries may be a consequence of genetic factors that favor or protect against IBD or PSC (Table 16.10). The frequency of PSC among first degree relatives is 0.7%, and it is 1.5% among siblings [376]. Three percent of patients with PSC have first degree relatives with PSC, and this occurrence is almost 100-fold greater than in the general population [376]. The risk of PSC in first degree relatives is independent of the presence of IBD, and the genetic factors associated with PSC have been different than those associated with IBD by high resolution typing of *DRB1* and *DQB1* loci [319]. These observations support a genetic basis for PSC, and they suggest a complex genetic disease that lacks a single genetic determinant.

PSC has been associated with HLA DRB1*03 and HLA B8 [377, 378], and haplotypes containing *DRB3*0101-DRB1*0301* and *DRB3*0101-DRB1*1301* have been proposed as risk factors for the disease [318] (Table 16.10). Furthermore, the haplotype containing *DRB1*04-DQB1*0501* has been associated with protection from the disease [318, 378]. Genome wide association studies have found the strongest associations with PSC near *HLA-B* at chromosome 6p21, and it has also implicated alleles outside the HLA complex at chromosome 13q31 [12, 336].

HLA associations with HLA B8 and HLA DRB1*13 have been identified as risk factors for PSC in patients listed for liver transplantation, and HLA DRB1*04 has been protective [321] (Table 16.10). African Americans were at greater risk for liver transplantation than European Americans (odds ratio, 1.323; 95% CI: 1.221–1.438), and they had HLA B8 more commonly than the HLA B8-DRB1*03 linkage disequilibrium found in European Americans. These observations introduced the possibility that refinements in HLA typing might be able to distinguish ethnic differences in susceptibility to PSC. Such differences might explain in part regional variations in the occurrence of PSC and support future studies designed to discover triggering antigens in different age groups, ethnic populations, and geographical regions.

Table 16.10 Risk factors for primary sclerosing cholangitis

Risk factor	Presumed mechanism	Evidence
Non-smoking	Smoking may be protective against IBD [327, 371] Actions uncertain [327]	More non-smokers in PSC than controls [327–329, 371] Independent of protective effect on IBD [327, 371]
Tonsillectomy	Uncertain [329]	Statistical association in risk survey [329]
Intestinal microbiome	Reservoir of microbial agents, metabolic products, and activated immune cells affect systemic immune responses [32]	BEC express TLR4 and TLR9 [373] BEC respond to bacterial LPS [331, 373] BEC produce pro-inflammatory cytokines [331, 373] pANCA cross-react with microbial antigen [330] Commensal intestinal bacteria protective [332] Antibiotic therapy improves patients [374]
IBD	Disordered intestinal microbiome (dysbiosis) [32] Increased intestinal permeability to microbial antigens and gut-derived immune cells [32]	Present in 67–80% of patients with PSC [311, 316, 335] Different genetic risk factors than PSC [320] More frequent in men with or without PSC [312, 338] Increasing frequency in certain countries [308, 338, 339] May be basis for increasing frequency of PSC [338, 339]
Family history	Genetic predisposition with low penetrance [376]	PSC in 0.7% of FDRs and 1.5% of siblings [376] 3% of patients with PSC have FDRs with PSC [376]
Genetic predisposition	Complex genetic disease associated with susceptibility loci within and outside MHC [12, 322, 325]	Associated with HLA DRB1*03 and HLA B8 [377] HLA DRB1*04 protective [321, 378] *DRB3*0101-DRB1*0301* and *DRB3*0101-DRB1*1301* are susceptibility haplotypes [318] *DRB1*04-DQB1*0501* is protective haplotype [318] Associated with *HLA-B* locus at chromosome 6p21 and non-HLA alleles on chromosome 13q31 by GWAS [12]

BEC biliary epithelial cells, *FDRs* first degree relatives, *GWAS* genome-wide association studies, *HLA* human leukocyte antigen, *IBD* inflammatory bowel disease, *LPS* lipopolysaccharide, *MHC* major histocompatibility complex, *PSC* primary sclerosing cholangitis, *TLR* toll-like receptors
Numbers in brackets are references

16.4.8 Possible Epigenetic Changes Affecting Predisposition and Outcome

Patients with PSC have 21 miRNAs that are differentially expressed, and miR-200c is the principal distinguishing marker [379]. miR-200c is down-regulated in PSC compared to healthy individuals but up-regulated in patients with cholangiocarcinoma. The miRNAs associated with PSC may influence the actions of diverse regulatory genes that may include anti- and pro-inflammatory genes and tumor suppressors. Aberrant DNA methylation has been described in the genes of patients with cholangiocarcinoma and PSC [380], and these epigenetic changes might be clues to the mechanisms of malignant transformation in PSC and the identity of biomarkers that reflect this propensity [381]. The genes regulating the expression of the miRNAs are subject to epigenetic factors that may be influenced by inheritable traits or environmental cues, and these epigenetic changes could contribute to variations in disease behavior between individuals, populations or geographical regions.

16.5 Overview

Autoimmune hepatitis, PBC and PSC are rare chronic liver diseases (annual incidence, <50 cases per 100,000 persons), but they are persistent, progressive, and variably responsive to current management strategies. They can affect individuals in their most productive phases of life, and their societal costs may be high. Misdirected immune-mediated mechanisms and regulatory pathways have been implicated in their occurrence, and a constellation of genetic factors may influence susceptibility to the disease and outcome.

Variant (overlap) syndromes have also been described in which patients with autoimmune hepatitis may have features similar to those of PBC or PSC, and patients with PBC or PSC may have features similar to those of autoimmune hepatitis [5, 6]. The pathogenic bases for these variant syndromes are uncertain; diagnostic criteria have not been codified; and their inclusion within the classical disease categories based on their predominant component remains controversial [349]. These variant syndromes may confound epidemiological studies of the classical immune-mediated liver diseases. They may also re-shape the understanding of host-dependent mechanisms and pathogenic pathways of autoimmunity and help explain regional differences in the occurrence, clinical phenotype, and outcomes of autoimmune hepatitis, PBC and PSC.

Population-based epidemiological studies have indicated that autoimmune hepatitis, PBC, and PSC can occur with different frequencies in different geographical regions, ethnic groups, and age-ranges and that the incidence and prevalence of each disease may be increasing in certain regions. The etiological triggers for autoimmune hepatitis, PBC and PSC are uncertain, but the preferential emergence of these diseases in certain populations and their clustering in certain locations suggests that environmental and infectious agents are critical factors in genetically predisposed individuals.

Variations in the incidence of the disease in different regions and ethnic groups should direct investigations that define genetic susceptibility factors and etiological agents, and variations in prevalence should direct evaluations of management strategies that impact on immediate and long-term survival. Population-based studies have been lacking in developing countries, and they have also been deficient in describing the burden, distribution, and trends of autoimmune hepatitis and the variant syndromes world-wide. Epidemiological studies that fill these current gaps in knowledge are essential to design pertinent investigational protocols, appropriately allocate resources, and impel changes in healthcare policy and practice.

Acknowledgments This review did not receive financial support from a funding agency or institution, and Albert J. Czaja, MD has no conflict of interests to declare.

Table of Landmark Literature

Study title and authors	Study design	Summary results	Main limitations
Ngu JH et al. J Gastroenterol Hepatol 2010;25:1681–86	Population-based study of AIH in Canterbury, New Zealand	• Peak age in sixth decade • Ethnic-specificity	• Tertiary referral center over-representative
Gronbaek L, et al. J Hepatol 2014;60:612–17	Population-based study of AIH using Danish National Patient Registry	• Cirrhosis in 28% • Incidence increasing • Prognosis improving	• Uncertain uniformity of diagnostic criteria
Van Gerven NM, et al. Scand J Gastroenterol 2014;49:1245–54	Population-based study of AIH in the Netherlands	• Concurrent immune diseases in 26%	• Incomplete datasets • Diagnostic uncertainties
Sood S, et al. Gastroenterology 2004;127:470–5	Population-based studies of PBC in Victoria, Australia	• Victorians protected • Absent environmental trigger possible	• Inconsistent case finding methods used
Myers RP, et al. Hepatology 2009;50:1884–92	Population-based study of PBC in Calgary, Canada	• Increasing prevalence • Need for better therapy	• Risk factors unavailable • Incomplete datasets
Gershwin ME, et al. Hepatology 2005;42:1194–1202	Large case-controlled interview-based study of PBC	• Risk factors of family history, UTIs, past smoking, and HRT	• Patients highly selected • Dependent on patient's recall and understanding
Bambha K, et al. Gastroenterology 2003;125:1364–69	Population-based study of PSC in U.S. community	• Male predominance • 73% of PSC with IBD • Poor overall survival	• Uncertain case discovery
Molodecky NA, et al. Hepatology 2011;53:1590–99	Meta-analysis of 8 mainly population-based studies of PSC	• Incidence increasing	• Small number of studies • No prevalence data
Boonstra K, et al. Hepatology 2013;58:2045–55	Population-based study of PSC in the Netherlands	• Lower survival in tertiary referral centers • CRC increased	• Incomplete datasets • Uncertain case discovery

AIH autoimmune hepatitis, *CRC* colorectal cancer, *HRT* hormone replacement therapy, *IBD* inflammatory bowel disease, *PBC* primary biliary cholangitis, *PSC* primary sclerosing cholangitis, *UTIs* urinary tract infections

References

1. Czaja AJ. Autoimmune hepatitis in diverse ethnic populations and geographical regions. Expert Rev Gastroenterol Hepatol. 2013;7:365–85.
2. Czaja AJ. Review article: next-generation transformative advances in the pathogenesis and management of autoimmune hepatitis. Aliment Pharmacol Ther. 2017;46:920–37.
3. Kim WR, Brown RS Jr, Terrault NA, El-Serag H. Burden of liver disease in the United States: summary of a workshop. Hepatology. 2002;36:227–42.
4. Czaja AJ. Transitioning from idiopathic to explainable autoimmune hepatitis. Dig Dis Sci. 2015;60:2881–900.
5. Czaja AJ. The variant forms of autoimmune hepatitis. Ann Intern Med. 1996;125:588–98.
6. Czaja AJ. The overlap syndromes of autoimmune hepatitis. Dig Dis Sci. 2013;58:326–43.
7. Czaja AJ. Cholestatic phenotypes of autoimmune hepatitis. Clin Gastroenterol Hepatol. 2014;12:1430–8.
8. Oldstone MB. Molecular mimicry, microbial infection, and autoimmune disease: evolution of the concept. Curr Top Microbiol Immunol. 2005;296:1–17.
9. Bogdanos DP, Baum H, Grasso A, Okamoto M, Butler P, Ma Y, et al. Microbial mimics are major targets of crossreactivity with human pyruvate dehydrogenase in primary biliary cirrhosis. J Hepatol. 2004;40:31–9.
10. Czaja AJ. Autoimmune hepatitis. Part A: pathogenesis. Expert Rev Gastroenterol Hepatol. 2007;1:113–28.
11. Czaja AJ. Genetic factors affecting the occurrence, clinical phenotype, and outcome of autoimmune hepatitis. Clin Gastroenterol Hepatol. 2008;6:379–88.
12. Karlsen TH, Franke A, Melum E, Kaser A, Hov JR, Balschun T, et al. Genome-wide association analysis in primary sclerosing cholangitis. Gastroenterology. 2010;138:1102–11.
13. Hirschfield GM, Invernizzi P. Progress in the genetics of primary biliary cirrhosis. Semin Liver Dis. 2011;31:147–56.
14. Hirschfield GM, Chapman RW, Karlsen TH, Lammert F, Lazaridis KN, Mason AL. The genetics of complex cholestatic disorders. Gastroenterology. 2013;144:1357–74.
15. Berntsen NL, Klingenberg O, Juran BD, Benito de Valle M, Lindkvist B, Lazaridis KN, et al. Association between HLA haplotypes and increased serum levels of IgG4 in patients with primary sclerosing cholangitis. Gastroenterology. 2015;148:924–27.e2.
16. van Gerven NM, de Boer YS, Zwiers A, Verwer BJ, Drenth JP, van Hoek B, et al. HLA-DRB1*03:01 and HLA-DRB1*04:01 modify the presentation and outcome in autoimmune hepatitis type-1. Genes Immun. 2015;16:247–52.
17. Juran BD, Atkinson EJ, Schlicht EM, Fridley BL, Lazaridis KN. Primary biliary cirrhosis is associated with a genetic variant in the 3′ flanking region of the CTLA4 gene. Gastroenterology. 2008;135:1200–6.
18. Paladino N, Flores AC, Fainboim H, Schroder T, Cuarterolo M, Lezama C, et al. The most severe forms of type I autoimmune hepatitis are associated with genetically determined levels of TGF-beta1. Clin Immunol. 2010;134:305–12.
19. Mann DA. Epigenetics in liver disease. Hepatology. 2014;60:1418–25.
20. Jeffries MA, Sawalha AH. Autoimmune disease in the epigenetic era: how has epigenetics changed our understanding of disease and how can we expect the field to evolve? Expert Rev Clin Immunol. 2015;11:45–58.
21. Czaja AJ. Epigenetic changes and their implications in autoimmune hepatitis. Eur J Clin Investig. 2018;48:e12899.
22. Czaja AJ. Global disparities and their implications in the occurrence and outcome of autoimmune hepatitis. Dig Dis Sci. 2017;62:2277–92.
23. Pando M, Larriba J, Fernandez GC, Fainboim H, Ciocca M, Ramonet M, et al. Pediatric and adult forms of type I autoimmune hepatitis in Argentina: evidence for differential genetic predisposition. Hepatology. 1999;30:1374–80.

24. Smyk D, Mytilinaiou MG, Rigopoulou EI, Bogdanos DP. PBC triggers in water reservoirs, coal mining areas and waste disposal sites: from Newcastle to New York. Dis Markers. 2010;29:337–44.
25. Fainboim L, Canero Velasco MC, Marcos CY, Ciocca M, Roy A, Theiler G, et al. Protracted, but not acute, hepatitis A virus infection is strongly associated with HLA-DRB*1301, a marker for pediatric autoimmune hepatitis. Hepatology. 2001;33:1512–7.
26. Henao-Mejia J, Elinav E, Thaiss CA, Licona-Limon P, Flavell RA. Role of the intestinal microbiome in liver disease. J Autoimmun. 2013;46:66–73.
27. Barin JG, Tobias LD, Peterson DA. The microbiome and autoimmune disease: report from a Noel R. Rose Colloquium. Clin Immunol. 2015;159:183–8.
28. Chong CW, Ahmad AF, Lim YA, Teh CS, Yap IK, Lee SC, et al. Effect of ethnicity and socio-economic variation to the gut microbiota composition among pre-adolescent in Malaysia. Sci Rep. 2015;5:13338.
29. Francino MP. Antibiotics and the human gut microbiome: dysbioses and accumulation of resistances. Front Microbiol. 2015;6:1543.
30. Lin R, Zhou L, Zhang J, Wang B. Abnormal intestinal permeability and microbiota in patients with autoimmune hepatitis. Int J Clin Exp Pathol. 2015;8:5153–60.
31. Miller GE, Engen PA, Gillevet PM, Shaikh M, Sikaroodi M, Forsyth CB, et al. Lower neighborhood socioeconomic status associated with reduced diversity of the colonic microbiota in healthy adults. PLoS One. 2016;11:e0148952.
32. Czaja AJ. Factoring the intestinal microbiome into the pathogenesis of autoimmune hepatitis. World J Gastroenterol. 2016;22:9257–78.
33. Javierre BM, Hernando H, Ballestar E. Environmental triggers and epigenetic deregulation in autoimmune disease. Discov Med. 2011;12:535–45.
34. Canas CA, Canas F, Bonilla-Abadia F, Ospina FE, Tobon GJ. Epigenetics changes associated to environmental triggers in autoimmunity. Autoimmunity. 2016;49:1–11.
35. Heyn H, Moran S, Hernando-Herraez I, Sayols S, Gomez A, Sandoval J, et al. DNA methylation contributes to natural human variation. Genome Res. 2013;23:1363–72.
36. Morales LS, Lara M, Kington RS, Valdez RO, Escarce JJ. Socioeconomic, cultural, and behavioral factors affecting Hispanic health outcomes. J Health Care Poor Underserved. 2002;13:477–503.
37. Carrion AF, Ghanta R, Carrasquillo O, Martin P. Chronic liver disease in the Hispanic population of the United States. Clin Gastroenterol Hepatol. 2011;9:834–41.
38. Hurlburt KJ, McMahon BJ, Deubner H, Hsu-Trawinski B, Williams JL, Kowdley KV. Prevalence of autoimmune liver disease in Alaska Natives. Am J Gastroenterol. 2002;97:2402–7.
39. Haider AS, Kaye G, Thomson A. Autoimmune hepatitis in a demographically isolated area of Australia. Intern Med J. 2010;40:281–5.
40. Gronbaek L, Vilstrup H, Jepsen P. Autoimmune hepatitis in Denmark: incidence, prevalence, prognosis, and causes of death. A nationwide registry-based cohort study. J Hepatol. 2014;60:612–7.
41. Delgado JS, Vodonos A, Malnick S, Kriger O, Wilkof-Segev R, Delgado B, et al. Autoimmune hepatitis in southern Israel: a 15-year multicenter study. J Dig Dis. 2013;14:611–8.
42. van Gerven NM, Verwer BJ, Witte BI, van Erpecum KJ, van Buuren HR, Maijers I, et al. Epidemiology and clinical characteristics of autoimmune hepatitis in the Netherlands. Scand J Gastroenterol. 2014;49:1245–54.
43. Ngu JH, Bechly K, Chapman BA, Burt MJ, Barclay ML, Gearry RB, et al. Population-based epidemiology study of autoimmune hepatitis: a disease of older women? J Gastroenterol Hepatol. 2010;25:1681–6.
44. Boberg KM, Aadland E, Jahnsen J, Raknerud N, Stiris M, Bell H. Incidence and prevalence of primary biliary cirrhosis, primary sclerosing cholangitis, and autoimmune hepatitis in a Norwegian population. Scand J Gastroenterol. 1998;33:99–103.

45. Lee YM, Teo EK, Ng TM, Khor C, Fock KM. Autoimmune hepatitis in Singapore: a rare syndrome affecting middle-aged women. J Gastroenterol Hepatol. 2001;16:1384–9.
46. Primo J, Merino C, Fernandez J, Moles JR, Llorca P, Hinojosa J. [Incidence and prevalence of autoimmune hepatitis in the area of the Hospital de Sagunto (Spain)]. Gastroenterol Hepatol. 2004;27:239–43.
47. Primo J, Maroto N, Martinez M, Anton MD, Zaragoza A, Giner R, et al. Incidence of adult form of autoimmune hepatitis in Valencia (Spain). Acta Gastroenterol Belg. 2009;72:402–6.
48. Werner M, Prytz H, Ohlsson B, Almer S, Bjornsson E, Bergquist A, et al. Epidemiology and the initial presentation of autoimmune hepatitis in Sweden: a nationwide study. Scand J Gastroenterol. 2008;43:1232–40.
49. Deneau M, Jensen MK, Holmen J, Williams MS, Book LS, Guthery SL. Primary sclerosing cholangitis, autoimmune hepatitis, and overlap in Utah children: epidemiology and natural history. Hepatology. 2013;58:1392–400.
50. Griffiths L, Dyson JK, Jones DE. The new epidemiology of primary biliary cirrhosis. Semin Liver Dis. 2014;34:318–28.
51. Bjornsson ES, Ekbom A. Scandinavian epidemiological research in gastroenterology and hepatology. Scand J Gastroenterol. 2015;50:636–48.
52. Jimenez-Rivera C, Ling SC, Ahmed N, Yap J, Aglipay M, Barrowman N, et al. Incidence and characteristics of autoimmune hepatitis. Pediatrics. 2015;136:e1237–48.
53. Chung HV, Riley M, Ho JK, Leung B, Jevon GP, Arbour LT, et al. Retrospective review of pediatric and adult autoimmune hepatitis in two quaternary care centres in British Columbia: increased prevalence seen in British Columbia's First Nations community. Can J Gastroenterol. 2007;21:565–8.
54. Czaja AJ, Carpenter HA. Validation of scoring system for diagnosis of autoimmune hepatitis. Dig Dis Sci. 1996;41:305–14.
55. Alvarez F, Berg PA, Bianchi FB, Bianchi L, Burroughs AK, Cancado EL, et al. International Autoimmune Hepatitis Group report: review of criteria for diagnosis of autoimmune hepatitis. J Hepatol. 1999;31:929–38.
56. Czaja AJ. Performance parameters of the diagnostic scoring systems for autoimmune hepatitis. Hepatology. 2008;48:1540–8.
57. D'Souza R, Sinnott P, Glynn MJ, Sabin CA, Foster GR. An unusual form of autoimmune hepatitis in young Somalian men. Liver Int. 2005;25:325–30.
58. Zolfino T, Heneghan MA, Norris S, Harrison PM, Portmann BC, McFarlane IG. Characteristics of autoimmune hepatitis in patients who are not of European Caucasoid ethnic origin. Gut. 2002;50:713–7.
59. Gregorio GV, Portmann B, Karani J, Harrison P, Donaldson PT, Vergani D, et al. Autoimmune hepatitis/sclerosing cholangitis overlap syndrome in childhood: a 16-year prospective study. Hepatology. 2001;33:544–53.
60. Abdalian R, Dhar P, Jhaveri K, Haider M, Guindi M, Heathcote EJ. Prevalence of sclerosing cholangitis in adults with autoimmune hepatitis: evaluating the role of routine magnetic resonance imaging. Hepatology. 2008;47:949–57.
61. Lewin M, Vilgrain V, Ozenne V, Lemoine M, Wendum D, Paradis V, et al. Prevalence of sclerosing cholangitis in adults with autoimmune hepatitis: a prospective magnetic resonance imaging and histological study. Hepatology. 2009;50:528–37.
62. Perdigoto R, Carpenter HA, Czaja AJ. Frequency and significance of chronic ulcerative colitis in severe corticosteroid-treated autoimmune hepatitis. J Hepatol. 1992;14:325–31.
63. Czaja AJ, Carpenter HA, Santrach PJ, Moore SB, Taswell HF, Homburger HA. Evidence against hepatitis viruses as important causes of severe autoimmune hepatitis in the United States. J Hepatol. 1993;18:342–52.
64. Czaja AJ, Carpenter HA, Santrach PJ, Moore SB. Significance of HLA DR4 in type 1 autoimmune hepatitis. Gastroenterology. 1993;105:1502–7.
65. Czaja AJ, dos Santos RM, Porto A, Santrach PJ, Moore SB. Immune phenotype of chronic liver disease. Dig Dis Sci. 1998;43:2149–55.

66. Homberg JC, Abuaf N, Bernard O, Islam S, Alvarez F, Khalil SH, et al. Chronic active hepatitis associated with antiliver/kidney microsome antibody type 1: a second type of "autoimmune" hepatitis. Hepatology. 1987;7:1333–9.
67. Gregorio GV, Portmann B, Reid F, Donaldson PT, Doherty DG, McCartney M, et al. Autoimmune hepatitis in childhood: a 20-year experience. Hepatology. 1997;25:541–7.
68. Czaja AJ, Manns MP, Homburger HA. Frequency and significance of antibodies to liver/kidney microsome type 1 in adults with chronic active hepatitis. Gastroenterology. 1992;103:1290–5.
69. Czaja AJ. Performance parameters of the conventional serological markers for autoimmune hepatitis. Dig Dis Sci. 2011;56:545–54.
70. Ferucci ED, Choromanski TL, Hurlburt KJ, Livingston S, Plotnik J, Manns MP, et al. Autoimmune hepatitis in the Alaska Native population: autoantibody profile and HLA associations. Liver Int. 2014;34:1241–9.
71. Czaja AJ, Morshed SA, Parveen S, Nishioka M. Antibodies to single-stranded and double-stranded DNA in antinuclear antibody-positive type 1-autoimmune hepatitis. Hepatology. 1997;26:567–72.
72. Targan SR, Landers C, Vidrich A, Czaja AJ. High-titer antineutrophil cytoplasmic antibodies in type-1 autoimmune hepatitis. Gastroenterology. 1995;108:1159–66.
73. Parveen S, Morshed SA, Arima K, Nishioka M, Czaja AJ, Chow WC, et al. Antibodies to Ro/La, Cenp-B, and snRNPs antigens in autoimmune hepatitis of North America versus Asia: patterns of immunofluorescence, ELISA reactivities, and HLA association. Dig Dis Sci. 1998;43:1322–31.
74. Montano-Loza AJ, Shums Z, Norman GL, Czaja AJ. Prognostic implications of antibodies to Ro/SSA and soluble liver antigen in type 1 autoimmune hepatitis. Liver Int. 2012;32:85–92.
75. Umemura T, Zen Y, Hamano H, Ichijo T, Kawa S, Nakanuma Y, et al. IgG4 associated autoimmune hepatitis: a differential diagnosis for classical autoimmune hepatitis. Gut. 2007;56:1471–2.
76. Umemura T, Zen Y, Hamano H, Joshita S, Ichijo T, Yoshizawa K, et al. Clinical significance of immunoglobulin G4-associated autoimmune hepatitis. J Gastroenterol. 2011;46(Suppl 1):48–55.
77. Chung H, Watanabe T, Kudo M, Maenishi O, Wakatsuki Y, Chiba T. Identification and characterization of IgG4-associated autoimmune hepatitis. Liver Int. 2010;30:222–31.
78. Yada N, Kudo M, Chung H, Watanabe T. Autoimmune hepatitis and immunoglobulin g4-associated autoimmune hepatitis. Dig Dis. 2013;31:415–20.
79. Umemura T, Zen Y, Hamano H, Kawa S, Nakanuma Y, Kiyosawa K. Immunoglobin G4-hepatopathy: association of immunoglobin G4-bearing plasma cells in liver with autoimmune pancreatitis. Hepatology. 2007;46:463–71.
80. Zhao XY, Rakhda MI, Wang TI, Jia JD. Immunoglobulin G4-associated de novo autoimmune hepatitis after liver transplantation for chronic hepatitis B- and C-related cirrhosis and hepatocellular carcinoma: a case report with literature review. Transplant Proc. 2013;45:824–7.
81. Ishizu Y, Ishigami M, Kuzuya T, Honda T, Hayashi K, Nakano I, et al. Immunoglobulin G4-associated autoimmune hepatitis later complicated by autoimmune pancreatitis: a case report. Hepatol Res. 2016;46:601–6.
82. Jeannin P, Lecoanet S, Delneste Y, Gauchat JF, Bonnefoy JY. IgE versus IgG4 production can be differentially regulated by IL-10. J Immunol. 1998;160:3555–61.
83. Meiler F, Klunker S, Zimmermann M, Akdis CA, Akdis M. Distinct regulation of IgE, IgG4 and IgA by T regulatory cells and toll-like receptors. Allergy. 2008;63:1455–63.
84. Zen Y, Fujii T, Harada K, Kawano M, Yamada K, Takahira M, et al. Th2 and regulatory immune reactions are increased in immunoglobin G4-related sclerosing pancreatitis and cholangitis. Hepatology. 2007;45:1538–46.
85. Asrani SK, Larson JJ, Yawn B, Therneau TM, Kim WR. Underestimation of liver-related mortality in the United States. Gastroenterology. 2013;145:375–82. e2
86. Verma S, Torbenson M, Thuluvath PJ. The impact of ethnicity on the natural history of autoimmune hepatitis. Hepatology. 2007;46:1828–35.

87. Lim KN, Casanova RL, Boyer TD, Bruno CJ. Autoimmune hepatitis in African Americans: presenting features and response to therapy. Am J Gastroenterol. 2001;96:3390–4.
88. Wong RJ, Corley DA. Survival differences by race/ethnicity and treatment for localized hepatocellular carcinoma within the United States. Dig Dis Sci. 2009;54:2031–9.
89. Mathur AK, Osborne NH, Lynch RJ, Ghaferi AA, Dimick JB, Sonnenday CJ. Racial/ethnic disparities in access to care and survival for patients with early-stage hepatocellular carcinoma. Arch Surg. 2010;145:1158–63.
90. Mathur AK, Sonnenday CJ, Merion RM. Race and ethnicity in access to and outcomes of liver transplantation: a critical literature review. Am J Transplant. 2009;9:2662–8.
91. Mathur AK, Schaubel DE, Gong Q, Guidinger MK, Merion RM. Racial and ethnic disparities in access to liver transplantation. Liver Transpl. 2010;16:1033–40.
92. Yu JC, Neugut AI, Wang S, Jacobson JS, Ferrante L, Khungar V, et al. Racial and insurance disparities in the receipt of transplant among patients with hepatocellular carcinoma. Cancer. 2010;116:1801–9.
93. Harvin JA, Van Buren G, Tsao K, Cen P, Ko TC, Wray CJ. Hepatocellular carcinoma survival in uninsured and underinsured patients. J Surg Res. 2011;166:189–93.
94. Siegel AB, McBride RB, El-Serag HB, Hershman DL, Brown RS Jr, Renz JF, et al. Racial disparities in utilization of liver transplantation for hepatocellular carcinoma in the United States, 1998–2002. Am J Gastroenterol. 2008;103:120–7.
95. Hoeroldt B, McFarlane E, Dube A, Basumani P, Karajeh M, Campbell MJ, et al. Long-term outcomes of patients with autoimmune hepatitis managed at a nontransplant center. Gastroenterology. 2011;140:1980–9.
96. Roberts SK, Therneau TM, Czaja AJ. Prognosis of histological cirrhosis in type 1 autoimmune hepatitis. Gastroenterology. 1996;110:848–57.
97. Gupta R, Agarwal SR, Jain M, Malhotra V, Sarin SK. Autoimmune hepatitis in the Indian subcontinent: 7 years experience. J Gastroenterol Hepatol. 2001;16:1144–8.
98. Montano-Loza AJ, Carpenter HA, Czaja AJ. Predictive factors for hepatocellular carcinoma in type 1 autoimmune hepatitis. Am J Gastroenterol. 2008;103:1944–51.
99. Park SZ, Nagorney DM, Czaja AJ. Hepatocellular carcinoma in autoimmune hepatitis. Dig Dis Sci. 2000;45:1944–8.
100. Yeoman AD, Al-Chalabi T, Karani JB, Quaglia A, Devlin J, Mieli-Vergani G, et al. Evaluation of risk factors in the development of hepatocellular carcinoma in autoimmune hepatitis: implications for follow-up and screening. Hepatology. 2008;48:863–70.
101. Findor JA, Sorda JA, Daruich JR, Manero EF. Familial association in autoimmune liver disease. Medicina (B Aires). 2002;62:241–4.
102. Wang P, Su H, Underhill J, Blackmore LJ, Longhi MS, Grammatikopoulos T, et al. Autoantibody and human leukocyte antigen profiles in children with autoimmune liver disease and their first-degree relatives. J Pediatr Gastroenterol Nutr. 2014;58:457–62.
103. Strettell MD, Donaldson PT, Thomson LJ, Santrach PJ, Moore SB, Czaja AJ, et al. Allelic basis for HLA-encoded susceptibility to type 1 autoimmune hepatitis. Gastroenterology. 1997;112:2028–35.
104. de Boer YS, van Gerven NM, Zwiers A, Verwer BJ, van Hoek B, van Erpecum KJ, et al. Genome-wide association study identifies variants associated with autoimmune hepatitis type 1. Gastroenterology. 2014;147:443–52.
105. Czaja AJ, Strettell MD, Thomson LJ, Santrach PJ, Moore SB, Donaldson PT, et al. Associations between alleles of the major histocompatibility complex and type 1 autoimmune hepatitis. Hepatology. 1997;25:317–23.
106. Yoshizawa K, Ota M, Katsuyama Y, Ichijo T, Matsumoto A, Tanaka E, et al. Genetic analysis of the HLA region of Japanese patients with type 1 autoimmune hepatitis. J Hepatol. 2005;42:578–84.
107. Yoshizawa K, Umemura T, Ota M. Genetic background of autoimmune hepatitis in Japan. J Gastroenterol. 2011;46(Suppl 1):42–7.
108. Qiu DK, Ma X. Relationship between human leukocyte antigen-DRB1 and autoimmune hepatitis type I in Chinese patients. J Gastroenterol Hepatol. 2003;18:63–7.

109. Vazquez-Garcia MN, Alaez C, Olivo A, Debaz H, Perez-Luque E, Burguete A, et al. MHC class II sequences of susceptibility and protection in Mexicans with autoimmune hepatitis. J Hepatol. 1998;28:985–90.
110. Lim YS, Oh HB, Choi SE, Kwon OJ, Heo YS, Lee HC, et al. Susceptibility to type 1 autoimmune hepatitis is associated with shared amino acid sequences at positions 70–74 of the HLA-DRB1 molecule. J Hepatol. 2008;48:133–9.
111. Fainboim L, Marcos Y, Pando M, Capucchio M, Reyes GB, Galoppo C, et al. Chronic active autoimmune hepatitis in children. Strong association with a particular HLA-DR6 (DRB1*1301) haplotype. Hum Immunol. 1994;41:146–50.
112. Goldberg AC, Bittencourt PL, Mougin B, Cancado EL, Porta G, Carrilho F, et al. Analysis of HLA haplotypes in autoimmune hepatitis type 1: identifying the major susceptibility locus. Hum Immunol. 2001;62:165–9.
113. Czaja AJ, Souto EO, Bittencourt PL, Cancado EL, Porta G, Goldberg AC, et al. Clinical distinctions and pathogenic implications of type 1 autoimmune hepatitis in Brazil and the United States. J Hepatol. 2002;37:302–8.
114. Fortes Mdel P, Machado IV, Gil G, Fernandez-Mestre M, Dagher L, Leon RV, et al. Genetic contribution of major histocompatibility complex class II region to type 1 autoimmune hepatitis susceptibility in Venezuela. Liver Int. 2007;27:1409–16.
115. Padilla M, Mayorga R, Carrasco F, Bedregal T, Bobadilla F, Rondon C, et al. Liver transplantation for autoimmune hepatitis in Peru: outcomes and recurrence. Ann Hepatol. 2012;11:222–7.
116. Duarte-Rey C, Pardo AL, Rodriguez-Velosa Y, Mantilla RD, Anaya JM, Rojas-Villarraga A. HLA class II association with autoimmune hepatitis in Latin America: a meta-analysis. Autoimmun Rev. 2009;8:325–31.
117. Schreuder GM, Hurley CK, Marsh SG, Lau M, Maiers M, Kollman C, et al. The HLA dictionary 2001: a summary of HLA-A, -B, -C, -DRB1/3/4/5, -DQB1 alleles and their association with serologically defined HLA-A, -B, -C, -DR, and -DQ antigens. Hum Immunol. 2001;62:826–49.
118. Vento S, Garofano T, Di Perri G, Dolci L, Concia E, Bassetti D. Identification of hepatitis A virus as a trigger for autoimmune chronic hepatitis type 1 in susceptible individuals. Lancet. 1991;337:1183–7.
119. Huppertz HI, Treichel U, Gassel AM, Jeschke R, Meyer zum Buschenfelde KH. Autoimmune hepatitis following hepatitis A virus infection. J Hepatol. 1995;23:204–8.
120. Tabak F, Ozdemir F, Tabak O, Erer B, Tahan V, Ozaras R. Autoimmune hepatitis induced by the prolonged hepatitis A virus infection. Ann Hepatol. 2008;7:177–9.
121. Elfaramawy AA, Elhossiny RM, Abbas AA, Aziz HM. HLA-DRB1 as a risk factor in children with autoimmune hepatitis and its relation to hepatitis A infection. Ital J Pediatr. 2010;36:73.
122. Djilali-Saiah I, Renous R, Caillat-Zucman S, Debray D, Alvarez F. Linkage disequilibrium between HLA class II region and autoimmune hepatitis in pediatric patients. J Hepatol. 2004;40:904–9.
123. Djilali-Saiah I, Fakhfakh A, Louafi H, Caillat-Zucman S, Debray D, Alvarez F. HLA class II influences humoral autoimmunity in patients with type 2 autoimmune hepatitis. J Hepatol. 2006;45:844–50.
124. Bittencourt PL, Goldberg AC, Cancado EL, Porta G, Carrilho FJ, Farias AQ, et al. Genetic heterogeneity in susceptibility to autoimmune hepatitis types 1 and 2. Am J Gastroenterol. 1999;94:1906–13.
125. Goldberg AC, Bittencourt PL, Oliveira LC, Ramasawmy R, Marin ML, Palacios SA, et al. Autoimmune hepatitis in Brazil: an overview. Scand J Immunol. 2007;66:208–16.
126. Ma Y, Bogdanos DP, Hussain MJ, Underhill J, Bansal S, Longhi MS, et al. Polyclonal T-cell responses to cytochrome P450IID6 are associated with disease activity in autoimmune hepatitis type 2. Gastroenterology. 2006;130:868–82.
127. Czaja AJ, Kruger M, Santrach PJ, Moore SB, Manns MP. Genetic distinctions between types 1 and 2 autoimmune hepatitis. Am J Gastroenterol. 1997;92:2197–200.

128. Manns MP, Griffin KJ, Sullivan KF, Johnson EF. LKM-1 autoantibodies recognize a short linear sequence in P450IID6, a cytochrome P-450 monooxygenase. J Clin Invest. 1991;88:1370–8.
129. Kerkar N, Choudhuri K, Ma Y, Mahmoud A, Bogdanos DP, Muratori L, et al. Cytochrome P4502D6(193–212): a new immunodominant epitope and target of virus/self cross-reactivity in liver kidney microsomal autoantibody type 1-positive liver disease. J Immunol. 2003;170:1481–9.
130. Agarwal K, Jones DE, Daly AK, James OF, Vaidya B, Pearce S, et al. CTLA-4 gene polymorphism confers susceptibility to primary biliary cirrhosis. J Hepatol. 2000;32:538–41.
131. Agarwal K, Czaja AJ, Jones DE, Donaldson PT. Cytotoxic T lymphocyte antigen-4 (CTLA-4) gene polymorphisms and susceptibility to type 1 autoimmune hepatitis. Hepatology. 2000;31:49–53.
132. Mells GF, Kaser A, Karlsen TH. Novel insights into autoimmune liver diseases provided by genome-wide association studies. J Autoimmun. 2013;46:41–54.
133. Bittencourt PL, Palacios SA, Cancado EL, Porta G, Carrilho FJ, Laudanna AA, et al. Cytotoxic T lymphocyte antigen-4 gene polymorphisms do not confer susceptibility to autoimmune hepatitis types 1 and 2 in Brazil. Am J Gastroenterol. 2003;98:1616–20.
134. Tang J, Zhou C, Zhang ZJ, Zheng SS. Association of polymorphisms in non-classic MHC genes with susceptibility to autoimmune hepatitis. Hepatobiliary Pancreat Dis Int. 2012;11:125–31.
135. Djilali-Saiah I, Ouellette P, Caillat-Zucman S, Debray D, Kohn JI, Alvarez F. CTLA-4/CD 28 region polymorphisms in children from families with autoimmune hepatitis. Hum Immunol. 2001;62:1356–62.
136. Hiraide A, Imazeki F, Yokosuka O, Kanda T, Kojima H, Fukai K, et al. Fas polymorphisms influence susceptibility to autoimmune hepatitis. Am J Gastroenterol. 2005;100:1322–9.
137. Agarwal K, Czaja AJ, Donaldson PT. A functional Fas promoter polymorphism is associated with a severe phenotype in type 1 autoimmune hepatitis characterized by early development of cirrhosis. Tissue Antigens. 2007;69:227–35.
138. Cookson S, Constantini PK, Clare M, Underhill JA, Bernal W, Czaja AJ, et al. Frequency and nature of cytokine gene polymorphisms in type 1 autoimmune hepatitis. Hepatology. 1999;30:851–6.
139. Li S, Huang X, Zhong H, Chen Z, Peng Q, Deng Y, et al. Tumour necrosis factor alpha (TNF-alpha) genetic polymorphisms and the risk of autoimmune liver disease: a meta-analysis. J Genet. 2013;92:617–28.
140. Vogel A, Strassburg CP, Manns MP. Genetic association of vitamin D receptor polymorphisms with primary biliary cirrhosis and autoimmune hepatitis. Hepatology. 2002;35:126–31.
141. Fan L, Tu X, Zhu Y, Zhou L, Pfeiffer T, Feltens R, et al. Genetic association of vitamin D receptor polymorphisms with autoimmune hepatitis and primary biliary cirrhosis in the Chinese. J Gastroenterol Hepatol. 2005;20:249–55.
142. Migita K, Nakamura M, Abiru S, Jiuchi Y, Nagaoka S, Komori A, et al. Association of STAT4 polymorphisms with susceptibility to type-1 autoimmune hepatitis in the Japanese population. PLoS One. 2013;8:e71382.
143. Sanchez-Urdazpal L, Czaja AJ, van Hoek B, Krom RA, Wiesner RH. Prognostic features and role of liver transplantation in severe corticosteroid-treated autoimmune chronic active hepatitis. Hepatology. 1992;15:215–21.
144. Czaja AJ, Carpenter HA. Distinctive clinical phenotype and treatment outcome of type 1 autoimmune hepatitis in the elderly. Hepatology. 2006;43:532–8.
145. Czaja AJ. Clinical features, differential diagnosis and treatment of autoimmune hepatitis in the elderly. Drugs Aging. 2008;25:219–39.
146. Seki T, Kiyosawa K, Inoko H, Ota M. Association of autoimmune hepatitis with HLA-Bw54 and DR4 in Japanese patients. Hepatology. 1990;12:1300–4.
147. Seki T, Ota M, Furuta S, Fukushima H, Kondo T, Hino K, et al. HLA class II molecules and autoimmune hepatitis susceptibility in Japanese patients. Gastroenterology. 1992;103:1041–7.

148. Nakamura K, Yoneda M, Yokohama S, Tamori K, Sato Y, Aso K, et al. Efficacy of ursodeoxycholic acid in Japanese patients with type 1 autoimmune hepatitis. J Gastroenterol Hepatol. 1998;13:490–5.
149. Miyake Y, Iwasaki Y, Takaki A, Kobashi H, Sakaguchi K, Shiratori Y. Clinical features of Japanese elderly patients with type 1 autoimmune hepatitis. Intern Med. 2007;46:1945–9.
150. Abe M, Mashiba T, Zeniya M, Yamamoto K, Onji M, Tsubouchi H. Present status of autoimmune hepatitis in Japan: a nationwide survey. J Gastroenterol. 2011;46:1136–41.
151. Pratt AJ, MacRae IJ. The RNA-induced silencing complex: a versatile gene-silencing machine. J Biol Chem. 2009;284:17897–901.
152. Ambros V. microRNAs: tiny regulators with great potential. Cell. 2001;107:823–6.
153. Migita K, Komori A, Kozuru H, Jiuchi Y, Nakamura M, Yasunami M, et al. Circulating microRNA profiles in patients with type-1 autoimmune hepatitis. PLoS One. 2015;10:e0136908.
154. Han L, Witmer PD, Casey E, Valle D, Sukumar S. DNA methylation regulates MicroRNA expression. Cancer Biol Ther. 2007;6:1284–8.
155. Tang JT, Wang JL, Du W, Hong J, Zhao SL, Wang YC, et al. MicroRNA 345, a methylation-sensitive microRNA is involved in cell proliferation and invasion in human colorectal cancer. Carcinogenesis. 2011;32:1207–15.
156. Fisher L, Fisher A. Vitamin D and parathyroid hormone in outpatients with noncholestatic chronic liver disease. Clin Gastroenterol Hepatol. 2007;5:513–20.
157. Miroliaee A, Nasiri-Toosi M, Khalilzadeh O, Esteghamati A, Abdollahi A, Mazloumi M. Disturbances of parathyroid hormone-vitamin D axis in non-cholestatic chronic liver disease: a cross-sectional study. Hepatol Int. 2010;4:634–40.
158. Stokes CS, Volmer DA, Grunhage F, Lammert F. Vitamin D in chronic liver disease. Liver Int. 2013;33:338–52.
159. Efe C, Kav T, Aydin C, Cengiz M, Imga NN, Purnak T, et al. Low serum vitamin D levels are associated with severe histological features and poor response to therapy in patients with autoimmune hepatitis. Dig Dis Sci. 2014;59:3035–42.
160. Holick MF. Vitamin D deficiency. N Engl J Med. 2007;357:266–81.
161. Ohyama Y, Yamasaki T. Eight cytochrome P450s catalyze vitamin D metabolism. Front Biosci. 2004;9:3007–18.
162. Lemire JM. Immunomodulatory role of 1,25-dihydroxyvitamin D3. J Cell Biochem. 1992;49:26–31.
163. Adams JS, Hewison M. Unexpected actions of vitamin D: new perspectives on the regulation of innate and adaptive immunity. Nat Clin Pract Endocrinol Metab. 2008;4:80–90.
164. Luong KV, Nguyen LT. The role of vitamin D in autoimmune hepatitis. J Clin Med Res. 2013;5:407–15.
165. Provvedini DM, Tsoukas CD, Deftos LJ, Manolagas SC. 1,25-dihydroxyvitamin D3 receptors in human leukocytes. Science. 1983;221:1181–3.
166. Bhalla AK, Amento EP, Clemens TL, Holick MF, Krane SM. Specific high-affinity receptors for 1,25-dihydroxyvitamin D3 in human peripheral blood mononuclear cells: presence in monocytes and induction in T lymphocytes following activation. J Clin Endocrinol Metab. 1983;57:1308–10.
167. Barbour GL, Coburn JW, Slatopolsky E, Norman AW, Horst RL. Hypercalcemia in an anephric patient with sarcoidosis: evidence for extrarenal generation of 1,25-dihydroxyvitamin D. N Engl J Med. 1981;305:440–3.
168. Adams JS, Sharma OP, Gacad MA, Singer FR. Metabolism of 25-hydroxyvitamin D3 by cultured pulmonary alveolar macrophages in sarcoidosis. J Clin Invest. 1983;72:1856–60.
169. Kim S, Shevde NK, Pike JW. 1,25-dihydroxyvitamin D3 stimulates cyclic vitamin D receptor/retinoid X receptor DNA-binding, co-activator recruitment, and histone acetylation in intact osteoblasts. J Bone Miner Res. 2005;20:305–17.
170. Gershwin ME, Ansari AA, Mackay IR, Nakanuma Y, Nishio A, Rowley MJ, et al. Primary biliary cirrhosis: an orchestrated immune response against epithelial cells. Immunol Rev. 2000;174:210–25.

171. Lindor KD, Gershwin ME, Poupon R, Kaplan M, Bergasa NV, Heathcote EJ. AASLD Practice Guidelines. Primary biliary cirrhosis. Hepatology. 2009;50:291–308.
172. Lindgren S, Glaumann H, Almer S, Bergquist A, Bjornsson E, Broome U, et al. Transitions between variant forms of primary biliary cirrhosis during long-term follow-up. Eur J Intern Med. 2009;20:398–402.
173. Lofgren J, Jarnerot G, Danielsson D, Hemdal I. Incidence and prevalence of primary biliary cirrhosis in a defined population in Sweden. Scand J Gastroenterol. 1985;20:647–50.
174. Prince MI, Chetwynd A, Craig WL, Metcalf JV, James OF. Asymptomatic primary biliary cirrhosis: clinical features, prognosis, and symptom progression in a large population based cohort. Gut. 2004;53:865–70.
175. Podda M, Selmi C, Lleo A, Moroni L, Invernizzi P. The limitations and hidden gems of the epidemiology of primary biliary cirrhosis. J Autoimmun. 2013;46:81–7.
176. Chong VH, Telisinghe PU, Jalihal A. Primary biliary cirrhosis in Brunei Darussalam. Hepatobiliary Pancreat Dis Int. 2010;9:622–8.
177. Remmel T, Remmel H, Uibo R, Salupere V. Primary biliary cirrhosis in Estonia. With special reference to incidence, prevalence, clinical features, and outcome. Scand J Gastroenterol. 1995;30:367–71.
178. Metcalf JV, Bhopal RS, Gray J, Howel D, James OF. Incidence and prevalence of primary biliary cirrhosis in the city of Newcastle upon Tyne, England. Int J Epidemiol. 1997;26:830–6.
179. James OF, Bhopal R, Howel D, Gray J, Burt AD, Metcalf JV. Primary biliary cirrhosis once rare, now common in the United Kingdom? Hepatology. 1999;30:390–4.
180. Kim WR, Lindor KD, Locke GR 3rd, Therneau TM, Homburger HA, Batts KP, et al. Epidemiology and natural history of primary biliary cirrhosis in a US community. Gastroenterology. 2000;119:1631–6.
181. Myers RP, Shaheen AA, Fong A, Burak KW, Wan A, Swain MG, et al. Epidemiology and natural history of primary biliary cirrhosis in a Canadian health region: a population-based study. Hepatology. 2009;50:1884–92.
182. Lleo A, Jepsen P, Morenghi E, Carbone M, Moroni L, Battezzati PM, et al. Evolving trends in female to male incidence and male mortality of primary biliary cholangitis. Sci Rep. 2016;6:25906.
183. Pla X, Vergara M, Gil M, Dalmau B, Cistero B, Bella RM, et al. Incidence, prevalence and clinical course of primary biliary cirrhosis in a Spanish community. Eur J Gastroenterol Hepatol. 2007;19:859–64.
184. Triger DR, Berg PA, Rodes J. Epidemiology of primary biliary cirrhosis. Liver. 1984;4:195–200.
185. Mao TK, Lian ZX, Selmi C, Ichiki Y, Ashwood P, Ansari AA, et al. Altered monocyte responses to defined TLR ligands in patients with primary biliary cirrhosis. Hepatology. 2005;42:802–8.
186. Kikuchi K, Lian ZX, Yang GX, Ansari AA, Ikehara S, Kaplan M, et al. Bacterial CpG induces hyper-IgM production in CD27(+) memory B cells in primary biliary cirrhosis. Gastroenterology. 2005;128:304–12.
187. Honda Y, Yamagiwa S, Matsuda Y, Takamura M, Ichida T, Aoyagi Y. Altered expression of TLR homolog RP105 on monocytes hypersensitive to LPS in patients with primary biliary cirrhosis. J Hepatol. 2007;47:404–11.
188. Shimoda S, Harada K, Niiro H, Shirabe K, Taketomi A, Maehara Y, et al. Interaction between Toll-like receptors and natural killer cells in the destruction of bile ducts in primary biliary cirrhosis. Hepatology. 2011;53:1270–81.
189. Yurkovetskiy L, Burrows M, Khan AA, Graham L, Volchkov P, Becker L, et al. Gender bias in autoimmunity is influenced by microbiota. Immunity. 2013;39:400–12.
190. Markle JG, Frank DN, Mortin-Toth S, Robertson CE, Feazel LM, Rolle-Kampczyk U, et al. Sex differences in the gut microbiome drive hormone-dependent regulation of autoimmunity. Science. 2013;339:1084–8.

191. Chavhan GB, Roberts E, Moineddin R, Babyn PS, Manson DE. Primary sclerosing cholangitis in children: utility of magnetic resonance cholangiopancreatography. Pediatr Radiol. 2008;38:868–73.
192. Kerkar N, Miloh T. Sclerosing cholangitis: pediatric perspective. Curr Gastroenterol Rep. 2010;12:195–202.
193. Roberts EA. Autoimmune hepatitis from the paediatric perspective. Liver Int. 2011;31:1424–31.
194. Watson RG, Angus PW, Dewar M, Goss B, Sewell RB, Smallwood RA. Low prevalence of primary biliary cirrhosis in Victoria, Australia. Melbourne Liver Group. Gut. 1995;36:927–30.
195. Inoue K, Hirohara J, Nakano T, Seki T, Sasaki H, Higuchi K, et al. Prediction of prognosis of primary biliary cirrhosis in Japan. Liver. 1995;15:70–7.
196. Liu H, Liu Y, Wang L, Xu D, Lin B, Zhong R, et al. Prevalence of primary biliary cirrhosis in adults referring hospital for annual health check-up in Southern China. BMC Gastroenterol. 2010;10:100.
197. Delgado J, Sperber AD, Novack V, Delgado B, Edelman L, Gaspar N, et al. The epidemiology of primary biliary cirrhosis in southern Israel. Isr Med Assoc J. 2005;7:717–21.
198. Sood S, Gow PJ, Christie JM, Angus PW. Epidemiology of primary biliary cirrhosis in Victoria, Australia: high prevalence in migrant populations. Gastroenterology. 2004;127:470–5.
199. Myszor M, James OF. The epidemiology of primary biliary cirrhosis in north-east England: an increasingly common disease? Q J Med. 1990;75:377–85.
200. Ilyas JA, O'Mahony CA, Vierling JM. Liver transplantation in autoimmune liver diseases. Best Pract Res Clin Gastroenterol. 2011;25:765–82.
201. Invernizzi P. Geoepidemiology of autoimmune liver diseases. J Autoimmun. 2010;34:J300–6.
202. Abu-Mouch S, Selmi C, Benson GD, Kenny TP, Invernizzi P, Zuin M, et al. Geographic clusters of primary biliary cirrhosis. Clin Dev Immunol. 2003;10:127–31.
203. Howel D, Fischbacher CM, Bhopal RS, Gray J, Metcalf JV, James OF. An exploratory population-based case-control study of primary biliary cirrhosis. Hepatology. 2000;31:1055–60.
204. Parikh-Patel A, Gold EB, Worman H, Krivy KE, Gershwin ME. Risk factors for primary biliary cirrhosis in a cohort of patients from the united states. Hepatology. 2001;33:16–21.
205. Gershwin ME, Selmi C, Worman HJ, Gold EB, Watnik M, Utts J, et al. Risk factors and comorbidities in primary biliary cirrhosis: a controlled interview-based study of 1032 patients. Hepatology. 2005;42:1194–202.
206. Prince MI, Ducker SJ, James OF. Case-control studies of risk factors for primary biliary cirrhosis in two United Kingdom populations. Gut. 2010;59:508–12.
207. Liang Y, Yang Z, Zhong R. Smoking, family history and urinary tract infection are associated with primary biliary cirrhosis: a meta-analysis. Hepatol Res. 2011;41:572–8.
208. Smyk DS, Rigopoulou EI, Muratori L, Burroughs AK, Bogdanos DP. Smoking as a risk factor for autoimmune liver disease: what we can learn from primary biliary cirrhosis. Ann Hepatol. 2012;11:7–14.
209. Lammert C, Nguyen DL, Juran BD, Schlicht E, Larson JJ, Atkinson EJ, et al. Questionnaire based assessment of risk factors for primary biliary cirrhosis. Dig Liver Dis. 2013;45:589–94.
210. Corpechot C, Chretien Y, Chazouilleres O, Poupon R. Demographic, lifestyle, medical and familial factors associated with primary biliary cirrhosis. J Hepatol. 2010;53:162–9.
211. Zein CO, Beatty K, Post AB, Logan L, Debanne S, McCullough AJ. Smoking and increased severity of hepatic fibrosis in primary biliary cirrhosis: a cross validated retrospective assessment. Hepatology. 2006;44:1564–71.
212. Corpechot C, Gaouar F, Chretien Y, Johanet C, Chazouilleres O, Poupon R. Smoking as an independent risk factor of liver fibrosis in primary biliary cirrhosis. J Hepatol. 2012;56:218–24.
213. Costenbader KH, Karlson EW. Cigarette smoking and autoimmune disease: what can we learn from epidemiology? Lupus. 2006;15:737–45.

214. Glossop JR, Dawes PT, Mattey DL. Association between cigarette smoking and release of tumour necrosis factor alpha and its soluble receptors by peripheral blood mononuclear cells in patients with rheumatoid arthritis. Rheumatology (Oxford). 2006;45:1223–9.
215. Arnson Y, Shoenfeld Y, Amital H. Effects of tobacco smoke on immunity, inflammation and autoimmunity. J Autoimmun. 2010;34:J258–65.
216. Juran BD, Lazaridis KN. Environmental factors in primary biliary cirrhosis. Semin Liver Dis. 2014;34:265–72.
217. Whetzel CA, Corwin EJ, Klein LC. Disruption in Th1/Th2 immune response in young adult smokers. Addict Behav. 2007;32:1–8.
218. Harada K, Van de Water J, Leung PS, Coppel RL, Ansari A, Nakanuma Y, et al. In situ nucleic acid hybridization of cytokines in primary biliary cirrhosis: predominance of the Th1 subset. Hepatology. 1997;25:791–6.
219. Montano-Loza AJ, Thandassery RB, Czaja AJ. Targeting hepatic fibrosis in autoimmune hepatitis. Dig Dis Sci. 2016;61:3118–39.
220. Kroening PR, Barnes TW, Pease L, Limper A, Kita H, Vassallo R. Cigarette smoke-induced oxidative stress suppresses generation of dendritic cell IL-12 and IL-23 through ERK-dependent pathways. J Immunol. 2008;181:1536–47.
221. Bae HR, Leung PS, Tsuneyama K, Valencia JC, Hodge DL, Kim S, et al. Chronic expression of interferon-gamma leads to murine autoimmune cholangitis with a female predominance. Hepatology. 2016;64:1189–201.
222. Bluhm AL, Weinstein J, Sousa JA. Free radicals in tobacco smoke. Nature. 1971;229:500.
223. Pryor WA, Stone K. Oxidants in cigarette smoke. Radicals, hydrogen peroxide, peroxynitrate, and peroxynitrite. Ann N Y Acad Sci. 1993;686:12–27; discussion 27–8.
224. Amano K, Leung PS, Rieger R, Quan C, Wang X, Marik J, et al. Chemical xenobiotics and mitochondrial autoantigens in primary biliary cirrhosis: identification of antibodies against a common environmental, cosmetic, and food additive, 2-octynoic acid. J Immunol. 2005;174:5874–83.
225. Czaja AJ. Nature and implications of oxidative and nitrosative stresses in autoimmune hepatitis. Dig Dis Sci. 2016;61:2784–803.
226. Triger DR. Primary biliary cirrhosis: an epidemiological study. Br Med J. 1980;281:772–5.
227. Ala A, Stanca CM, Bu-Ghanim M, Ahmado I, Branch AD, Schiano TD, et al. Increased prevalence of primary biliary cirrhosis near Superfund toxic waste sites. Hepatology. 2006;43:525–31.
228. Walden HR, Kirby JA, Yeaman SJ, Gray J, Jones DE, Palmer JM. Xenobiotic incorporation into pyruvate dehydrogenase complex can occur via the exogenous lipoylation pathway. Hepatology. 2008;48:1874–84.
229. Yeaman SJ, Kirby JA, Jones DE. Autoreactive responses to pyruvate dehydrogenase complex in the pathogenesis of primary biliary cirrhosis. Immunol Rev. 2000;174:238–49.
230. Hamlyn AN, Macklon AF, James O. Primary biliary cirrhosis: geographical clustering and symptomatic onset seasonality. Gut. 1983;24:940–5.
231. Czaja AJ. Drug-induced autoimmune-like hepatitis. Dig Dis Sci. 2011;56:958–76.
232. Menon KV, Angulo P, Boe GM, Lindor KD. Safety and efficacy of estrogen therapy in preventing bone loss in primary biliary cirrhosis. Am J Gastroenterol. 2003;98:889–92.
233. Alvaro D, Invernizzi P, Onori P, Franchitto A, De Santis A, Crosignani A, et al. Estrogen receptors in cholangiocytes and the progression of primary biliary cirrhosis. J Hepatol. 2004;41:905–12.
234. Guattery JM, Faloon WW. Effect of estradiol upon serum enzymes in primary biliary cirrhosis. Hepatology. 1987;7:737–42.
235. McNally RJ, James PW, Ducker S, James OF. Seasonal variation in the patient diagnosis of primary biliary cirrhosis: further evidence for an environmental component to etiology. Hepatology. 2011;54:2099–103.
236. McNally RJ, Ducker S, James OF. Are transient environmental agents involved in the cause of primary biliary cirrhosis? Evidence from space-time clustering analysis. Hepatology. 2009;50:1169–74.

237. Xu L, Shen Z, Guo L, Fodera B, Keogh A, Joplin R, et al. Does a betaretrovirus infection trigger primary biliary cirrhosis? Proc Natl Acad Sci U S A. 2003;100:8454–9.
238. Selmi C, Balkwill DL, Invernizzi P, Ansari AA, Coppel RL, Podda M, et al. Patients with primary biliary cirrhosis react against a ubiquitous xenobiotic-metabolizing bacterium. Hepatology. 2003;38:1250–7.
239. Kaplan MM. Novosphingobium aromaticivorans: a potential initiator of primary biliary cirrhosis. Am J Gastroenterol. 2004;99:2147–9.
240. Olafsson S, Gudjonsson H, Selmi C, Amano K, Invernizzi P, Podda M, et al. Antimitochondrial antibodies and reactivity to N. aromaticivorans proteins in Icelandic patients with primary biliary cirrhosis and their relatives. Am J Gastroenterol. 2004;99:2143–6.
241. Padgett KA, Selmi C, Kenny TP, Leung PS, Balkwill DL, Ansari AA, et al. Phylogenetic and immunological definition of four lipoylated proteins from Novosphingobium aromaticivorans, implications for primary biliary cirrhosis. J Autoimmun. 2005;24:209–19.
242. Zabiegala B, Urbanowicz M, Namiesnik J, Gorecki T. Spatial and seasonal patterns of benzene, toluene, ethylbenzene, and xylenes in the Gdansk, Poland and surrounding areas determined using radiello passive samplers. J Environ Qual. 2010;39:896–906.
243. Tiwari V, Hanai Y, Masunaga S. Ambient levels of volatile organic compounds in the vicinity of petrochemical industrial area of Yokohama, Japan. Air Qual Atmos Health. 2010;3:65–75.
244. Wang JJ, Yang GX, Zhang WC, Lu L, Tsuneyama K, Kronenberg M, et al. *Escherichia coli* infection induces autoimmune cholangitis and anti-mitochondrial antibodies in non-obese diabetic (NOD).B6 (Idd10/Idd18) mice. Clin Exp Immunol. 2014;175:192–201.
245. Haydon GH, Neuberger J. PBC: an infectious disease? Gut. 2000;47:586–8.
246. Kumagi T, Abe M, Ikeda Y, Hiasa Y. Infection as a risk factor in the pathogenesis of primary biliary cirrhosis: pros and cons. Dis Markers. 2010;29:313–21.
247. Koutsoumpas AL, Kriese S, Rigopoulou EI. Popular and unpopular infectious agents linked to primary biliary cirrhosis. Auto Immun Highlights. 2012;3:95–104.
248. Mattner J, Savage PB, Leung P, Oertelt SS, Wang V, Trivedi O, et al. Liver autoimmunity triggered by microbial activation of natural killer T cells. Cell Host Microbe. 2008;3:304–15.
249. Mohammed JP, Mattner J. Autoimmune disease triggered by infection with alphaproteobacteria. Expert Rev Clin Immunol. 2009;5:369–79.
250. Mason AL, Xu L, Guo L, Munoz S, Jaspan JB, Bryer-Ash M, et al. Detection of retroviral antibodies in primary biliary cirrhosis and other idiopathic biliary disorders. Lancet. 1998;351:1620–4.
251. Xu L, Sakalian M, Shen Z, Loss G, Neuberger J, Mason A. Cloning the human betaretrovirus proviral genome from patients with primary biliary cirrhosis. Hepatology. 2004;39:151–6.
252. Selmi C, Ross SR, Ansari AA, Invernizzi P, Podda M, Coppel RL, et al. Lack of immunological or molecular evidence for a role of mouse mammary tumor retrovirus in primary biliary cirrhosis. Gastroenterology. 2004;127:493–501.
253. Wang W, Indik S, Wasilenko ST, Faschinger A, Carpenter EJ, Tian Z, et al. Frequent proviral integration of the human betaretrovirus in biliary epithelium of patients with autoimmune and idiopathic liver disease. Aliment Pharmacol Ther. 2015;41:393–405.
254. Lytvyak E, Montano-Loza AJ, Mason AL. Combination antiretroviral studies for patients with primary biliary cirrhosis. World J Gastroenterol. 2016;22:349–60.
255. Hopf U, Moller B, Stemerowicz R, Lobeck H, Rodloff A, Freudenberg M, et al. Relation between *Escherichia coli* R(rough)-forms in gut, lipid A in liver, and primary biliary cirrhosis. Lancet. 1989;2:1419–22.
256. Bogdanos DP, Baum H, Butler P, Rigopoulou EI, Davies ET, Ma Y, et al. Association between the primary biliary cirrhosis specific anti-sp100 antibodies and recurrent urinary tract infection. Dig Liver Dis. 2003;35:801–5.
257. Burroughs AK, Rosenstein IJ, Epstein O, Hamilton-Miller JM, Brumfitt W, Sherlock S. Bacteriuria and primary biliary cirrhosis. Gut. 1984;25:133–7.
258. Smyk DS, Bogdanos DP, Kriese S, Billinis C, Burroughs AK, Rigopoulou EI. Urinary tract infection as a risk factor for autoimmune liver disease: from bench to bedside. Clin Res Hepatol Gastroenterol. 2012;36:110–21.

259. Butler P, Hamilton-Miller JM, McIntyre N, Burroughs AK. Natural history of bacteriuria in women with primary biliary cirrhosis and the effect of antimicrobial therapy in symptomatic and asymptomatic groups. Gut. 1995;36:931–4.
260. Varyani FK, West J, Card TR. An increased risk of urinary tract infection precedes development of primary biliary cirrhosis. BMC Gastroenterol. 2011;11:95.
261. Mason A, Xu L, Neuberger J. Proof of principal studies to assess the role of the human betaretrovirus in patients with primary biliary cirrhosis. Am J Gastroenterol. 2004;99:2499–500.
262. Johal H, Scott GM, Jones R, Camaris C, Riordan S, Rawlinson WD. Mouse mammary tumour virus-like virus (MMTV-LV) is present within the liver in a wide range of hepatic disorders and unrelated to nuclear p53 expression or hepatocarcinogenesis. J Hepatol. 2009;50:548–54.
263. Morshed SA, Nishioka M, Saito I, Komiyama K, Moro I. Increased expression of Epstein-Barr virus in primary biliary cirrhosis patients. Gastroenterol Jpn. 1992;27:751–8.
264. Vilagut L, Pares A, Vinas O, Vila J, Jimenez de Anta MT, Rodes J. Antibodies to mycobacterial 65-kD heat shock protein cross-react with the main mitochondrial antigens in patients with primary biliary cirrhosis. Eur J Clin Investig. 1997;27:667–72.
265. Nilsson HO, Taneera J, Castedal M, Glatz E, Olsson R, Wadstrom T. Identification of *Helicobacter pylori* and other *Helicobacter* species by PCR, hybridization, and partial DNA sequencing in human liver samples from patients with primary sclerosing cholangitis or primary biliary cirrhosis. J Clin Microbiol. 2000;38:1072–6.
266. Abdulkarim AS, Petrovic LM, Kim WR, Angulo P, Lloyd RV, Lindor KD. Primary biliary cirrhosis: an infectious disease caused by Chlamydia pneumoniae? J Hepatol. 2004;40:380–4.
267. Berg CP, Kannan TR, Klein R, Gregor M, Baseman JB, Wesselborg S, et al. Mycoplasma antigens as a possible trigger for the induction of antimitochondrial antibodies in primary biliary cirrhosis. Liver Int. 2009;29:797–809.
268. Shapira Y, Agmon-Levin N, Renaudineau Y, Porat-Katz BS, Barzilai O, Ram M, et al. Serum markers of infections in patients with primary biliary cirrhosis: evidence of infection burden. Exp Mol Pathol. 2012;93:386–90.
269. Tsuji K, Watanabe Y, Van De Water J, Nakanishi T, Kajiyama G, Parikh-Patel A, et al. Familial primary biliary cirrhosis in Hiroshima. J Autoimmun. 1999;13:171–8.
270. Selmi C, Mayo MJ, Bach N, Ishibashi H, Invernizzi P, Gish RG, et al. Primary biliary cirrhosis in monozygotic and dizygotic twins: genetics, epigenetics, and environment. Gastroenterology. 2004;127:485–92.
271. Mantaka A, Koulentaki M, Chlouverakis G, Enele-Melono JM, Darivianaki A, Tzardi M, et al. Primary biliary cirrhosis in a genetically homogeneous population: disease associations and familial occurrence rates. BMC Gastroenterol. 2012;12:110.
272. Nakamura M, Nishida N, Kawashima M, Aiba Y, Tanaka A, Yasunami M, et al. Genome-wide association study identifies TNFSF15 and POU2AF1 as susceptibility loci for primary biliary cirrhosis in the Japanese population. Am J Hum Genet. 2012;91:721–8.
273. Liu X, Invernizzi P, Lu Y, Kosoy R, Lu Y, Bianchi I, et al. Genome-wide meta-analyses identify three loci associated with primary biliary cirrhosis. Nat Genet. 2010;42:658–60.
274. Mells GF, Floyd JA, Morley KI, Cordell HJ, Franklin CS, Shin SY, et al. Genome-wide association study identifies 12 new susceptibility loci for primary biliary cirrhosis. Nat Genet. 2011;43:329–32.
275. Gulamhusein AF, Juran BD, Lazaridis KN. Genome-wide association studies in primary biliary cirrhosis. Semin Liver Dis. 2015;35:392–401.
276. Jones DE, Watt FE, Metcalf JV, Bassendine MF, James OF. Familial primary biliary cirrhosis reassessed: a geographically-based population study. J Hepatol. 1999;30:402–7.
277. Bittencourt PL, Farias AQ, Abrantes-Lemos CP, Goncalves LL, Goncalves PL, Magalhaes EP, et al. Prevalence of immune disturbances and chronic liver disease in family members of patients with primary biliary cirrhosis. J Gastroenterol Hepatol. 2004;19:873–8.
278. Brind AM, Bray GP, Portmann BC, Williams R. Prevalence and pattern of familial disease in primary biliary cirrhosis. Gut. 1995;36:615–7.
279. Yanagisawa M, Takagi H, Takahashi H, Uehara M, Otsuka T, Yuasa K, et al. Familial clustering and genetic background of primary biliary cirrhosis in Japan. Dig Dis Sci. 2010;55:2651–8.

280. Bach N, Schaffner F. Familial primary biliary cirrhosis. J Hepatol. 1994;20:698–701.
281. Lazaridis KN, Juran BD, Boe GM, Slusser JP, de Andrade M, Homburger HA, et al. Increased prevalence of antimitochondrial antibodies in first-degree relatives of patients with primary biliary cirrhosis. Hepatology. 2007;46:785–92.
282. Zografos TA, Gatselis N, Zachou K, Liaskos C, Gabeta S, Koukoulis GK, et al. Primary biliary cirrhosis-specific autoantibodies in first degree relatives of Greek primary biliary cirrhosis patients. World J Gastroenterol. 2012;18:4721–8.
283. Watt FE, James OF, Jones DE. Patterns of autoimmunity in primary biliary cirrhosis patients and their families: a population-based cohort study. Q J Med. 2004;97:397–406.
284. Gulamhusein AF, Juran BD, Atkinson EJ, McCauley B, Schlicht E, Lazaridis KN. Low incidence of primary biliary cirrhosis (PBC) in the first-degree relatives of PBC probands after 8 years of follow-up. Liver Int. 2016;36:1378–82.
285. Underhill JA, Donaldson PT, Doherty DG, Manabe K, Williams R. HLA DPB polymorphism in primary sclerosing cholangitis and primary biliary cirrhosis. Hepatology. 1995;21:959–62.
286. Jones DE, Donaldson PT. Genetic factors in the pathogenesis of primary biliary cirrhosis. Clin Liver Dis. 2003;7:841–64.
287. Webb GJ, Siminovitch KA, Hirschfield GM. The immunogenetics of primary biliary cirrhosis: a comprehensive review. J Autoimmun. 2015;64:42–52.
288. Cordell HJ, Han Y, Mells GF, Li Y, Hirschfield GM, Greene CS, et al. International genome-wide meta-analysis identifies new primary biliary cirrhosis risk loci and targetable pathogenic pathways. Nat Commun. 2015;6:8019.
289. Hirschfield GM, Liu X, Xu C, Lu Y, Xie G, Lu Y, et al. Primary biliary cirrhosis associated with HLA, IL12A, and IL12RB2 variants. N Engl J Med. 2009;360:2544–55.
290. van Wanrooij RL, Zwiers A, Kraal G, Bouma G. Genetic variations in interleukin-12 related genes in immune-mediated diseases. J Autoimmun. 2012;39:359–68.
291. Lleo A, Zhang W, Zhao M, Tan Y, Bernuzzi F, Zhu B, et al. DNA methylation profiling of the X chromosome reveals an aberrant demethylation on CXCR3 promoter in primary biliary cirrhosis. Clin Epigenetics. 2015;7:61.
292. Tomiyama T, Yang GX, Zhao M, Zhang W, Tanaka H, Wang J, et al. The modulation of co-stimulatory molecules by circulating exosomes in primary biliary cirrhosis. Cell Mol Immunol. 2017;14:276–84.
293. Sydow JF, Cramer P. RNA polymerase fidelity and transcriptional proofreading. Curr Opin Struct Biol. 2009;19:732–9.
294. Tough DF, Prinjha RK. Immune disease-associated variants in gene enhancers point to BET epigenetic mechanisms for therapeutic intervention. Epigenomics. 2017;9:573–84.
295. Marra F, Tacke F. Roles for chemokines in liver disease. Gastroenterology. 2014;147:577–94.
296. Smigielska-Czepiel K, van den Berg A, Jellema P, van der Lei RJ, Bijzet J, Kluiver J, et al. Comprehensive analysis of miRNA expression in T-cell subsets of rheumatoid arthritis patients reveals defined signatures of naive and memory Tregs. Genes Immun. 2014;15:115–25.
297. Bartholomew LG, Cain JC, Woolner LB, Utz DC, Ferris DO. Sclerosing cholangitis: its possible association with Riedel's struma and fibrous retroperitonitis. Report of two cases. N Engl J Med. 1963;269:8–12.
298. Geubel AP, Baggenstoss AH, Summerskill WH. Responses to treatment can differentiate chronic active liver disease with cholangitic features from the primary biliary cirrhosis syndrome. Gastroenterology. 1976;71:444–9.
299. Wiesner RH, LaRusso NF. Clinicopathologic features of the syndrome of primary sclerosing cholangitis. Gastroenterology. 1980;79:200–6.
300. Ludwig J, Barham SS, LaRusso NF, Elveback LR, Wiesner RH, McCall JT. Morphologic features of chronic hepatitis associated with primary sclerosing cholangitis and chronic ulcerative colitis. Hepatology. 1981;1:632–40.
301. Chapman R, Fevery J, Kalloo A, Nagorney DM, Boberg KM, Shneider B, et al. Diagnosis and management of primary sclerosing cholangitis. Hepatology. 2010;51:660–78.
302. Lindor KD, Kowdley KV, Harrison ME. ACG Clinical Guideline: primary sclerosing cholangitis. Am J Gastroenterol. 2015;110:646–59.

303. Lunder AK, Hov JR, Borthne A, Gleditsch J, Johannesen G, Tveit K, et al. Prevalence of sclerosing cholangitis detected by magnetic resonance cholangiography in patients with long-term inflammatory bowel disease. Gastroenterology. 2016;151:660–69.e4.
304. Angulo P, Maor-Kendler Y, Lindor KD. Small-duct primary sclerosing cholangitis: a long-term follow-up study. Hepatology. 2002;35:1494–500.
305. Lindkvist B, Benito de Valle M, Gullberg B, Bjornsson E. Incidence and prevalence of primary sclerosing cholangitis in a defined adult population in Sweden. Hepatology. 2010;52:571–7.
306. Boonstra K, Beuers U, Ponsioen CY. Epidemiology of primary sclerosing cholangitis and primary biliary cirrhosis: a systematic review. J Hepatol. 2012;56:1181–8.
307. Jepsen P, Gronbaek L, Vilstrup H. Worldwide incidence of autoimmune liver disease. Dig Dis. 2015;33(Suppl 2):2–12.
308. Boonstra K, Weersma RK, van Erpecum KJ, Rauws EA, Spanier BW, Poen AC, et al. Population-based epidemiology, malignancy risk, and outcome of primary sclerosing cholangitis. Hepatology. 2013;58:2045–55.
309. Card TR, Solaymani-Dodaran M, West J. Incidence and mortality of primary sclerosing cholangitis in the UK: a population-based cohort study. J Hepatol. 2008;48:939–44.
310. Kingham JG, Kochar N, Gravenor MB. Incidence, clinical patterns, and outcomes of primary sclerosing cholangitis in South Wales, United Kingdom. Gastroenterology. 2004;126:1929–30.
311. Bambha K, Kim WR, Talwalkar J, Torgerson H, Benson JT, Therneau TM, et al. Incidence, clinical spectrum, and outcomes of primary sclerosing cholangitis in a United States community. Gastroenterology. 2003;125:1364–9.
312. Toy E, Balasubramanian S, Selmi C, Li CS, Bowlus CL. The prevalence, incidence and natural history of primary sclerosing cholangitis in an ethnically diverse population. BMC Gastroenterol. 2011;11:83.
313. Kaplan GG, Laupland KB, Butzner D, Urbanski SJ, Lee SS. The burden of large and small duct primary sclerosing cholangitis in adults and children: a population-based analysis. Am J Gastroenterol. 2007;102:1042–9.
314. Escorsell A, Pares A, Rodes J, Solis-Herruzo JA, Miras M, de la Morena E. Epidemiology of primary sclerosing cholangitis in Spain. Spanish Association for the Study of the Liver. J Hepatol. 1994;21:787–91.
315. Berdal JE, Ebbesen J, Rydning A. [Incidence and prevalence of autoimmune liver diseases]. Tidsskr Nor Laegeforen. 1998;118:4517–9.
316. Molodecky NA, Kareemi H, Parab R, Barkema HW, Quan H, Myers RP, et al. Incidence of primary sclerosing cholangitis: a systematic review and meta-analysis. Hepatology. 2011;53:1590–9.
317. Norris S, Kondeatis E, Collins R, Satsangi J, Clare M, Chapman R, et al. Mapping MHC-encoded susceptibility and resistance in primary sclerosing cholangitis: the role of MICA polymorphism. Gastroenterology. 2001;120:1475–82.
318. Donaldson PT, Norris S. Evaluation of the role of MHC class II alleles, haplotypes and selected amino acid sequences in primary sclerosing cholangitis. Autoimmunity. 2002;35:555–64.
319. Karlsen TH, Boberg KM, Vatn M, Bergquist A, Hampe J, Schrumpf E, et al. Different HLA class II associations in ulcerative colitis patients with and without primary sclerosing cholangitis. Genes Immun. 2007;8:275–8.
320. Karlsen TH, Hampe J, Wiencke K, Schrumpf E, Thorsby E, Lie BA, et al. Genetic polymorphisms associated with inflammatory bowel disease do not confer risk for primary sclerosing cholangitis. Am J Gastroenterol. 2007;102:115–21.
321. Bowlus CL, Li CS, Karlsen TH, Lie BA, Selmi C. Primary sclerosing cholangitis in genetically diverse populations listed for liver transplantation: unique clinical and human leukocyte antigen associations. Liver Transpl. 2010;16:1324–30.
322. Hov JR, Lleo A, Selmi C, Woldseth B, Fabris L, Strazzabosco M, et al. Genetic associations in Italian primary sclerosing cholangitis: heterogeneity across Europe defines a critical role for HLA-C. J Hepatol. 2010;52:712–7.

323. Juran BD, Atkinson EJ, Schlicht EM, Larson JJ, Ellinghaus D, Franke A, et al. Genetic polymorphisms of matrix metalloproteinase 3 in primary sclerosing cholangitis. Liver Int. 2011;31:785–91.
324. Friedrich K, Rupp C, Hov JR, Steinebrunner N, Weiss KH, Stiehl A, et al. A frequent PNPLA3 variant is a sex specific disease modifier in PSC patients with bile duct stenosis. PLoS One. 2013;8:e58734.
325. Liu JZ, Hov JR, Folseraas T, Ellinghaus E, Rushbrook SM, Doncheva NT, et al. Dense genotyping of immune-related disease regions identifies nine new risk loci for primary sclerosing cholangitis. Nat Genet. 2013;45:670–5.
326. Spurkland A, Saarinen S, Boberg KM, Mitchell S, Broome U, Caballeria L, et al. HLA class II haplotypes in primary sclerosing cholangitis patients from five European populations. Tissue Antigens. 1999;53:459–69.
327. Loftus EV Jr, Sandborn WJ, Tremaine WJ, Mahoney DW, Zinsmeister AR, Offord KP, et al. Primary sclerosing cholangitis is associated with nonsmoking: a case-control study. Gastroenterology. 1996;110:1496–502.
328. van Erpecum KJ, Smits SJ, van de Meeberg PC, Linn FH, Wolfhagen FH, vanBerge-Henegouwen GP, et al. Risk of primary sclerosing cholangitis is associated with nonsmoking behavior. Gastroenterology. 1996;110:1503–6.
329. Mitchell SA, Thyssen M, Orchard TR, Jewell DP, Fleming KA, Chapman RW. Cigarette smoking, appendectomy, and tonsillectomy as risk factors for the development of primary sclerosing cholangitis: a case control study. Gut. 2002;51:567–73.
330. Terjung B, Sohne J, Lechtenberg B, Gottwein J, Muennich M, Herzog V, et al. p-ANCAs in autoimmune liver disorders recognise human beta-tubulin isotype 5 and cross-react with microbial protein FtsZ. Gut. 2010;59:808–16.
331. Mueller T, Beutler C, Pico AH, Shibolet O, Pratt DS, Pascher A, et al. Enhanced innate immune responsiveness and intolerance to intestinal endotoxins in human biliary epithelial cells contributes to chronic cholangitis. Liver Int. 2011;31:1574–88.
332. Tabibian JH, O'Hara SP, Trussoni CE, Tietz PS, Splinter PL, Mounajjed T, et al. Absence of the intestinal microbiota exacerbates hepatobiliary disease in a murine model of primary sclerosing cholangitis. Hepatology. 2016;63:185–96.
333. Fausa O, Schrumpf E, Elgjo K. Relationship of inflammatory bowel disease and primary sclerosing cholangitis. Semin Liver Dis. 1991;11:31–9.
334. Schrumpf E, Fausa O, Kolmannskog F, Elgjo K, Ritland S, Gjone E. Sclerosing cholangitis in ulcerative colitis. A follow-up study. Scand J Gastroenterol. 1982;17:33–9.
335. Talwalkar JA, Lindor KD. Primary sclerosing cholangitis. Inflamm Bowel Dis. 2005;11:62–72.
336. Melum E, Franke A, Schramm C, Weismuller TJ, Gotthardt DN, Offner FA, et al. Genome-wide association analysis in primary sclerosing cholangitis identifies two non-HLA susceptibility loci. Nat Genet. 2011;43:17–9.
337. Saich R, Chapman R. Primary sclerosing cholangitis, autoimmune hepatitis and overlap syndromes in inflammatory bowel disease. World J Gastroenterol. 2008;14:331–7.
338. Jussila A, Virta LJ, Kautiainen H, Rekiaro M, Nieminen U, Farkkila MA. Increasing incidence of inflammatory bowel diseases between 2000 and 2007: a nationwide register study in Finland. Inflamm Bowel Dis. 2012;18:555–61.
339. Vind I, Riis L, Jess T, Knudsen E, Pedersen N, Elkjaer M, et al. Increasing incidences of inflammatory bowel disease and decreasing surgery rates in Copenhagen City and County, 2003–2005: a population-based study from the Danish Crohn colitis database. Am J Gastroenterol. 2006;101:1274–82.
340. Culver EL, Chapman RW. Systematic review: management options for primary sclerosing cholangitis and its variant forms—IgG4-associated cholangitis and overlap with autoimmune hepatitis. Aliment Pharmacol Ther. 2011;33:1273–91.
341. Luth S, Kanzler S, Frenzel C, Kasper HU, Dienes HP, Schramm C, et al. Characteristics and long-term prognosis of the autoimmune hepatitis/primary sclerosing cholangitis overlap syndrome. J Clin Gastroenterol. 2009;43:75–80.

342. Oliveira EM, Oliveira PM, Becker V, Dellavance A, Andrade LE, Lanzoni V, et al. Overlapping of primary biliary cirrhosis and small duct primary sclerosing cholangitis: first case report. J Clin Med Res. 2012;4:429–33.
343. McNair AN, Moloney M, Portmann BC, Williams R, McFarlane IG. Autoimmune hepatitis overlapping with primary sclerosing cholangitis in five cases. Am J Gastroenterol. 1998;93:777–84.
344. Burak KW, Urbanski SJ, Swain MG. A case of coexisting primary biliary cirrhosis and primary sclerosing cholangitis: a new overlap of autoimmune liver diseases. Dig Dis Sci. 2001;46:2043–7.
345. Abdo AA, Bain VG, Kichian K, Lee SS. Evolution of autoimmune hepatitis to primary sclerosing cholangitis: a sequential syndrome. Hepatology. 2002;36:1393–9.
346. Kingham JG, Abbasi A. Co-existence of primary biliary cirrhosis and primary sclerosing cholangitis: a rare overlap syndrome put in perspective. Eur J Gastroenterol Hepatol. 2005;17:1077–80.
347. Czaja AJ. Frequency and nature of the variant syndromes of autoimmune liver disease. Hepatology. 1998;28:360–5.
348. Kaya M, Angulo P, Lindor KD. Overlap of autoimmune hepatitis and primary sclerosing cholangitis: an evaluation of a modified scoring system. J Hepatol. 2000;33:537–42.
349. Boberg KM, Chapman RW, Hirschfield GM, Lohse AW, Manns MP, Schrumpf E. Overlap syndromes: the International Autoimmune Hepatitis Group (IAIHG) position statement on a controversial issue. J Hepatol. 2011;54:374–85.
350. Beuers U, Boberg KM, Chapman RW, Chazouilleres O, Invernizzi P, Jones DEJ, et al. EASL Clinical Practice Guidelines: management of cholestatic liver diseases. J Hepatol. 2009;51:237–67.
351. Bjornsson E, Chari S, Silveira M, Gossard A, Takahashi N, Smyrk T, et al. Primary sclerosing cholangitis associated with elevated immunoglobulin G4: clinical characteristics and response to therapy. Am J Ther. 2011;18:198–205.
352. Okazaki K, Uchida K, Koyabu M, Miyoshi H, Ikeura T, Takaoka M. IgG4 cholangiopathy: current concept, diagnosis, and pathogenesis. J Hepatol. 2014;61:690–5.
353. Naitoh I, Zen Y, Nakazawa T, Ando T, Hayashi K, Okumura F, et al. Small bile duct involvement in IgG4-related sclerosing cholangitis: liver biopsy and cholangiography correlation. J Gastroenterol. 2011;46:269–76.
354. Deshpande V, Sainani NI, Chung RT, Pratt DS, Mentha G, Rubbia-Brandt L, et al. IgG4-associated cholangitis: a comparative histological and immunophenotypic study with primary sclerosing cholangitis on liver biopsy material. Mod Pathol. 2009;22:1287–95.
355. Deshpande V, Zen Y, Chan JK, Yi EE, Sato Y, Yoshino T, et al. Consensus statement on the pathology of IgG4-related disease. Mod Pathol. 2012;25:1181–92.
356. Stone JH, Zen Y, Deshpande V. IgG4-related disease. N Engl J Med. 2012;366:539–51.
357. Ohara H, Okazaki K, Tsubouchi H, Inui K, Kawa S, Kamisawa T, et al. Clinical diagnostic criteria of IgG4-related sclerosing cholangitis 2012. J Hepatobiliary Pancreat Sci. 2012;19:536–42.
358. Ghazale A, Chari ST, Zhang L, Smyrk TC, Takahashi N, Levy MJ, et al. Immunoglobulin G4-associated cholangitis: clinical profile and response to therapy. Gastroenterology. 2008;134:706–15.
359. Boonstra K, Culver EL, de Buy Wenniger LM, van Heerde MJ, van Erpecum KJ, Poen AC, et al. Serum immunoglobulin G4 and immunoglobulin G1 for distinguishing immunoglobulin G4-associated cholangitis from primary sclerosing cholangitis. Hepatology. 2014;59:1954–63.
360. Dastis SN, Latinne D, Sempoux C, Geubel AP. Ulcerative colitis associated with IgG4 cholangitis: similar features in two HLA identical siblings. J Hepatol. 2009;51:601–5.
361. Narula N, Vasudev M, Marshall JK. IgG(4)-related sclerosing disease: a novel mimic of inflammatory bowel disease. Dig Dis Sci. 2010;55:3047–51.
362. Mendes FD, Jorgensen R, Keach J, Katzmann JA, Smyrk T, Donlinger J, et al. Elevated serum IgG4 concentration in patients with primary sclerosing cholangitis. Am J Gastroenterol. 2006;101:2070–5.

363. Oh HC, Kim MH, Lee KT, Lee JK, Moon SH, Song TJ, et al. Clinical clues to suspicion of IgG4-associated sclerosing cholangitis disguised as primary sclerosing cholangitis or hilar cholangiocarcinoma. J Gastroenterol Hepatol. 2010;25:1831–7.
364. Feldstein AE, Perrault J, El-Youssif M, Lindor KD, Freese DK, Angulo P. Primary sclerosing cholangitis in children: a long-term follow-up study. Hepatology. 2003;38:210–7.
365. Miloh T, Arnon R, Shneider B, Suchy F, Kerkar N. A retrospective single-center review of primary sclerosing cholangitis in children. Clin Gastroenterol Hepatol. 2009;7:239–45.
366. Takikawa H, Takamori Y, Tanaka A, Kurihara H, Nakanuma Y. Analysis of 388 cases of primary sclerosing cholangitis in Japan; presence of a subgroup without pancreatic involvement in older patients. Hepatol Res. 2004;29:153–9.
367. Tanaka A, Takikawa H. Geoepidemiology of primary sclerosing cholangitis: a critical review. J Autoimmun. 2013;46:35–40.
368. Kochhar R, Goenka MK, Das K, Nagi B, Bhasin DK, Chawla YK, et al. Primary sclerosing cholangitis: an experience from India. J Gastroenterol Hepatol. 1996;11:429–33.
369. Ang TL, Fock KM, Ng TM, Teo EK, Chua TS, Tan JY. Clinical profile of primary sclerosing cholangitis in Singapore. J Gastroenterol Hepatol. 2002;17:908–13.
370. Hiatt RA, Kaufman L. Epidemiology of inflammatory bowel disease in a defined northern California population. West J Med. 1988;149:541–6.
371. Boonstra K, de Vries EM, van Geloven N, van Erpecum KJ, Spanier M, Poen AC, et al. Risk factors for primary sclerosing cholangitis. Liver Int. 2016;36:84–91.
372. Rutgeerts P, D'Haens G, Hiele M, Geboes K, Vantrappen G. Appendectomy protects against ulcerative colitis. Gastroenterology. 1994;106:1251–3.
373. Karrar A, Broome U, Sodergren T, Jaksch M, Bergquist A, Bjornstedt M, et al. Biliary epithelial cell antibodies link adaptive and innate immune responses in primary sclerosing cholangitis. Gastroenterology. 2007;132:1504–14.
374. Tabibian JH, Weeding E, Jorgensen RA, Petz JL, Keach JC, Talwalkar JA, et al. Randomised clinical trial: vancomycin or metronidazole in patients with primary sclerosing cholangitis—a pilot study. Aliment Pharmacol Ther. 2013;37:604–12.
375. Tabibian JH, Talwalkar JA, Lindor KD. Role of the microbiota and antibiotics in primary sclerosing cholangitis. Biomed Res Int. 2013;2013:389537.
376. Bergquist A, Lindberg G, Saarinen S, Broome U. Increased prevalence of primary sclerosing cholangitis among first-degree relatives. J Hepatol. 2005;42:252–6.
377. Schrumpf E, Fausa O, Forre O, Dobloug JH, Ritland S, Thorsby E. HLA antigens and immunoregulatory T cells in ulcerative colitis associated with hepatobiliary disease. Scand J Gastroenterol. 1982;17:187–91.
378. Czaja AJ, Santrach PJ, Breanndan Moore S. Shared genetic risk factors in autoimmune liver disease. Dig Dis Sci. 2001;46:140–7.
379. Bernuzzi F, Marabita F, Lleo A, Carbone M, Mirolo M, Marzioni M, et al. Serum microRNAs as novel biomarkers for primary sclerosing cholangitis and cholangiocarcinoma. Clin Exp Immunol. 2016;185:61–71.
380. Timmer MR, Beuers U, Fockens P, Ponsioen CY, Rauws EA, Wang KK, et al. Genetic and epigenetic abnormalities in primary sclerosing cholangitis-associated cholangiocarcinoma. Inflamm Bowel Dis. 2013;19:1789–97.
381. Andresen K, Boberg KM, Vedeld HM, Honne H, Hektoen M, Wadsworth CA, et al. Novel target genes and a valid biomarker panel identified for cholangiocarcinoma. Epigenetics. 2012;7:1249–57.

The Epidemiology of Rare Hereditary Metabolic Liver Diseases

17

Marinos Pericleous, Claire Kelly, Aftab Ala, and Michael L. Schilsky

17.1 Introduction

A rare disease is defined by the European Health Commission as a disorder occurring in less than 5 per 10,000 individuals in the population whereas the United States definition sets a numerical maximum of fewer than 200,000 affected individuals in the country [1, 2]. A disease is defined as ultra-rare if less than 1 person per 50,000 people is affected [2]. The medical and socioeconomic impact of rare diseases is quite significant as there may be as many as 30 million people who live with a rare disease in the US and another 3.5 million in the UK [3, 4]. There are over 100 individual liver diseases, and it is estimated that more than 29 million people in the European Union and more than 30 million Americans suffer from liver disease [5, 6]. This chapter discusses the epidemiology of four rare metabolic liver disorders encountered by gastroenterologists and hepatologists: Wilson disease, lysosomal acid lipase deficiency, α1-antitrypsin deficiency and HFE-related hereditary hemochromatosis. The OMIM database codes (online Mendelian inheritance in man) have been included for each disease as these have been used extensively in the literature especially in relation to genotype-phenotype characterization.

M. Pericleous · C. Kelly · A. Ala
Department of Gastroenterology and Hepatology, Royal Surrey County Hospital, Guildford, Surrey, UK

Department of Clinical and Experimental Medicine, University of Surrey, Guildford, Surrey, UK

M. L. Schilsky (✉)
Divisions of Digestive Disease and Transplantation and Immunology, Departments of Medicine and Surgery, Yale University, New Haven, CT, USA
e-mail: michael.schilsky@yale.edu

R. J. Wong, R. G. Gish (eds.), *Clinical Epidemiology of Chronic Liver Diseases*,
https://doi.org/10.1007/978-3-319-94355-8_17

17.1.1 Wilson Disease (OMIM #277900)

Wilson disease (WD) was initially described as pseudosclerosis by the German neurologist Carl Westphal in 1883, and similar descriptions exist in the literature by William Gowers and Adolph Strümpell in 1888 and 1898 respectively [7]. The condition was named after the American born and British trained neurologist Samuel Alexander Kinnier Wilson who in 1912 presented a series of 13 patients with progressive lenticular degeneration with associated liver cirrhosis [8]. WD is an inherited autosomal recessive condition characterized by ineffective copper metabolism [9]. The specific association between WD and excess copper deposition in tissues such as the brain and the liver came much later in 1948 [10]. The deposition of copper in various organs explains the neuropsychiatric and hepatic manifestations of this disease. The molecular defect for WD has been mapped to chromosome 13 (13q14.3) and encodes ATP7B, a copper transporting ATPase that is mainly expressed in hepatocytes [11–17]. The gene, *ATP7B*, is approximately 80 kb and contains 21 exons that encode an approximately 7.5 kb transcript. ATP7B functions in copper homeostasis to facilitate transport of copper into bile, and in WD, there is a reduction in biliary copper transport and pathologic copper accumulation. The ATP7B gene was cloned in 1993 [18]. To date, over 500 unique ATP7B mutations have been described [19, 20].

The true worldwide prevalence of WD has not been fully elucidated, and several studies suggest there may be a range of disease prevalence. Most studies on mutation analysis focus on a limited number of mutations, especially His1069Glu, which is the commonest, especially in European populations. Similarly, Arg778Leu, R778L, A874V, and N1270S appear to be the commonest mutation in Asian regions [21, 22]. Many patients are compound heterozygotes and mutation frequency varies depending on the population/country being studied [23, 24].

Scheinberg et al. used published data from East Germany, USA and Japan to estimate a disease prevalence of 30 per million individuals and a carrier frequency of 1:90 [25]. A similar carrier frequency was described by Kim et al. for a Korean population, who estimated the disease incidence to be 1:30,778 [26]. Riley et al. reported a carrier frequency of 1:139 with a disease incidence of 1:58,823 [27]. Using the prevalence by Scheinberg et al., and the expectation that 2000 patients should be identified in UK's 60,000,000 population, Coffey et al. explored screening using molecular sequencing in a series of 181 patients with WD. Following identification of 116 mutations, they suggested that within the population, the likelihood of inheriting two mutated *ATP7B* alleles to be around 1 in 7026 [28]. The marked discrepancy between the genetic prevalence and the number of clinically diagnosed cases of WD may be due to a number of reasons including reduced penetrance of ATP7B mutations and failure to diagnose patients with this eminently treatable disorder. There may also be instances where WD may be mistaken for autoimmune hepatitis and/or other liver diseases that are found synchronous to WD which may be unrelated. These observations could lead to not only a delay in WD diagnosis but eventually lead to a particularly severe and pronounced WD.

Olivarez et al. carried out newborn screening in a U.S. Caucasian population for the His1069Glu mutation. The mutation was found in 0.285% of babies with an estimated heterozygote frequency of 0.855% and WD frequency of approximately 1 in 55,000 births [29].

The disease prevalence of WD is much higher in certain areas of the world. The highest prevalence reported was in a village on the Greek island Crete outside Heraklion where 1 in 15 babies born were affected by WD. This has been attributed to consanguinity. The estimated carrier frequency was 1:11 [30]. High prevalence for WD has also been found in the Far East. In 1999, Ohura et al. screened 2789 Japanese children for low ceruloplasmin levels using dry blood-spot (DBS) testing and found the incidence to be 1 in 40,000 and prevalence to be ~1:1500 [31]. Using DBS testing for screening in a Korean sample, Hahn et al. report a prevalence of ~1:3600. The combined mutation frequency for R778L, A874V, and N1270S for a Korean population was found to be 2%. These mutations are believed to constitute 54.2% of Korean WD patients and the estimated prevalence was found to be ~1:3000 [22]. Mak et al. analysed the p.L770L/p.R778L status of 660 Hong Kong Chinese patients and found a prevalence of ~1:5400 [32]. In Sardinia, the prevalence is believed to be ~1:7000 [33].

Other areas appear to have a low prevalence of WD. Park et al. identified WD patients clinically in Scotland and reported a much lower estimated prevalence of 4 patients per million [34]. Low prevalence of ~1:250,000 and 1:38,168 births have been reported in Swedish [35] and Irish [36] cohorts, respectively, although the true prevalence of WD in the UK is not known.

Historically, WD was not considered to have gender preponderance. Lau et al. studied a population of 37 Chinese patients and found no significant gender differences [37]. Emre et al. reported the outcomes in 17 patients who underwent liver transplantation including nine males and eight females [38]. In a large Austrian series of 229 patients, Beinhardt et al. identified 110 male and 119 female patients [39]. In a much larger Polish registry study, Litwin et al. registered 627 patients, 337 men and 290 women, eluding to a significantly different predilection of WD for male individuals [40]. In his pediatric series of 283 Japanese children, Takeshi Saito found a slight difference with 158 male and 125 female patients (44.2%).

Copper accumulation begins after birth and children may present as early as ages 3–5, but more often after the first decade of life. The age of presentation depends on the extent of copper accumulation. It is generally recognized that patients with predominantly hepatic involvement present earlier and are at a higher risk for hepatic decompensation and liver failure; a smaller percentage present with acute liver failure (ALF). Children more often present with hepatic disease [41]. Acute severe liver disease secondary to WD can present with very high bilirubin and normal/low alkaline phosphatase (ALP). A high bilirubin (mg/dL) to alkaline phosphatase (IU/L) ratio (>2.0) and an AST:ALT ratio >2.2 have a high sensitivity and specificity in diagnosing a patient with fulminant liver failure due to WD [42, 43]. Serum uric acid levels may be low. Extrahepatic manifestations of WD may involve the kidneys (renal tubular acidosis and renal calculi), heart (cardiomyopathy and arrhythmias), the bone marrow and red blood cells (hemolytic anemia) and the joints/bones (premature arthritis, arthralgia, chondrocalcinosis). The neurological manifestations of WD include dystonia, dysarthria, cerebellar dysfunction (including dysdiadochokinesis, ataxia, nystagmus, intention tremor, staccato speech, hypotonia), basal ganglia dysfunction, peripheral neuropathy and seizures. The psychiatric and behavioral manifestations of WD include falling behind with school, hallucinations, personality and behavioural changes, deliberate self-harm, depression/mania/bipolar disorder, euphoria, anxiety, apathy, mood changes, suicidal ideation, memory impairment, hypersexuality, paranoia, disinhibition, schizophrenia/psychosis, catatonia, delusions and obsessive compulsive disorder.

In the pediatric series by Saito et al. from Japan, the mean age of presentation was 12 years (range 4–30). Patients with hepatic involvement had higher mortality [44]. Similarly, in his case series of 87 children with predominantly hepatic WD, Walshe described a mean age of presentation of 11 years (range 5–22) [45]. Children who are identified through screening of a family proband are often asymptomatic [41].

In their patient series of adult and pediatric cases, Beinhardt et al. and Litwin et al. reported a mean age of symptomatic presentation of 22.1 and 26.3 years, respectively, with patient age ranging from 6 to 61 years. Unlike children with WD, older patients will more commonly present with neuropsychiatric instead of hepatic symptoms (and therefore present later in life) [40]. Most of these patients are males. Ala and Schilsky first described the notion of later onset WD which appears to be frequently overlooked in the diagnostic algorithm of evaluating a patient with WD. They reported two septuagenarian siblings presenting with WD [46]. Specific molecular studies demonstrated compound heterozygosity for disease specific identical *ATP7B* mutations E1064A and H1069Q in both these patients. These observations were later confirmed by Ferenci et al. and raise the question of the degree of penetrance for these and other *ATP7B* mutations [47]. Environmental and extragenic factors appear to be pivotal determinants of disease phenotype. We suggest that WD must be considered at all ages in patients with hepatic disease, neurological disease, or psychiatric symptoms. While in most cases, the diagnosis can be made by a combination of clinical and biochemical testing, none of the available tests is specific for the diagnosis of Wilson disease. Clinical symptoms may be absent in a large proportion of patients. A diagnostic algorithm based on all available tests was proposed by the Working Party at the Eighth International Meeting on Wilson's disease, Leipzig 2001 [48, 49]. The Leipzig score was developed to guide clinicians as to whether further testing is needed or whether the diagnosis is established. Following this meeting the scoring system was supported by the European Association for the Study of the Liver (EASL) and the EASL Clinical Guidelines. A score of 4 or above is required to establish the diagnosis of Wilson Disease. If after all the testing is complete the score is below 4, then an alternative diagnosis needs to be considered. The Leipzig scoring system has now been validated in both adult and pediatric patients with Wilson Disease.

Some postulate that female patients may have delayed manifestation of neuropsychiatric symptoms, possibly due to the protective effect of estrogens and differences in iron metabolism [40]. However, since a higher number of female patients will present with the hepatic sequelae of WD [40, 41] it is possible that they are identified with the liver disease prior to what might have been a later presentation with neuropsychiatric symptoms. More men were reported to be symptomatic at diagnosis than women [40] and, just like children, adults with hepatic symptoms present at a younger age compared to those presenting with neuropsychiatric symptoms [39].

The treatment of WD is primarily pharmacological while liver transplantation may be considered for patients with decompensated liver disease or acute liver failure. The pharmacological management of WD involves two phases, the initial phase of de-coppering of body tissues and blood using potent chelators and the maintenance phase where accumulation of excess copper is prevented primarily by inhibition of intestinal absorption. The chelators of choice are D-penicillamine, trientine and tetrathiomolybdate (under study), while zinc salts are mainly recommended for the maintenance phase [48, 50]. The primary chelator traditionally used is D-penicillamine. However, many patients may not tolerate the extended adverse effect profile initially, or will develop late complications. Trientine can be used for patients intolerant of D-penicillamine or can be considered for primary therapy for certain patients such as those with neurological manifestations, although paradoxical early worsening has been reported with ~10–25% with both. Tetrathiomolybdate is a novel chelator with promising results in prospective clinical trials, especially for patients with neurological WD [51–53]. For the more severe hepatic disease, zinc and chelators have been used synergistically, but there are no data comparing outcomes [54, 55]. A diet low in copper is also recommended but is not sufficient for therapy alone.

The first liver transplantation for WD took place in 1971 [56]. The modified Wilson index (King's score) that uses laboratory data on patients can be used as a predictive model for liver transplantation for adult and pediatric patients with WD [57]. Transplantation is curative for patients with hepatic WD. However, there is an ongoing debate about its indication in patients with neuropsychiatric disease [58, 59]. The long-term outcomes appear to be excellent and similar for both adults and children. Arnon et al. evaluated 170 children and 400 adults and reported the 1- and 5-year survival rates to be 90.1% and 89%, respectively, in children, and 88.3% and 86%, respectively, in adults. These rates were not found to be significantly different [60]. Smaller case series showed slightly worse survival rates. Weiss et al. reported transplantation outcomes in 19 patients (mean age 29.3 years) with 1- and 5-year survival rates of 78% and 65% respectively. Schilsky et al. examined the outcomes in 55 patients (mean age 17.4 years, range 8–51) and reported a 1-year survival rate of 79% [61]. Over the last few years, the number of liver transplants for WD does not appear to have changed significantly, and these trends are depicted in Fig. 17.1.

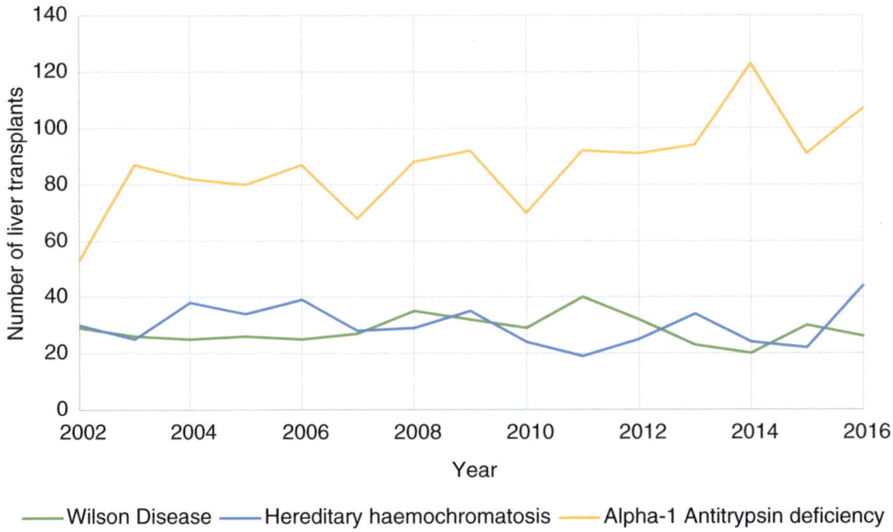

Fig. 17.1 Trends in orthotopic liver transplantation in the United States according to the United Network for Organ Sharing (UNOS) database related to WD, HH, A1AT

17.1.2 Lysosomal Acid Lipase Deficiency (OMIM #278000)

Wolman disease (WoD) and cholesteryl ester storage disorder (CESD) are two disease entities that lie on the spectrum of lysosomal acid lipase deficiency (LALd) which was described more than 55 years ago [62]. Acid lipase deficiency was demonstrated in patient fibroblasts in 1972 and the lipase gene (LIPA) was identified in 1994 [63, 64]. Human lysosomal acid lipase (LAL) was purified in small amounts in 1985 [65]. LAL is involved in the intra-lysosomal hydrolysis of cholesteryl esters (CE) and triglycerides (TG) [66]. WoD is regarded as the infantile form of the disease and patients exhibit none or less than 1–2% of the LAL enzyme activity. CESD describes the same disease in patients who still retain some LAL activity of up to 12% [67–88]. Patients will often present with abdominal distension due to hepatosplenomegaly, malnutrition, dyslipidemia, general gastrointestinal disturbances, elevated liver enzymes and, in severe cases, abnormal liver function tests (LFTs) [67–88]. Patients are often misdiagnosed as suffering from nonalcoholic fatty liver disease (NAFLD), nonalcoholic steatohepatitis (NASH), cryptogenic cirrhosis or Fredrickson type IIa and IIb hyperlipoproteinemia [68, 88, 89].

The prevalence of the disease has been estimated by Reiner et al. to be between 1:40,000–300,000 depending on geographical and ethnic background [66]. More than 100 mutations have been identified to date, the commonest being the exon 8 splice junction mutation (c.894G>A); E8SJM [70, 82, 90–97]. The carrier frequency of the E8SJM allele in a cohort of 1152 in Germany was found to be 1 in 200 with a homozygote frequency of 25 per million [98]. Scott et al. evaluated the allele frequency by analysing 8000 multi-ethnic blood samples in New York and Dallas and reported the c.894G>A allele frequency for the Caucasian, Hispanic, Ashkenazi Jewish and Asian populations to be 1 in 298 (prevalence ~0.8 in 100,000), 1 in 296 (prevalence ~0.8 in 100,000), 1 in 500 (prevalence ~0.3 in 100,000) and 1 in 1000 (prevalence ~0.1 in 100,000), respectively [99]. The overall, prevalence was estimated to be approximately 1 in 130,000 (95% CI: ~1 in 90,000–1 in 170,000) [99]. Combination of the data with the German cohort estimated a much higher carrier frequency of 1 in 242; prevalence of ~1.2 WoD was found to be 1 in 528,000; incidence was 1 in 704,000 births [100]. Valles-Ayoub et al. studied 162 samples for the LIPA Exon 4 p.G87V (ggc>gtc, alternative numbering p.G66V) mutation in an Iranian and Iraqi-Jewish community in the Los Angeles area. The mutation incidence was reported to be 1 in 4200 in this cohort [101]. Overall, there are very limited data for the epidemiology of this ultra-rare liver disease.

Several treatment modalities have been used for the management of LALd, including statins, ezetimibe, cholestyramine, low-fat diets, liver transplantation and stem-cell transplantation. More recently, enzyme replacement therapy with sebelipase alfa has been used with good results [102–105]. Eight clinical trials have explored the efficacy of sebelipase alfa in humans and these are listed in Table 17.1 [102–104, 106–108]. The long-term outcomes from liver transplantation or medical therapy have not been fully established [109].

The largest of these clinical trials is the phase 3 ARISE study by Burton et al. which examined the effectiveness of sebelipase alfa in a cohort of 66 adults and children for 36 weeks. Statistically significant improvements in most endpoints were observed including normalization of alanine and aspartate aminotransferase

Table 17.1 Summary of clinical trials using enzyme replacement therapy related to LALd

Name of trial	Phase	Author	Type of patients	n	Status
LAL-CL01 NCT01307098	I–II	Balwani et al. [102]	Adults	9	Completed
LAL-CL04 NCT01488097 (extension of LAL-CL01)	II	Valayannopoulos et al. [104]	Adults	8	Ongoing
LAL-CL03 NCT01371825 **VITAL**	II–III	Jones et al. [160]	Infants	9	Ongoing
LAL-CL02 NCT01757184 **ARISE**	III	Burton et al. [103]	Children and adults	66	Ongoing
LAL-CL06 NCT02112994	II	Alexion Pharma [161]	Children (>8 months) and adults	30	Ongoing
LAL-CL08 NCT02193867	II	Friedman et al. [162]	Infants <8 months	10	Ongoing
LAL-1-NH01 NCT01358370	Observational	Jones et al. [106]	Children and adults	35	Completed
LAL-2-NH01 NCT01528917	Observational	Burton et al. [107]	Children and adults	49	Completed

levels, improvement of low and high density lipoproteins, reduction in hepatic steatosis and reduction in the spleen volume [103]. Though long-term data are not yet available, sebelipase alfa appears to be safe and well tolerated for the management of LALd.

17.1.3 A1-Antitrypsin Deficiency (OMIM #107400)

This condition was first described by Laurell et al. in 1963 in relation to emphysematous pulmonary changes [110] while its association with liver disease was defined in 1969 [111]. A1-antitrypsin belongs in the superfamily of serine protease inhibitors (SERPINs) and physiologically it inhibits the proteolytic degradation of neutrophil elastin. Therefore, deficiency of α1-antitrypsin (A1AD) leads to an imbalance in the levels of elastin in various tissues, causing structural abnormalities in the organs involved, mainly the lungs and liver. Whereas in the lungs the damage is induced by the uncontrolled destruction of elastin due to the loss of function of α1-antitrypsin, the damage observed in the liver is via the mechanism of toxic accumulation of an aggregated and polymerized form of α1-antitrypsin in the hepatocytes. The extent of tissue damage is determined by the amounts expressed of α1-antitrypsin and the extent of proteosomal degradation [112]. For these reasons the disease has a variable genotype to phenotype expression. Smoking and occupational exposure have been identified as risk factors which can accelerate the development of lung disease [113, 114]. Thus, the interplay between endogenous and exogenous factors can determine the outcome in A1AD [115].

The SERPINA1 gene which encodes for the 52 kDa α1-antitrypsin glycoprotein has been located on chromosome 14 (q31–32.3) [116]. The disease is inherited in an autosomal recessive condition with co-dominant expression (each allele contributes to 50% of the circulating enzyme). While there are over 100 identified alleles which can predispose to A1AD, three alleles, M, S and Z, are most frequently encountered and can determine the phenotypic outcome of the disease [117]. These alleles are given letters based on older methods for protein separation by isoelectric focusing protein electrophoresis. PiMM phenotype is normal while PiZZ is associated with the highest risk of developing disease, including severe liver injury and hepatocellular carcinoma [118–120]. The PiZZ is believed to be found in 98% of patients with A1AD [121]. PiSS has not been associated with lung disease. Currently, diagnostic genotyping has significantly influenced how we differentiate between these types and can be used to identify specific alleles by utilizing polymerase chain reaction and molecular gene sequencing.

The prevalence of A1AD has been estimated using population-based screening studies as well as indirect epidemiological genetic studies using the Hardy-Weinberg Equilibrium principle. While it was previously assumed that A1AD was a disease of white Caucasians, a plethora of non-Caucasian countries have reported several cases. de Serres et al. used data from 69 countries in an attempt to estimate the prevalence of five phenotypic types of A1AD. The world prevalence of each phenotype was found to be PiMS (2.8%), PiMZ (0.6%), PiSS (0.6%), PiSZ (0.2%) and

PiZZ (0.004%) [122]. While PiS and PiZ are moderately-highly encountered in European countries (or those colonized by Europeans), both alleles are rare in Asians and aboriginals. The PiS allele was found to be high in Sub-Saharan countries and Southern Europe. The highest prevalence of the PiZ allele was reported in Northern European countries. The same group reviewed the data from an additional 25 countries 2 years later. The highest prevalence of PiZZ and PiSS phenotypes was reported in an area covering Brazil, Ecuador and Peru. The disease was found to be absent in Amerindians [123]. More data by Blanco et al. from 224 cohorts (65 countries) confirm that most homozygous PiZZ patients are European or from European descent living in North America. The same authors identify that the Pi*Z mutation must have occurred in Sweden approximately 2000 years ago [121].

Screening studies are also useful in elucidating the epidemiology of a rare disease. A large prospective Swedish study screened 200,000 newborns for A1AD and identified 1 PiS (prevalence 1:200,000), 122 PiZ (prevalence 1:1639), and 48 PiSZ (prevalence 1:4166) infants. The total prevalence was ~1:1170 [124]. O'Brien et al. screened 107,038 newborns in the US and identified 21 patients (prevalence 1:5097) [125]. Silverman et al. screened 20,000 blood samples in the US and found 7 PiZ patients (prevalence 1:2857) [126]. Spence et al. screened 11,081 specimens from newborns and found 3 PiS patients estimating an incidence for the disease of 1:2019 in Caucasians and 1:3694 in the general population. Stoller et al. combined data from the largest US screening studies into a cohort of 138,119 patients and estimated a PiZZ prevalence in the US of 1:4455 [127]. In addition Stoller et al. looked at the screening results from 23 selected smaller studies from several European countries, the USA, Africa, Saudi Arabia and Japan. Just as in the aforementioned studies by de Serres et al., the heterogeneity in geographical distribution and dispersity of allele frequency were once again highlighted. PiZ and PiS appears to be more prevalent in Western and Southwestern European countries, respectively. These striking differences between the distributions of PIS and PIZ have also been demonstrated in a study of 21 European countries (75,390 individuals) by Blanco et al. [128]. Currently, the exercise of mass screening in newborns and other individuals is generally discouraged unless performed in a high-risk area. A more targeted screening approached is preferred following risk stratification [121].

Gender predilection in A1AD has not been widely reported. A large registry study of 929 patients identified a male preponderance for both PiZZ (male 56%, female 45%) and PiSZ (male 55%; female 45%) phenotypes [129]. The AlphaNet cohort includes 646 patients with COPD on augmentation therapy. Pardinas-Gutierrez et al. reported equal numbers of male and female patients in this AlphaNet cohort [130].

A1AD usually involves the lungs and, less commonly, extrapulmonary sites such as the liver and skin. Reports of A1AD manifesting as vascultis, inflammatory bowel disease, and glomerulonephritis can also be found in the literature even though these are far less common. Emphysema due to A1AD commonly represents symptoms of classic chronic obstructive pulmonary diseases (COPD) including dyspnea, purulent phlegm, wheezing and recurrent chest infections. In contrast to COPD secondary to smoking, A1AD lung disease often occurs at a younger age.

Patients may also present with secondary pneumothorax and bronchiectasis. Hepatic manifestations are commonly seen in patients with mutations in the M and Z alleles. In neonatal cases, patients not uncommonly present with neonatal hepatitis, jaundice and cirrhosis. Adult patients may show manifestation of chronic hepatitis, cirrhosis and hepatocellular carcinoma (more common in male patients). The most common dermatological presentation is necrotizing panniculitis.

The treatment of A1AD involves supportive care and pharmacological treatment. Smoking cessation is advised and so is optimization of pulmonary therapy for emphysema. Perhaps the most effective treatment, but mainly for those with lung disease, is intravenous augmentation therapy with pooled human alpha-1 antitrypsin. Weekly infusions are required for carefully-selected patients with a particular focus on the effectiveness of therapy on lung function. Most studies describing augmentation therapy do not focus on the impact on hepatic disease, and this remains largely unexplored and experimental [131, 132]. For patients with hepatic disease, liver transplantation is a curative option. Approximately 1% of all adult liver transplants were for A1AD and the number of liver transplants appears to be decreasing for the pediatric population [133]. Overall, the number of liver transplants for A1AD is increasing (Fig. 17.1).

Since protein handling and proteosomal degradation are involved in the pathogenesis and the phenotypic severity of the disease, the role of molecular chaperones has been considered for the management of hepatic A1AD in recent years. One such chaperone is carbamazepine which is of particular interest and is currently being investigated in a phase 2 multicenter trial [134]. Other future therapies are aimed at reducing hepatic protein production and accumulation, either by anti-sense or microRNA technologies. The role of these modalities remains to be determined.

17.1.4 HFE-Related Hereditary Hemochromatosis (OMIM #235200)

Hereditary hemochromatosis (HH) is the commonest inherited genetic disease in Europe, especially in populations from Northern European descent [135]. The condition is autosomal recessive and is caused by mutations on the HFE gene on the short arm of chromosome 6. The gene was identified approximately 20 years ago but the close association of HFE to the locus of HLA-A3 on chromosome 6 was discovered 40 years ago [136, 137]. The commonest mutation is a cysteine-for-tyrosine substitution at amino acid position 282 (C282Y). This is regarded as the major HFE-associated polymorphism. The minor HFE-associated polymorphism involves a substitution of aspartate for histidine at amino acid position 63 (H63D). Rarer HFE polymorphisms such as Ser65Cys (S65C) have also been reported [138]. HFE mutations lead to excessive iron absorption from the gut and unregulated intracellular iron accumulation, especially in hepatocytes. The clinical presentation can be described by the triad of liver disease, diabetes mellitus, and skin pigmentation. This clinical trial is a feature of late disease. Not uncommonly, patients may present with arthralgia, arthritis, hypogonadism, hypopituitarism, dilated cardiomyopathy and hepatocellular carcinoma. Iron-overload states can also predispose individuals to infections including *Listeria monocytogenes*, *Yersinia enterocolitica* and *Vibrio vulnificus* [139].

Population-based studies provide an insight into the frequency of HFE mutations in the general population. In a large study in the United States Steinberg et al. genotyped 5171 specimens from the third National Health and Nutrition Examination Survey (NHANES III) DNA bank [140]. Homozygosity for C282Y/C282Y and H63D/H63D was found to occur in 0.26% and 1.89%, respectively, in the U.S. population. C282Y/H63D heterozygosity was observed in 1.97% of individuals. The homozygous C282Y/C282Y mutation frequency was considerably higher in non-Hispanic whites (0.30%), compared to non-Hispanic blacks (0.06%) and Mexican-Americans (0.03%) [140]. Similarly, the homozygous H63D/H63D mutation was higher in non-Hispanic whites (2.15%), compared to non-Hispanic blacks (0.32%) and Mexican-Americans (1.08%) [140]. Heterozygosity for C282Y/H63D was also higher in non-Hispanic whites (2.35%), compared to non-Hispanic blacks (0.06%) and Mexican-Americans (0.19%) [140]. In a much larger study in U.S. primary care, Adams et al. analyzed the genotypes and iron profiles of 99,711 individuals. As previously reported, the authors found much higher carrier frequencies for non-Hispanic whites. Specifically, homozygosity for C282Y/C282Y was reported in 0.44% of whites, compared to 0.11% in Native Americans, 0.027% in Mexican-Americans, 0.014 in blacks, 0.012% in Pacific islanders and 0.000039% in patients of Asian origin. Homozygosity for H63D/H63D was reported in 2.40% of whites, compared to 1.3% of Native Americans, 1.1% of Mexican-Americans, 0.089% of blacks, 0.20% of Pacific islanders and 0.20% of patients of Asian origin [141]. In a meta-analysis of 36 studies focused on European and Northern American countries, the genotypes of 127,613 individuals were analyzed. The population carrier allelic frequency of Cys282Tyr was found to be 6.2% with an estimated C282Y/C282Y homozygosity of 0.38% (1:260) [138]. Prevalence appears to be lower in the countries of Southern Europe. Similarly, the carrier allelic frequency for His63Asp was on average much higher (14%) with less geographic variation [138]. The Ser65Cys polymorphism is found in approximately 0.5% of the population. Asberg et al. screened 65,238 Norwegian blood samples and found the prevalence of the C282Y/C282Y to be at least 0.68% [142].

Several studies looked at the prevalence of HFE mutations in patients with recognised HH. A meta-analysis included 2802 patients with phenotypic HH from 32 studies and found that 80.6% were C282Y/C282Y homozygous and 5.3% compound heterozygous C282Y/H63D [138]. The studies were primarily focused on patients with European ancestry. Although this meta-analysis does not report the frequency of H63D homozygosity, this was found to be 0–1.5% by other authors [136, 143–147]. The remaining patients are believed to be heterozygotes for C282Y, H63D or S65C or to have other non-HFE related iron overload due to other hereditary pathology including juvenile hemochromatosis, Transferrin receptor 2 disorder, ferroportin disease, hereditary hyperferritinemia-cataract syndrome, H-ferritin disorder and aceruloplasminemia [139].

The genotype-to-phenotype relationship of HH is challenging to elucidate due to variable disease penetrance as well as the heterogeneous research methodology used in different studies. Furthermore, the definition used for confirmed diagnosis of HH appears to vary between studies. A large population study of 41,000 individuals in the U.S. by Beutler et al. identified 152 patients with homozygous C282Y/C282Y genotype, out of which only 1 patient had clinically diagnosable HH (penetrance 0.67%) [148]. In a similar European study of 3011 individuals, Olynyk et al. identified 16 homozygous C282Y/C282Y patients and described clinical disease in half of them [149]. In a French study of 352 patients, penetrance was reported to be 15.8% [150]. In a recent meta-analysis of 19 studies, the penetrance of C282Y/C282Y homozygous disease was 13.5% [138]. Penetrance appears to be higher for C282Y/C282Y homozygous patients identified through family screening compared to population studies [138]. Patients who are C282Y/H63D compound heterozygotes appear to have an estimated disease penetrance of 0.5–1.5% [144, 151] and may only develop clinic disease when there is an additional compound hepatic insult [151].

Large studies have shown that homozygosity for C282Y appears to be more common in female patients [141, 152]. However, a smaller study by Steinberg et al. reported a higher number of homozygous male patients compared to females (5 vs. 3 patients) [140]. Men display more frequent biochemical and symptomatic HH compared to females, possibly due to the physiological iron loss during menstruation, the effect of estrogen and the gender-specific HFH genetic modifiers [135]. In their Australian cohort of 31,192 patients with northern European ancestry, Allen et al. found 29.2% of patients with phenotypic HH (males 28% vs. females 1.2%) [152]. Aguilar-Martinez et al. also reported higher prevalence and earlier diagnosis in men with C282Y/C282Y homozygosity (19% vs. 13%).

The treatment of HH depends on symptoms and status of iron overload. Dietary restrictions are not often required and patients with HH should be advised not to take any supplementary iron or extra vitamin C. Excessive consumption of agents which have been shown to reduce iron absorption such as oxalates, tannates, oxalates, calcium and phosphate is not required in patients who are being treated with therapeutic phlebotomy. The consumption of alcohol is discouraged.

Patients without iron overload or organ involvement do not require treatment and systematic monitoring is advised. Patients with iron overload or organ involvement will require treatment. Therapeutic phlebotomy remains the simplest and most economical method of removing excess iron. Ferritin levels can be used to dictate the frequency of phlebotomy as discussed in published guidance [138, 153]. Erythrocytapheresis has been described as a treatment for patients with symptomatic HH and involves the removal of red blood cells (RBC) from patients' blood (apheresis) and the return of the erythropenic plasma to the body. Probably the biggest advantage of erythrocytapheresis over therapeutic phebotomy is the fact that much larger amounts of RBC can be removed per single procedure. A phase 3 trial compared phlebotomy vs. erythrocytapheresis in 38 C282Y/C282Y homozygous patients. The authors reported significantly lower mean number of procedures required in the erythrocytapheresis group and the treatments were found to be equally cost-effective [154]. However, the treatment remains expensive and the technique largely unavailable.

Patients who are intolerant or have contraindications to phlebotomy (e.g., significant anemia) or in cases where phlebotomy is not possible (e.g., poor intravenous access) should be considered for iron chelation therapy. Historically, deferoxamine and deferiprone had been used with good clinical and biochemical responses; however, therapy remains expensive and potentially toxic [155, 156]. Deferasirox is another chelator which has been evaluated in a Phase 1/2 trial. Despite the encouraging initial results, the study had to be terminated due to poor recruitment [157]. A subsequent phase 2 study with 10 patients receiving deferasirox demonstrated good efficacy and acceptable adverse effect profile [158]. More studies on more patients are required to appreciate the merits and long-term outcomes of chelation therapy with deferasirox.

Liver transplantation is an option for the treatment of HH and in the more recent era has comparable 1-, 3- and 5-year survival rates compared to other indications for liver transplantation [159]. Figure 17.1 shows the transplantation trends in the U.S. which remain unchanged over several years. There also may be occasional patients that require dual organ transplant, heart and liver, if they have severe cardiomyopathy and liver disease. These results could, however, be biased as patients with HH and cirrhosis have a significantly higher risk of hepatocellular carcinoma, and may undergo transplant on the basis of having tumor and not for decompensated liver failure due to HH per se. Therefore, transplantation outcomes should not only be analyzed in the context of HH as the indication for transplantation, but also from the angle of development of hepatocellular carcinoma.

In conclusion, we have described four mainly genetically determined rare metabolic liver diseases and the growing awareness, knowledge and expertise in epidemiology about these. There are clear variations in genotype and phenotype, better diagnosis through improved molecular biology techniques, improving management repertoire through international multicenter clinical trials and liver transplantation which may be curative and lifesaving in some patients.

Summary Table of Landmark Literature

Wilson disease		
Study title and authors	Study design	Summary results
Progressive lenticular degeneration: a familial nervous disease associated with cirrhosis of the liver. Samuel Alexander Kinnier Wilson, *Brain 1912: 34; 295–509*	Case series	13 patients with progressive lenticular degeneration with associated liver cirrhosis
La dégénérescence hépato-lenticulaire (Maladie de Wilson—Pseudo-sclérose). Hall HC, *Masson, Paris, 1921* Scheinberg IH, Gitlin D. Deficiency of ceruloplasmin in patients with hepatolenticular degeneration (Wilson's disease). *Science 1952, 116:484–5* Biochemical abnormalities in Wilson's disease. Bearn AG and Kunkel HG, *J Clin Invest, 1952, 31:616*	Case Control study	Pattern of inheritance described as autosomal recessive Caeruloplasmin deficiency as a phenotypic marker that can be used for disease screening

(continued)

Wilson disease		
Study title and authors	Study design	Summary results
Assignment of the gene for Wilson disease to chromosome 13: linkage to the esterase D locus. Frydman M et al., Proc Natl Acad Sci U S A. 1985;82(6):1819–21	Linkage analysis	Localization of disease locus to chromosome 13
Isolation of a candidate gene for Menkes disease and evidence that it encodes a copper-transporting ATPase. Vulpe C et al., *Nat Genet. 1993;3(1):7–13* Isolation of a candidate gene for Menkes disease that encodes a potential heavy metal binding protein. Chelly J et al., *Nat Genet. 1993;3(1):14–9*	Gene isolation and sequencing	The gene for Menkes disease encodes a copper-transporting P-type ATPase
The Wilson disease gene is a putative copper transporting P-type ATPase similar to the Menkes gene. Bull PC et al., *Nat Genet. 1993;5(4):327–37*	Gene isolation and sequencing	The gene for Wilson disease encodes a copper-transporting P-type ATPase
Isolation of a partial candidate gene for Menkes disease by positional cloning. Mercer JF et al., *Nat Genet. 1993;3(1):20–5* Mapping, cloning and genetic characterization of the region containing the Wilson disease gene. Petrukhin K et al., *Nat Genet. 1993;5(4):338–43* The Wilson disease gene is a copper transporting ATPase with homology to the Menkes disease gene. Tanzi RE et al., *Nat Genet. 1993;5(4):344–50*	Gene isolation, sequencing, linkage disequilibrium and haplotype analysis	ATP7B gene is identified as the gene for Wilson disease. Specific mutations begin to be recognised
Isolation and characterization of a human liver cDNA as a candidate gene for Wilson disease. Yamaguchi Y et al., *Biochem Biophys Res Commun* 1993;197:271–7 Characterization of the Wilson disease gene encoding a P-type copper transporting ATPase: genomic organization, alternative splicing, and structure/function predictions. Petrukhin K et al., *Hum Mol Genet. 1994;3(9):1647–56*	Screening of cDNA clones, genomic organization, alternative splicing	Identification of disease-specific mutations and ATP7B polymorphisms and prediction of structure/function features of WD protein

Note: These studies were collectively limited by the small number of patients included due to the rarity of the condition

A1-Antitrypsin deficiency (A1AD)		
Study title and authors	Study design/method	Summary results
The electrophoretic alpha-1-globulin pattern of serum in alpha-1-antitrypsin deficiency. Laurell C-B et al., *Scand J Clin Lab Invest 1963, 15:132–140*	Serum protein electrophoresis	Absence of the α1-globulin peak in many patients with COPD noticed

A1-Antitrypsin deficiency (A1AD)		
Study title and authors	Study design/ method	Summary results
Cirrhosis associated with alpha-1-antitrypsin deficiency: a previously unrecognized inherited disorder. Sharp HL et al., *J Lab Clin Med 1969, 73:934–939*	Observational study	A1AD is associated with liver disease and cirrhosis
Liver disease in alpha1-antitrypsin deficiency detected by screening of 200,000 infants. Tomas Sveger, *N Engl J Med 1976; 294:1316–1321*	Prospective study	Liver disease has been associated with the PiZ and PiSZ phenotypes. Approximately 8% of patients developed clinically significant liver disease
α1-Antitrypsin deficiency in 26-year-old subjects. Piitulainen E et al., *Chest* 2005, 128:2076–2081	Case-control study	Interplay of exogenous and endogenous factors will determine phenotype and outcomes
Performance of enhanced liver fibrosis plasma markers in asymptomatic individuals with ZZ a1-antitrypsin deficiency. Janciauskiene S et al., *Eur J Gastroenterol Hepatol 2011, 23:716–720*	Case-control study	The enhanced liver fibrosis plasma markers are useful in identifying PiZZ young adults who are at risk of developing significant liver disease
Characteristics of hepatocellular carcinoma in a murine model of alpha-1-antitrypsin deficiency. Marcus NY et al., *Hepatol Res. 2010, 40:641–653* Analyses of hepatocellular proliferation in a mouse model of alpha-1-antitrypsin deficiency. Rudnick DA et al., *Hepatology. 2004, 39:1048–1055*	Animal studies	Association of the homozygous PiZZ phenotype with HCC

Note: These studies were collectively limited by the small number of patients included due to the rarity of the condition

Abbreviations: *COPD* chronic obstructive pulmonary disease, *ELF* enhanced liver fibrosis, *HCC* hepatocellular carcinoma

Hereditary haemochromatosis		
Study title and authors	Study design/method	Summary results
Association of HLA-A3 and HLA-B14 antigens with idiopathic haemochromatosis. Simon M et al., *Gut 1976, 17:332–334*	Case series with determination of histocompatibility antigens	Idiopathic haemochromatosis is a genetic condition and the responsible gene may be localized to the region of the histocompatibility complex
A novel MHC class I-like gene is mutated in patients with hereditary haemo*chromatosis. Feder JN* et al. *Nat Genet 1996;13:399–408*	Disequilibrium and full haplotype analysis	Identification of gene for most common form of hereditary hemochromatosis. Close association of HLA-H (renamed later as HFE) to the locus of HLA-A3 on chromosome 6 and identification of pathogenic mutations of this gene and corresponding change in HFE protein that potentially leads to disease

(continued)

Hereditary haemochromatosis		
Study title and authors	Study design/method	Summary results
Hemochromatosis and iron-overload screening in a racially diverse population. Adams PC et al., N Engl J Med 2005;352:1769–1778 Iron-overload-related disease in HFE hereditary hemochromatosis. Allen KJ et al., N Engl J Med 2008, 358:221–230 Screening for hemochromatosis: high prevalence and low morbidity in an unselected population of 65,238 persons. Asberg A et al., Scand J Gastroenterol 2001, 36:1108–1115 Penetrance of 845G–>A (C282Y) HFE hereditary haemochromatosis mutation in the USA. Beutler E et al., *Lancet 2002, 359:211–218*	Population studies with a pooled cohort of 235,663 people	The prevalence of C282Y homozygosity in the general population is 1:146–333
European association for the study of the liver. EASL clinical practice guidelines for HFE hemochromatosis. *Journal of Hepatology 2010, 53:3–22*	Meta-analysis of 2802 patients with phenotypic HH from 32 studies	80.6% of patients are C282Y/C282Y homozygotes and 5.3% compound heterozygotes (C282Y/H63D)

Abbreviations: *HH* hereditary haemochromatosis

Lysosomal acid lipase deficiency		
Study title and authors	Study design/method	Summary results/milestone
Primary familial xanthomatosis with involvement and calcification of the adrenals. Report of two more cases in siblings of a previously described infant. Wolman, M. et al., *Pediatrics, 1961. 28: p. 742–57*	Observational study	Moshe Wolman describes the first case series of three siblings with Wolman disease
Lipid accumulation and acid lipase deficiency in fibroblasts from a family with Wolman's disease, and their apparent correction in vitro. Kyriakides EC et al., *J Lab Clin Med, 1972. 80(6): p. 810–6*	Case control study measuring acid lipase activity of cultured fibroblasts	Acid lipase deficiency is demonstrated in fibroblasts
Genomic organization of the human lysosomal acid lipase gene (LIPA). Aslanidis, C et al., *Genomics, 1994. 20(2): p. 329–31*	Gene isolation, sequencing and linkage	The lipase gene(LIPA) is assigned to locus 10q23.2q23.3

Lysosomal acid lipase deficiency		
Study title and authors	Study design/method	Summary results/milestone
Lysosomal acid lipase/cholesteryl ester hydrolase. Purification and properties of the form secreted by fibroblasts in microcarrier culture. Sando GM et al. *J Biol Chem, 1985. 260(28): p. 15186–93*	Enzyme purification, structural analysis and ascertainment of catalytic properties of the human enzyme	Human LAL is purified in small amounts
Wolman disease/cholesteryl ester storage disease: efficacy of plant-produced human lysosomal acid lipase in mice. Du H et al., J Lipid Res, 2008. 49(8): p. 1646–57	Animal study	Enzyme replacement therapy effective in the murine model
Clinical effect and safety profile of recombinant human lysosomal acid lipase in patients with cholesteryl ester storage disease. Balwani M et al., *Hepatology, 2013. 58(3): p. 950–7* Sebelipase alfa over 52 weeks reduces serum transaminases, liver volume and improves serum lipids in patients with lysosomal acid lipase deficiency. Valayannopoulos V et al., *J Hepatol, 2014. 61(5): p. 1135–42*	Phase I–II interventional trial	Enzyme replacement therapy is tried successfully on humans
A phase 3 trial of sebelipase alfa in lysosomal acid lipase deficiency. Burton BK et al., *N Engl J Med, 2015. 373(11): p. 1010–20*	Phase III interventional trial	Enzyme replacement therapy has been shown to successfully normalise ALT and AST levels, improve LDL and HDL, reduce hepatic steatosis and reduce spleen volume

Abbreviations: *ALT* alanine aminotransferase, *AST* aspartate aminotransferase, *LDL* low-density lipoprotein, *HDL* high-density lipoprotein

References

1. Kim WR, Brown RS Jr, Terrault NA, El-Serag H. Burden of liver disease in the United States: summary of a workshop. Hepatology. 2002;36(1):227–42.
2. Directorate-General ECHCP. Useful information on rare diseases from an EU perspective. 2004. http://ec.europa.eu/health/ph_information/documents/ev20040705_rd05_en.pdf.
3. National Institutes of Health. National Institutes of Health website. Office of Rare Disease Research. http://rarediseases.info.nih.gov/AboutUs.aspx. Accessed 12 Dec 2015.
4. website RDU. Rare disease UK website. http://www.raredisease.org.uk. Accessed 12 Dec 2015.
5. Lowdown TL. American Liver Foundation. The Liver Lowdown—liver disease: the big picture. 2013. http://www.liverfoundation.org/education/liverlowdown/ll1013/bigpicture. Accessed 21 Mar 2017.
6. EASL. HEPAMAP. A roadmap for hepatology research in Europe: an overview for policy makers. 2013. http://www.easl.eu/medias/EASLimg/News/3f9dd90221ef292_file.pdf.

7. Robertson WM. Wilson's disease. Arch Neurol. 2000;57(2):276–7.
8. Compston A. Progressive lenticular degeneration: a familial nervous disease associated with cirrhosis of the liver, by S. A. Kinnier Wilson, (From the National Hospital, and the Laboratory of the National Hospital, Queen Square, London) Brain 1912: 34; 295–509. Brain. 2009;132(Pt 8):1997–2001.
9. Bearn AG, Kunkel HG. Abnormalities of copper metabolism in Wilson's disease and their relationship to the aminoaciduria. J Clin Invest. 1954;33(3):400–9.
10. Cumings JN. The copper and iron content of brain and liver in the normal and in hepato-lenticular degeneration. Brain. 1948;71(Pt 4):410–5.
11. Frydman M, Bonne-Tamir B, Farrer LA, et al. Assignment of the gene for Wilson disease to chromosome 13: linkage to the esterase D locus. Proc Natl Acad Sci U S A. 1985;82(6):1819–21.
12. Vulpe C, Levinson B, Whitney S, Packman S, Gitschier J. Isolation of a candidate gene for Menkes disease and evidence that it encodes a copper-transporting ATPase. Nat Genet. 1993;3(1):7–13.
13. Chelly J, Tumer Z, Tonnesen T, et al. Isolation of a candidate gene for Menkes disease that encodes a potential heavy metal binding protein. Nat Genet. 1993;3(1):14–9.
14. Bull PC, Thomas GR, Rommens JM, Forbes JR, Cox DW. The Wilson disease gene is a putative copper transporting P-type ATPase similar to the Menkes gene. Nat Genet. 1993;5(4):327–37.
15. Mercer JF, Livingston J, Hall B, et al. Isolation of a partial candidate gene for Menkes disease by positional cloning. Nat Genet. 1993;3(1):20–5.
16. Petrukhin K, Fischer SG, Pirastu M, et al. Mapping, cloning and genetic characterization of the region containing the Wilson disease gene. Nat Genet. 1993;5(4):338–43.
17. Tanzi RE, Petrukhin K, Chernov I, et al. The Wilson disease gene is a copper transporting ATPase with homology to the Menkes disease gene. Nat Genet. 1993;5(4):344–50.
18. Yamaguchi Y, Heiny ME, Gitlin JD. Isolation and characterization of a human liver cDNA as a candidate gene for Wilson disease. Biochem Biophys Res Commun. 1993;197(1):271–7.
19. Kenney SM, Cox DW. Sequence variation database for the Wilson disease copper transporter, ATP7B. Hum Mutat. 2007;28(12):1171–7.
20. Petrukhin K, Lutsenko S, Chernov I, Ross BM, Kaplan JH, Gilliam TC. Characterization of the Wilson disease gene encoding a P-type copper transporting ATPase: genomic organization, alternative splicing, and structure/function predictions. Hum Mol Genet. 1994;3(9):1647–56.
21. Liu Y, Zhou H, Guo H, Bai Y. Genetic and clinical analysis in a cohort of patients with Wilson's disease in southwestern China. Arch Med Res. 2015;46(2):164–9.
22. Park HD, Ki CS, Lee SY, Kim JW. Carrier frequency of the R778L, A874V, and N1270S mutations in the ATP7B gene in a Korean population. Clin Genet. 2009;75(4):405–7.
23. Ala A, Walker AP, Ashkan K, Dooley JS, Schilsky ML. Wilson's disease. Lancet. 2007;369(9559):397–408.
24. Gomes A, Dedoussis GV. Geographic distribution of ATP7B mutations in Wilson disease. Ann Hum Biol. 2016;43(1):1–8.
25. Scheinberg IH, Sternlieb I. Wilson's disease. In: Smith Jr LH, editor. Major problems in internal medicine. Philadelphia, PA: WB Saunders; 1984.
26. Kim GH, Yang JY, Park JY, Lee JJ, Kim JH, Yoo HW. Estimation of Wilson's disease incidence and carrier frequency in the Korean population by screening ATP7B major mutations in newborn filter papers using the SYBR green intercalator method based on the amplification refractory mutation system. Genet Test. 2008;12(3):395–9.
27. Reilly M, Daly L, Hutchinson M. An epidemiological study of Wilson's disease in the Republic of Ireland. J Neurol Neurosurg Psychiatry. 1993;56(3):298–300.
28. Coffey AJ, Durkie M, Hague S, et al. A genetic study of Wilson's disease in the United Kingdom. Brain. 2013;136(Pt 5):1476–87.
29. Olivarez L, Caggana M, Pass KA, Ferguson P, Brewer GJ. Estimate of the frequency of Wilson's disease in the US Caucasian population: a mutation analysis approach. Ann Hum Genet. 2001;65(Pt 5):459–63.

30. Dedoussis GV, Genschel J, Sialvera TE, et al. Wilson disease: high prevalence in a mountainous area of Crete. Ann Hum Genet. 2005;69(Pt 3):268–74.
31. Ohura T, Abukawa D, Shiraishi H, et al. Pilot study of screening for Wilson disease using dried blood spots obtained from children seen at outpatient clinics. J Inherit Metab Dis. 1999;22(1):74–80.
32. Mak CM, Lam CW, Tam S, et al. Mutational analysis of 65 Wilson disease patients in Hong Kong Chinese: identification of 17 novel mutations and its genetic heterogeneity. J Hum Genet. 2008;53(1):55–63.
33. Loudianos G, Dessi V, Lovicu M, et al. Molecular characterization of Wilson disease in the Sardinian population—evidence of a founder effect. Hum Mutat. 1999;14(4):294–303.
34. Park RH, McCabe P, Fell GS, Russell RI. Wilson's disease in Scotland. Gut. 1991;32(12):1541–5.
35. Olsson C, Waldenstrom E, Westermark K, Landegre U, Syvanen AC. Determination of the frequencies of ten allelic variants of the Wilson disease gene (ATP7B), in pooled DNA samples. Eur J Hum Genet. 2000;8(12):933–8.
36. O'Brien M, Reilly M, Sweeney B, Walsh C, Hutchinson M. Epidemiology of Wilson's disease in Ireland. Mov Disord. 2014;29(12):1567–8.
37. Lau JY, Lai CL, Wu PC, Pan HY, Lin HJ, Todd D. Wilson's disease: 35 years' experience. Q J Med. 1990;75(278):597–605.
38. Emre S, Atillasoy EO, Ozdemir S, et al. Orthotopic liver transplantation for Wilson's disease: a single-center experience. Transplantation. 2001;72(7):1232–6.
39. Beinhardt S, Leiss W, Stattermayer AF, et al. Long-term outcomes of patients with Wilson disease in a large Austrian cohort. Clin Gastroenterol Hepatol. 2014;12(4):683–9.
40. Litwin T, Gromadzka G, Czlonkowska A. Gender differences in Wilson's disease. J Neurol Sci. 2012;312(1–2):31–5.
41. Schilsky ML. Wilson disease: Clinical manifestations, diagnosis, and natural history: UpToDate; 2015.
42. Korman JD, Volenberg I, Balko J, et al. Screening for Wilson disease in acute liver failure: a comparison of currently available diagnostic tests. Hepatology. 2008;48(4):1167–74.
43. Polson J, Lee WM. American Association for the Study of Liver D. AASLD position paper: the management of acute liver failure. Hepatology. 2005;41(5):1179–97.
44. Saito T. Presenting symptoms and natural history of Wilson disease. Eur J Pediatr. 1987;146(3):261–5.
45. Walshe JM. Wilson's disease presenting with features of hepatic dysfunction: a clinical analysis of eighty-seven patients. Q J Med. 1989;70(263):253–63.
46. Ala A, Borjigin J, Rochwarger A, Schilsky M. Wilson disease in septuagenarian siblings: Raising the bar for diagnosis. Hepatology. 2005;41(3):668–70.
47. Ferenci P, Czlonkowska A, Merle U, et al. Late-onset Wilson's disease. Gastroenterology. 2007;132(4):1294–8.
48. European Association for Study of Liver. EASL clinical practice guidelines: Wilson's disease. J Hepatol. 2012;56(3):671–85.
49. 8th International Conference on Wilson Disease and Menkes Disease. Leipzig, Germany, April 16–18, 2001. Abstracts. Z Gastroenterol. 2001;39(3):245–60.
50. Roberts EA, Schilsky ML, American Association for Study of Liver Diseases. Diagnosis and treatment of Wilson disease: an update. Hepatology. 2008;47(6):2089–111.
51. Brewer GJ, Hedera P, Kluin KJ, et al. Treatment of Wilson disease with ammonium tetrathiomolybdate: III. Initial therapy in a total of 55 neurologically affected patients and follow-up with zinc therapy. Arch Neurol. 2003;60(3):379–85.
52. Weiss KH, Askari FK, Ferenci P, et al. WTX101 in patients newly diagnosed with Wilson disease: final results of a global, prospective phase 2 trial [abstract & oral presentation]. EASL Meeting, Amsterdam, 2017.
53. Weiss KH, Askari FK, Czlonkowska A, et al. Bis-choline tetrathiomolybdate in patients with Wilson's disease: an open-label, multicentre, phase 2 study. Lancet Gastroenterol Hepatol. 2017;2(12):869–76.

54. Brewer GJ, Askari F, Dick RB, et al. Treatment of Wilson's disease with tetrathiomolybdate: V. Control of free copper by tetrathiomolybdate and a comparison with trientine. Transl Res. 2009;154(2):70–7.
55. Brewer GJ, Askari F, Lorincz MT, et al. Treatment of Wilson disease with ammonium tetrathiomolybdate: IV. Comparison of tetrathiomolybdate and trientine in a double-blind study of treatment of the neurologic presentation of Wilson disease. Arch Neurol. 2006;63(4):521–7.
56. DuBois RS, Rodgerson DO, Martineau G, et al. Orthotopic liver transplantation for Wilson's disease. Lancet. 1971;1(7698):505–8.
57. Dhawan A, Taylor RM, Cheeseman P, De Silva P, Katsiyiannakis L, Mieli-Vergani G. Wilson's disease in children: 37-year experience and revised King's score for liver transplantation. Liver Transpl. 2005;11(4):441–8.
58. Weiss KH, Schafer M, Gotthardt DN, et al. Outcome and development of symptoms after orthotopic liver transplantation for Wilson disease. Clin Transpl. 2013;27(6):914–22.
59. Schilsky ML. Wilson disease: treatment and prognosis: UpToDate; 2015.
60. Arnon R, Annunziato R, Schilsky M, et al. Liver transplantation for children with Wilson disease: comparison of outcomes between children and adults. Clin Transpl. 2011;25(1):E52–60.
61. Schilsky ML, Scheinberg IH, Sternlieb I. Liver transplantation for Wilson's disease: indications and outcome. Hepatology. 1994;19(3):583–7.
62. Wolman M, Sterk VV, Gatt S, Frenkel M. Primary familial xanthomatosis with involvement and calcification of the adrenals. Report of two more cases in siblings of a previously described infant. Pediatrics. 1961;28:742–57.
63. Kyriakides EC, Paul B, Balint JA. Lipid accumulation and acid lipase deficiency in fibroblasts from a family with Wolman's disease, and their apparent correction in vitro. J Lab Clin Med. 1972;80(6):810–6.
64. Aslanidis C, Klima H, Lackner KJ, Schmitz G. Genomic organization of the human lysosomal acid lipase gene (LIPA). Genomics. 1994;20(2):329–31.
65. Sando GN, Rosenbaum LM. Human lysosomal acid lipase/cholesteryl ester hydrolase. Purification and properties of the form secreted by fibroblasts in microcarrier culture. J Biol Chem. 1985;260(28):15186–93.
66. Reiner Z, Guardamagna O, Nair D, et al. Lysosomal acid lipase deficiency—an under-recognized cause of dyslipidaemia and liver dysfunction. Atherosclerosis. 2014;235(1):21–30.
67. Bernstein DL, Hulkova H, Bialer MG, Desnick RJ. Cholesteryl ester storage disease: review of the findings in 135 reported patients with an underdiagnosed disease. J Hepatol. 2013;58(6):1230–43.
68. Fouchier SW, Defesche JC. Lysosomal acid lipase A and the hypercholesterolaemic phenotype. Curr Opin Lipidol. 2013;24(4):332–8.
69. Grabowski GA, Charnas L, Du H. Lysosomal acid lipase deficiencies: the Wolman disease/cholesteryl ester storage disease spectrum. In: Valle DS, ALB BV, Kinzler KW, Antonarakis SE, Ballabio A, editors. Metabolic and molecular bases of inherited disease. 8th ed. New York, NY: McGraw-Hill; 2012.
70. Seedorf U, Wiebusch H, Muntoni S, et al. A novel variant of lysosomal acid lipase (Leu336-->Pro) associated with acid lipase deficiency and cholesterol ester storage disease. Arterioscler Thromb Vasc Biol. 1995;15(6):773–8.
71. Anderson RA, Bryson GM, Parks JS. Lysosomal acid lipase mutations that determine phenotype in Wolman and cholesterol ester storage disease. Mol Genet Metab. 1999;68(3):333–45.
72. Beaudet AL, Ferry GD, Nichols BL Jr, Rosenberg HS. Cholesterol ester storage disease: clinical, biochemical, and pathological studies. J Pediatr. 1977;90(6):910–4.
73. Besley GT, Broadhead DM, Lawlor E, et al. Cholesterol ester storage disease in an adult presenting with sea-blue histiocytosis. Clin Genet. 1984;26(3):195–203.
74. Burke JA, Schubert WK. Deficient activity of acid lipase in cholesterol-ester storage disease. J Lab Clin Med. 1971;78(6):988–9.
75. Crocker AC, Vawter GF, Neuhauser EB, Rosowsky A. Wolman's disease: three new patients with a recently described lipidosis. Pediatrics. 1965;35:627–40.

76. D'Agostino D, Bay L, Gallo G, Chamoles N. Cholesterol ester storage disease: clinical, biochemical, and pathological studies of four new cases. J Pediatr Gastroenterol Nutr. 1988;7(3):446–50.
77. Dalgic B, Sari S, Gunduz M, et al. Cholesteryl ester storage disease in a young child presenting as isolated hepatomegaly treated with simvastatin. Turk J Pediatr. 2006;48(2):148–51.
78. Di Bisceglie AM, Ishak KG, Rabin L, Hoeg JM. Cholesteryl ester storage disease: hepatopathology and effects of therapy with lovastatin. Hepatology. 1990;11(5):764–72.
79. Dincsoy HP, Rolfes DB, McGraw CA, Schubert WK. Cholesterol ester storage disease and mesenteric lipodystrophy. Am J Clin Pathol. 1984;81(2):263–9.
80. Edelstein RA, Filling-Katz MR, Pentchev P, et al. Cholesteryl ester storage disease: a patient with massive splenomegaly and splenic abscess. Am J Gastroenterol. 1988;83(6):687–92.
81. Elleder M, Chlumska A, Ledvinova J, Poupetova H. Testis—a novel storage site in human cholesteryl ester storage disease. Autopsy report of an adult case with a long-standing subclinical course complicated by accelerated atherosclerosis and liver carcinoma. Virchows Arch. 2000;436(1):82–7.
82. Fasano T, Pisciotta L, Bocchi L, et al. Lysosomal lipase deficiency: molecular characterization of eleven patients with Wolman or cholesteryl ester storage disease. Mol Genet Metab. 2012;105(3):450–6.
83. Hill SC, Hoeg JM, Dwyer AJ, Vucich JJ, Doppman JL. CT findings in acid lipase deficiency: Wolman disease and cholesteryl ester storage disease. J Comput Assist Tomogr. 1983;7(5):815–8.
84. Kunnert B, Pohlandt K, Ruschke I, Keller E. [Cholesterol ester storage disease and sea-blue histiocytes]. Zentralb Allg Pathol. 1987;133(6):517–25.
85. Marshall WC, Ockenden BG, Fosbrooke AS, Cumings JN. Wolman's disease. A rare lipidosis with adrenal calcification. Arch Dis Child. 1969;44(235):331–41.
86. Tylki-Szymanska A, Maciejko D, Wozniewicz B, Muszynska B. Two cases of cholesteryl ester storage disease (CESD) acid lipase deficiency. Hepatogastroenterology. 1987;34(3):98–9.
87. Young EP, Patrick AD. Deficiency of acid esterase activity in Wolman's disease. Arch Dis Child. 1970;45(243):664–8.
88. Zhang B, Porto AF. Cholesteryl ester storage disease: protean presentations of lysosomal acid lipase deficiency. J Pediatr Gastroenterol Nutr. 2013;56(6):682–5.
89. Kostner GM, Hadorn B, Roscher A, Zechner R. Plasma lipids and lipoproteins of a patient with cholesteryl ester storage disease. J Inherit Metab Dis. 1985;8(1):9–12.
90. Ameis D, Brockmann G, Knoblich R, et al. A 5′ splice-region mutation and a dinucleotide deletion in the lysosomal acid lipase gene in two patients with cholesteryl ester storage disease. J Lipid Res. 1995;36(2):241–50.
91. Redonnet-Vernhet I, Chatelut M, Basile JP, Salvayre R, Levade T. Cholesteryl ester storage disease: relationship between molecular defects and in situ activity of lysosomal acid lipase. Biochem Mol Med. 1997;62(1):42–9.
92. Redonnet-Vernhet I, Chatelut M, Salvayre R, Levade T. A novel lysosomal acid lipase gene mutation in a patient with cholesteryl ester storage disease. Hum Mutat. 1998;11(4):335–6.
93. Gasche C, Aslanidis C, Kain R, et al. A novel variant of lysosomal acid lipase in cholesteryl ester storage disease associated with mild phenotype and improvement on lovastatin. J Hepatol. 1997;27(4):744–50.
94. Klima H, Ullrich K, Aslanidis C, Fehringer P, Lackner KJ, Schmitz G. A splice junction mutation causes deletion of a 72-base exon from the mRNA for lysosomal acid lipase in a patient with cholesteryl ester storage disease. J Clin Invest. 1993;92(6):2713–8.
95. Pagani F, Garcia R, Pariyarath R, et al. Expression of lysosomal acid lipase mutants detected in three patients with cholesteryl ester storage disease. Hum Mol Genet. 1996;5(10):1611–7.
96. Muntoni S, Wiebusch H, Funke H, Ros E, Seedorf U, Assmann G. Homozygosity for a splice junction mutation in exon 8 of the gene encoding lysosomal acid lipase in a Spanish kindred with cholesterol ester storage disease (CESD). Hum Genet. 1995;95(5):491–4.
97. Valayannopoulos V, Mengel E, Brassier A, Grabowski G. Lysosomal acid lipase deficiency: expanding differential diagnosis. Mol Genet Metab. 2017;120(1–2):62–6.

98. Muntoni S, Wiebusch H, Jansen-Rust M, et al. Prevalence of cholesteryl ester storage disease. Arterioscler Thromb Vasc Biol. 2007;27(8):1866–8.
99. Scott SA, Liu B, Nazarenko I, et al. Frequency of the cholesteryl ester storage disease common LIPA E8SJM mutation (c.894G>A) in various racial and ethnic groups. Hepatology. 2013;58(3):958–65.
100. Meikle PJ, Hopwood JJ, Clague AE, Carey WF. Prevalence of lysosomal storage disorders. JAMA. 1999;281(3):249–54.
101. Valles-Ayoub Y, Esfandiarifard S, No D, et al. Wolman disease (LIPA p.G87V) genotype frequency in people of Iranian-Jewish ancestry. Genet Test Mol Biomarkers. 2011;15(6):395–8.
102. Balwani M, Breen C, Enns GM, et al. Clinical effect and safety profile of recombinant human lysosomal acid lipase in patients with cholesteryl ester storage disease. Hepatology. 2013;58(3):950–7.
103. Burton BK, Balwani M, Feillet F, et al. A phase 3 trial of sebelipase alfa in lysosomal acid lipase deficiency. N Engl J Med. 2015;373(11):1010–20.
104. Valayannopoulos V, Malinova V, Honzik T, et al. Sebelipase alfa over 52 weeks reduces serum transaminases, liver volume and improves serum lipids in patients with lysosomal acid lipase deficiency. J Hepatol. 2014;61(5):1135–42.
105. Du H, Cameron TL, Garger SJ, et al. Wolman disease/cholesteryl ester storage disease: efficacy of plant-produced human lysosomal acid lipase in mice. J Lipid Res. 2008;49(8):1646–57.
106. Jones SA, Valayannopoulos V, Schneider E, et al. Rapid progression and mortality of lysosomal acid lipase deficiency presenting in infants. Genet Med. 2016;18(5):452–8.
107. Burton BK, Deegan PB, Enns GM, et al. Clinical features of lysosomal acid lipase deficiency. J Pediatr Gastroenterol Nutr. 2015;61(6):619–25.
108. Jones SA, Brassier A, Hughes J, Plantaz D, Vara R, Breen C, Gargus JJ, Valayannopoulos V. Effect of sebelipase alfa on survival and liver function in infants with rapidly progressive lysosomal acid lipase deficiency: 2-year follow-up data. Mol Genet Metab. 2016;117(2):S63.
109. Pericleous M, Kelly C, Wang T, Livingstone C, Ala A. Wolman's disease and cholesteryl ester storage disorder: the phenotypic spectrum of lysosomal acid lipase deficiency. Lancet Gastroenterol Hepatol. 2017;2:670–9.
110. Laurell CB, Eriksson S. The electrophoretic α;1-globulin pattern of serum in α;1-antitrypsin deficiency. Scand J Clin Lab Invest. 1963;15(2):132–40.
111. Sharp HL, Bridges RA, Krivit W, Freier EF. Cirrhosis associated with alpha-1-antitrypsin deficiency: a previously unrecognized inherited disorder. J Lab Clin Med. 1969;73(6):934–9.
112. Teckman JH, Mangalat N. Alpha-1 antitrypsin and liver disease: mechanisms of injury and novel interventions. Expert Rev Gastroenterol Hepatol. 2015;9(2):261–8.
113. Janus ED, Phillips NT, Carrell RW. Smoking, lung function, and alpha 1-antitrypsin deficiency. Lancet. 1985;1(8421):152–4.
114. Mayer AS, Stoller JK, Bucher Bartelson B, James Ruttenber A, Sandhaus RA, Newman LS. Occupational exposure risks in individuals with PI*Z alpha(1)-antitrypsin deficiency. Am J Respir Crit Care Med. 2000;162(2 Pt 1):553–8.
115. Piitulainen E, Carlson J, Ohlsson K, Sveger T. Alpha1-antitrypsin deficiency in 26-year-old subjects: lung, liver, and protease/protease inhibitor studies. Chest. 2005;128(4):2076–81.
116. Crowther DC, Belorgey D, Miranda E, Kinghorn KJ, Sharp LK, Lomas DA. Practical genetics: alpha-1-antitrypsin deficiency and the serpinopathies. Eur J Hum Genet. 2004;12(3):167–72.
117. Fairbanks KD, Tavill AS. Liver disease in alpha 1-antitrypsin deficiency: a review. Am J Gastroenterol. 2008;103(8):2136–41; quiz 2142.
118. Marcus NY, Brunt EM, Blomenkamp K, et al. Characteristics of hepatocellular carcinoma in a murine model of alpha-1-antitrypsin deficiency. Hepatol Res. 2010;40(6):641–53.
119. Rudnick DA, Liao Y, An JK, Muglia LJ, Perlmutter DH, Teckman JH. Analyses of hepatocellular proliferation in a mouse model of alpha-1-antitrypsin deficiency. Hepatology. 2004;39(4):1048–55.
120. Janciauskiene S, Wallmark A, Piitulainen E, Kohnlein T, Welte T, Sveger T. Performance of enhanced liver fibrosis plasma markers in asymptomatic individuals with ZZ alpha1-antitrypsin deficiency. Eur J Gastroenterol Hepatol. 2011;23(8):716–20.

121. Blanco I, Bueno P, Diego I, et al. Alpha-1 antitrypsin Pi*Z gene frequency and Pi*ZZ genotype numbers worldwide: an update. Int J Chron Obstruct Pulmon Dis. 2017;12:561–9.
122. de Serres FJ, Blanco I, Fernandez-Bustillo E. PI S and PI Z alpha-1 antitrypsin deficiency worldwide. A review of existing genetic epidemiological data. Monaldi Arch Chest Dis. 2007;67(4):184–208.
123. de Serres FJ, Blanco I, Fernandez-Bustillo E. Estimates of PI*S and PI*Z Alpha-1 antitrypsin deficiency alleles prevalence in the Caribbean and North, Central and South America. Monaldi Arch Chest Dis. 2009;71(3):96–105.
124. Sveger T. Liver disease in alpha1-antitrypsin deficiency detected by screening of 200,000 infants. N Engl J Med. 1976;294(24):1316–21.
125. O'Brien ML, Buist NR, Murphey WH. Neonatal screening for alpha1-antitrypsin deficiency. J Pediatr. 1978;92(6):1006–10.
126. Silverman EK, Miletich JP, Pierce JA, et al. Alpha-1-antitrypsin deficiency. High prevalence in the St. Louis area determined by direct population screening. Am Rev Respir Dis. 1989;140(4):961–6.
127. Stoller JK, Aboussouan LS. A review of alpha1-antitrypsin deficiency. Am J Respir Crit Care Med. 2012;185(3):246–59.
128. Blanco I, de Serres FJ, Fernandez-Bustillo E, Lara B, Miravitlles M. Estimated numbers and prevalence of PI*S and PI*Z alleles of alpha1-antitrypsin deficiency in European countries. Eur Respir J. 2006;27(1):77–84.
129. Fahndrich S, Herr C, Greulich T, et al. Sex differences in alpha-1-antitrypsin deficiency lung disease-analysis from the German registry. COPD. 2015;12(Suppl 1):58–62.
130. Pardinas-Gutierrez MA, Mirsaeidi M, Sandhaus RA, Campos M. Gender differences in Alpha-1 antritrypsin deficiency [abstract A.43]. Am J Respir Crit Care Med. 2016;193:A1571.
131. McElvaney NG, Burdon J, Holmes M, et al. Long-term efficacy and safety of alpha1 proteinase inhibitor treatment for emphysema caused by severe alpha1 antitrypsin deficiency: an open-label extension trial (RAPID-OLE). Lancet Respir Med. 2017;5(1):51–60.
132. Chapman KR, Stockley RA, Dawkins C, Wilkes MM, Navickis RJ. Augmentation therapy for alpha1 antitrypsin deficiency: a meta-analysis. COPD. 2009;6(3):177–84.
133. Kemmer N, Kaiser T, Zacharias V, Neff GW. Alpha-1-antitrypsin deficiency: outcomes after liver transplantation. Transplant Proc. 2008;40(5):1492–4.
134. Silverman GA, Pak SC, Perlmutter DH. Disorders of protein misfolding: alpha-1-antitrypsin deficiency as prototype. J Pediatr. 2013;163(2):320–6.
135. Powell LW, Seckington RC, Deugnier Y. Haemochromatosis. Lancet. 2016;388(10045):706–16.
136. Feder JN, Gnirke A, Thomas W, et al. A novel MHC class I-like gene is mutated in patients with hereditary haemochromatosis. Nat Genet. 1996;13(4):399–408.
137. Simon M, Bourel M, Fauchet R, Genetet B. Association of HLA-A3 and HLA-B14 antigens with idiopathic haemochromatosis. Gut. 1976;17(5):332–4.
138. European Association for the Study of the Liver. EASL clinical practice guidelines for HFE hemochromatosis. J Hepatol. 2010;53(1):3–22.
139. Schrier SL, Bacon BR. Clinical manifestations and diagnosis of hereditary hemochromatosis. UpToDate; 2016. https://www.uptodate.com/contents/clinical-manifestations-and-diagnosis-of-hereditary-hemochromatosis?source=search_result&search=hereditary%20hemochromatosis&selectedTitle=1~96. Accessed 2 May 2017.
140. Steinberg KK, Cogswell ME, Chang JC, et al. Prevalence of C282Y and H63D mutations in the hemochromatosis (HFE) gene in the United States. JAMA. 2001;285(17):2216–22.
141. Adams PC, Reboussin DM, Barton JC, et al. Hemochromatosis and iron-overload screening in a racially diverse population. N Engl J Med. 2005;352(17):1769–78.
142. Asberg A, Hveem K, Thorstensen K, et al. Screening for hemochromatosis: high prevalence and low morbidity in an unselected population of 65,238 persons. Scand J Gastroenterol. 2001;36(10):1108–15.
143. Bacon BR. Diagnosis and management of hemochromatosis. Gastroenterology. 1997;113(3):995–9.

144. Beutler E, Gelbart T, West C, et al. Mutation analysis in hereditary hemochromatosis. Blood Cells Mol Dis. 1996;22(2):187–94; discussion 194a–b.
145. Jouanolle AM, Gandon G, Jezequel P, et al. Haemochromatosis and HLA-H. Nat Genet. 1996;14(3):251–2.
146. Jazwinska EC, Cullen LM, Busfield F, et al. Haemochromatosis and HLA-H. Nat Genet. 1996;14(3):249–51.
147. Carella M, D'Ambrosio L, Totaro A, et al. Mutation analysis of the HLA-H gene in Italian hemochromatosis patients. Am J Hum Genet. 1997;60(4):828–32.
148. Beutler E, Felitti VJ, Koziol JA, Ho NJ, Gelbart T. Penetrance of 845G-->A (C282Y) HFE hereditary haemochromatosis mutation in the USA. Lancet. 2002;359(9302):211–8.
149. Olynyk JK, Cullen DJ, Aquilia S, Rossi E, Summerville L, Powell LW. A population-based study of the clinical expression of the hemochromatosis gene. N Engl J Med. 1999;341(10):718–24.
150. Aguilar-Martinez P, Bismuth M, Blanc F, et al. The Southern French registry of genetic hemochromatosis: a tool for determining clinical prevalence of the disorder and genotype penetrance. Haematologica. 2010;95(4):551–6.
151. Walsh A, Dixon JL, Ramm GA, et al. The clinical relevance of compound heterozygosity for the C282Y and H63D substitutions in hemochromatosis. Clin Gastroenterol Hepatol. 2006;4(11):1403–10.
152. Allen KJ, Gurrin LC, Constantine CC, et al. Iron-overload-related disease in HFE hereditary hemochromatosis. N Engl J Med. 2008;358(3):221–30.
153. Bacon BR, Adams PC, Kowdley KV, Powell LW, Tavill AS, American Association for the Study of Liver Diseases. Diagnosis and management of hemochromatosis: 2011 practice guideline by the American Association for the Study of Liver Diseases. Hepatology. 2011;54(1):328–43.
154. Rombout-Sestrienkova E, Nieman FH, Essers BA, et al. Erythrocytapheresis versus phlebotomy in the initial treatment of HFE hemochromatosis patients: results from a randomized trial. Transfusion. 2012;52(3):470–7.
155. Rahko PS, Salerni R, Uretsky BF. Successful reversal by chelation therapy of congestive cardiomyopathy due to iron overload. J Am Coll Cardiol. 1986;8(2):436–40.
156. Nielsen P, Fischer R, Buggisch P, Janka-Schaub G. Effective treatment of hereditary haemochromatosis with desferrioxamine in selected cases. Br J Haematol. 2003;123(5):952–3.
157. Phatak P, Brissot P, Wurster M, et al. A phase 1/2, dose-escalation trial of deferasirox for the treatment of iron overload in HFE-related hereditary hemochromatosis. Hepatology. 2010;52(5):1671–779.
158. Cancado R, Melo MR, de Moraes Bastos R, et al. Deferasirox in patients with iron overload secondary to hereditary hemochromatosis: results of a 1-yr Phase 2 study. Eur J Haematol. 2015;95(6):545–50.
159. Yu L, Ioannou GN. Survival of liver transplant recipients with hemochromatosis in the United States. Gastroenterology. 2007;133(2):489–95.
160. Jones SA, Plantaz D, Vara R, et al. Effect of sebelipase alfa on survival and liver function in infants with rapidly progressive lysosomal acid lipase deficiency. Mol Genet Metab. 2015;114(2):S59.
161. US National Institutes of Health. ClinicalTrials.gov identifier NCT02112994. 2016.
162. US National Institutes of Health. ClinicalTrials.gov identifier NCT02193867. 2016. https://clinicaltrials.gov/ct2/results?term=NCT02193867&Search=Search. Accessed 18 Dec 2016.

Cryptogenic Cirrhosis 18

Zachary Henry, Curtis K. Argo, and Stephen H. Caldwell

Abstract

Cryptogenic cirrhosis (CC) is defined as the development of cirrhosis in the absence of a clear etiology of liver dysfunction. Over time, definitions of various forms of liver disease have been refined and improved so that the incidence of CC is in decline. With the advent of hepatitis C testing and better definitions of alcohol related liver disease these etiologies of cirrhosis have decreased their impact on the diagnosis of CC. Autoimmune hepatitis and non-alcoholic fatty liver disease (NAFLD), both of which can lose their characteristic histologic features with advancement to cirrhosis, have taken over as the primary explanations for developing CC, but even now as definitions and recognition of NAFLD improve these numbers are waning. Since CC is a diagnosis of exclusion, prospective investigations are challenging and thus study methodology has a large impact on how relevant data are interpreted. Herein we focus on how the diagnosis of CC is made, the liver diseases that have contributed most to this diagnosis over time, and how study design affects the results and interpretation of prior investigations.

Keywords

Cryptogenic cirrhosis · NAFLD · NASH · ASH · Autoimmune hepatitis · AIH · Hepatitis C · Cohort study · Case control · Epidemiology

Z. Henry (✉) · C. K. Argo · S. H. Caldwell
Division of GI/Hepatology, Department of Medicine, University of Virginia Medical Center, Charlottesville, VA, USA
e-mail: zhenry@virginia.edu; SHC5C@hscmail.mcc.virginia.edu

R. J. Wong, R. G. Gish (eds.), *Clinical Epidemiology of Chronic Liver Diseases*,
https://doi.org/10.1007/978-3-319-94355-8_18

18.1 Introduction

Cryptogenic cirrhosis (CC) is defined as cirrhosis arising in the absence of a clear etiology of chronic liver disease which makes it a difficult entity to define and investigate. The prevalence of CC is difficult to define due to this broad definition and is likely decreasing as emerging liver diseases such as nonalcoholic fatty liver disease (NAFLD) and nonalcoholic steatohepatitis (NASH) are better defined. In prior studies the prevalence of CC has ranged from 5% to 30%, but much of this data is retrospective and derived from single centers and thus subject to various biases [1–3]. Transplant databases have estimated the prevalence of CC to be approximately 10%, but these estimates frequently include CC in categories with "other" diagnoses, which further compromises ascertaining prevalence accurately [4, 5].

Over time the prevalence of CC is expected to decline as definitions of chronic liver diseases are refined and new liver diseases are discovered [1, 2, 4]. Alcohol-related liver disease is likely the oldest diagnosed liver disease, existing as long ago as 10,000 B.C. and commonplace in medical texts of the nineteenth century [6, 7]. In 1961 a group of diabetic patients were noted to have fatty liver outside of significant alcohol use, and some progressed to cirrhosis which at that time was referred to as "nutritional cirrhosis" [8]. In the 1960s and 1970s hepatitis B became better defined as a cause of chronic hepatitis as better serum tests enabled more reliable detection [9, 10]. Hepatitis C soon followed in the late 1980s and early 1990s [11–13]. Autoimmune hepatitis, originally called lupoid hepatitis, has gained improved diagnostic accuracy since its inception in the 1950s, but still remains a chief suspect in the quest to define CC [14, 15]. Over the last few decades NASH has grown in prominence in large part due to better definitions and improved recognition [16–19].

In this chapter we focus on the underlying liver diseases with the largest impact on development of CC, a diagnosis of exclusion (Table 18.1). In addition to a full biochemical work up for chronic liver diseases, careful attention to personal, family, and social histories is vital to find an accurate diagnosis (Table 18.2). In some cases, primarily when assessing alcohol intake or substance use history, it may also be important to speak with family members to comprehensively ascertain patient exposures potentially lost to recall bias. Assessing changes in physical stature over time, both prior to and following confirmed diagnosis of cirrhosis, may help to identify the possible underlying etiology of cirrhosis that may be masked by recent malnutrition and/or large volume ascites [20]. Medication exposure may also be difficult to discern as certain medications may cause drug-induced liver injury with long-term advanced fibrosis despite medication withdrawal [21, 22]. Histology may be very helpful in assessing for clues of underlying causes of CC, and a classification system was devised to help guide clinicians and pathologists in interpreting findings in the context of chronic liver disease of unclear etiology (Table 18.3) [15, 20, 23, 24].

Table 18.1 Disease associations with CC

Established associations
Nonalcoholic steatohepatitis
Autoimmune hepatitis
Occult viral hepatitis (hepatitis X)
Occult ethanol exposure
Less established but noted in some series
Occult biliary disease
Hepatic vascular disease
Celiac disease
Other associations
Mitochondriapathies
Familial Mediterranean fever
Systemic lupus erythematosus
Alstrom syndrome (celiopathy)
Abnormalities of apolipoprotein B with low-density-lipoprotein cholesterol
Short telomere syndromes
Keratin 18 mutations
Glutathione S-transferase mutations

Derived from Caldwell S. CC: what are we missing? Curr Gastroenterol Rep. 2010;12(1):40–48

Table 18.2 Key factors in determining the underlying diagnosis of CC

History
Prior fatty liver by imaging or biopsy: direct inquiry
Prior obesity, diabetes, or hyperlipidemia (cirrhosis causes loss of body fat/muscle mass)
Percutaneous exposures: blood or needles
Family history of liver disease
Personal or family history of autoimmune diseases
Careful assessment of cumulative ethanol exposure
Occupational history
Laboratory
Viral serologies
Autoantibodies
Immunoglobulin levels
Iron and copper indices
α-1-Antitrypsin level and phenotype
Celiac disease markers
Histology
Predominant type and distribution of inflammation, if present
Cellular ballooning
Mallory-Denk bodies
Glycogenated nuclei
Foci of macrosteatosis
Bile ductular proliferation
Apoptotic bodies

Derived from Caldwell S. CC: what are we missing? Curr Gastroenterol Rep. 2010;12(1):40–48

Table 18.3 Proposed classification system for CC

1. Cirrhosis with features of steatohepatitis including scattered foci of macrosteatosis, occasional ballooned hepatocytes with Mallory bodies, megamitochondria, and glycogenated nuclei, usually with a history of obesity and insulin-resistant syndrome. Family history of liver disease is common. Based on the existence of this late stage of NASH, stage 4 NASH should be further divided into:
(a) NASH with cirrhosis
(b) Cirrhosis with features of NASH
(c) Bland cirrhosis with risks for NASH (obesity, diabetes, hyperlipidemia)
2. Cirrhosis with features of autoimmune disease such as portal inflammation, plasma cells, or granulomas. Patients may have significant autoimmune score. Family history of autoimmune disease common
3. Occult viral infection such as postnecrotic hepatitis B or as-yet unidentified viral infection (non-B, non-C hepatitis or hepatitis X). Risk history may include prior blood transfusion, intravenous drug use, or other percutaneous exposure. Histologic characteristics possibly include predominant mononuclear inflammation, lymphoid follicles
4. Cirrhosis with lifelong history of significant alcohol consumption but with subthreshold consumption on a daily or weekly basis. Requires careful assessment of prior exposure including lifetime cumulative consumption. Less evidence of glycogenated nuclei and insulin receptor staining may distinguish NASH from ASH (see text)
5. Cirrhosis with features of biliary disease including proliferation of bile ductules and cholestasis
6. Bland cirrhosis: cirrhosis lacking other distinguishing features and without identifiable risks

Derived from Caldwell S. CC: what are we missing? Curr Gastroenterol Rep. 2010;12(1):40–48
ASH alcoholic steatohepatitis, *NASH* non-alcoholic steatohepatitis

18.2 The Impact of Study Methodology

Background in research methodology, particularly in defining disease definition, helps to inform about the changes in prevalence of CC diagnosis over time. Randomized, controlled trials are not helpful in evaluating underlying disease prevalence: strict diagnostic criteria are used to clearly define the study population with randomized implementation of a specific intervention. Instead, observational studies, including cohort and case control studies, better align associations of diagnoses and diagnostic tests with clinical outcomes. Nearly all cohort studies evaluating CC are retrospective, and thus understanding different types of study and research bias is critical to assessing the strengths and weaknesses of individual studies. Misclassification or information bias is a common flaw of retrospective cohort studies [25]. For example, in studies of alcoholic liver disease (ALD) patients may be misclassified as having CC when, as more history of alcohol exposure is known over time, their proper group assignment likely should have been ALD all along [1].

Observations from cohort studies often lead to a second generation of case control studies to more directly compare patient characteristics and outcomes between cases (in this instance CC) and controls (well defined chronic liver diseases) to show stronger associations with a particular disease entity. Significant bias can be introduced when attempting to study a less clearly defined condition such as CC. Selection bias may occur when patients included for analysis are not representative of the greater population; i.e., hospital-based populations have different characteristics than the general population thus overestimating certain health exposures [25]. In some studies of CC certain groups of patients may be excluded from the study focus findings within a specific group of patients. Unfortunately, this may result in a potentially important group being excluded, thus introducing selection bias. For a disease such as CC, a diagnosis of exclusion, selection bias may cause an important variable or group of patients to be misrepresented in either the control or case groups. Lastly, confounding variables are prevalent in studies of CC, mainly because the variable's association with CC is learned after the study was performed. In addition, because most studies of CC are retrospective, potential confounding variables may not have been collected at the time of diagnosis and thus cannot be controlled for during analysis. Naturally, as we learn more about specific disease processes over time some definitions may change and our understanding of pathophysiology may change the way a diagnosis is made. This may provide information to potentially control for confounding variables but given the fluid nature of CC diagnostic criteria, prior studies always require cautious consideration.

18.2.1 CC and NAFLD

Nonalcoholic fatty liver disease (NAFLD) has now become the most prominent form of chronic liver disease worldwide and is one of the leading indications for both liver transplant and simultaneous liver and kidney transplant in the United States [4, 5, 19, 26]. NAFLD appears to have the largest overlap with CC over the last 20–30 years. As definitions of ALD were refined and testing for hepatitis C was brought into mainstream practice, the influence of these two conditions in the setting of CC understandably waned [2, 7]. Over the same time period structured definitions and a more informative natural history of NAFLD and NASH led to the discovery of many clinical features that overlapped with CC [16–18, 27, 28]. There are much older reports suggesting that metabolic-related fatty liver disease may play a role in the development of a bland cirrhosis but the most significant breakthrough in making this connection came with an observational cohort series of NASH patients published in 1991 by Powell et al. [8, 29]. At that time NASH had a histologic definition that is similar to today's general definition [16], and the group rigorously excluded confounding disease processes such as ALD, drug-induced fatty liver disease, and other alternative causes of liver enzyme elevation. Their results from paired biopsy data revealed progression of NASH in some patients to bland, micronodular cirrhosis with loss of steatosis that implicated NASH as a potential significant cause of CC [29]. This produced a new hypothesis for development of CC and highlights the advantages of observational cohort studies as hypothesis generating. The study's methodology allowed the authors to set rigid criteria for NASH as well as other liver diseases to increase diagnostic confidence while allowing for adjustments with new diagnostic criteria over time.

Unfortunately, further assessment of this relationship becomes difficult given the hypothesis that clear evidence of the underlying etiology—steatosis and hepatocyte ballooning in the case of NASH—may deteriorate over time. There were case reports published confirming the findings of Powell et al. that NAFLD could progress to bland cirrhosis suggestive of CC; however, these singular studies unfortunately did not provide further insight into the degree of this relationship [30]. Further prospective cohort studies with larger sample sizes may certainly add more information but are time- and resource-consuming.

Case-control studies possess the advantage of allowing analysis of well-defined groups at the outset, thus pinpointing the similarities and differences between cases and controls via direct comparison. This methodology was successfully utilized in a study by Caldwell et al. in 1999 which compared 70 subjects with CC with control groups of subjects with NASH without cirrhosis, HCV-related cirrhosis, and primary biliary cholangitis (PBC)-related cirrhosis. The authors noted that many patients with CC had features similar to the NASH group, both clinically and histologically, and thus suggested that a significant portion of CC may develop from previously undiagnosed NASH [27]. Similarities in the AST:ALT ratios that suggested progression from NASH to CC [31] and a difference in age between the NASH and CC groups indicated a possible transition between these two entities, with the average age of the NASH group about 10 years less than the CC group. There were also overlapping metabolic features, including type 2 diabetes mellitus (T2DM) and obesity, between the NASH and CC groups that were not present in either the HCV cirrhosis or the PBC cirrhosis groups [27]. By isolating the groups in a case-control manner the similarities and differences between CC and the control groups are easier to evaluate. The authors did take a much more conservative approach to excluding ALD patients from analysis in order to reduce bias with that disease entity, but confounding data for autoimmune hepatitis (AIH) could still have been present given that this was not directly assessed.

A subsequent study employed slightly different methods in using age- and gender-matching of case and control groups composed of subjects drawn from their institution's liver transplant registry [32]. Because of the previous findings that NASH has significant association with T2DM and obesity, known NASH patients were excluded from the analysis, thus isolating CC for direct comparison to non-NASH etiologies. A weakness of this study is that the authors could no longer directly compare CC cases to NASH cirrhosis controls; however, it does provide a cleaner analysis for finding negative associations to other etiologies of liver disease. A strength of this study is that the control group subjects were selected randomly to provide a more representative sampling of the general population, thus minimizing selection bias. Remarkably, the authors found a significantly increased proportion of obesity and T2DM in the CC patients compared to the control groups, suggesting that CC is more similar to NASH than other causes of chronic liver disease and confirming the suspicions provoked by previous studies [32]. These results were further supported by similar findings of significant associations of T2DM and hypertriglyceridemia in obese patients with CC compared to lean patients with CC as well as obese or lean patients with HCV [33].

Further studies utilized similar methods to the case-control study design but employed patients undergoing liver transplantation (LT) as their main population of study [15, 23, 34–36]. This allowed complete examination of the histologic features of explanted livers in an attempt to define the underlying etiology of CC [23]. The authors noted that NASH and autoimmune hepatitis were the two largest groups of CC identified which is concordant with previous data [15, 27]. This particular study is unique in the CC literature in that the authors relied heavily on explant pathology to define their groups (NASH, AIH, other) and then attempted to associate clinical features with the presumed histologic diagnosis. Most previous studies have done the opposite where clinical features suggest a diagnosis and histology is subsequently defined based upon that diagnosis. The bias introduced by using histology as the defining feature post hoc relies upon the assumption that when patients develop cirrhosis they will maintain the features of their underlying disease. Unfortunately, prior studies showed that in many cases histology becomes unreliable once patients progress to cirrhosis. Since the study premise is based primarily on the underlying histology, significant bias is likely introduced [23]. Ideally for a study such as this there would be confirmatory data that patients with known NASH and/or AIH who progress to cirrhosis show similar features in their biopsies to patients with CC. Fortunately there was a follow up study some years later specifically evaluating histology in known NASH patients who progressed to cirrhosis noting many of the same histologic findings as Ayata and colleagues [37]. The difference in this study is that the investigators paired CC diagnoses histologically (termed non-specific cirrhosis by a blinded pathologist) to patients who had prior liver biopsies showing non-cirrhotic NASH. This overcomes the assumption that histologic features would be similar pre- and post-cirrhosis and confirmed that although steatosis deteriorates as NASH progresses to cirrhosis, other underlying features such as cellular ballooning and Mallory-Denk bodies (MDB) may remain. The authors also compared these results to a subgroup of patients with HCV-related cirrhosis to show that findings of cellular ballooning and MDB are much more frequent in NASH cirrhosis compared to viral etiologies and in the right clinical context more likely indicate prior NASH rather than viral cirrhosis [37].

The study by Ayata and colleagues also went on to note differences in the patients' post-transplant courses. While their initial histologic inclusion criteria may have biased their results, this does reveal the potentially important assessment of NASH recurrence post-transplant as confirmation of the relationship between CC and NASH. Earlier studies evaluated similar post-transplant changes as a potential corroborating factor related to the underlying etiology of liver disease, but these authors primarily focused on viral and autoimmune risk factors [2, 38]. In a study by Ong et al., a cohort of CC patients was monitored after LT for recurrence of NAFLD. They found that 25% of CC patients developed NAFLD in the post-transplant follow up period and suggested that these patients had higher risk of DM and obesity post-transplant [34]. Unfortunately, this cohort study of CC patients included relatively significant assumptions that likely biased their results, perhaps even leading away from identifying a more significant association. For example, of the 51 patients in the cohort, the majority did not have a post-LT liver biopsy and were therefore assumed to not have NAFLD, possibly biasing results towards not seeing differences. Excluding those patients completely from the analysis would have introduced a different bias simply because only biopsied patients from the CC cohort would be included. Other investigations have overcome this problem by only including patients with serial liver biopsies in the post-OLT period and one such study also included control groups with ALD as well as cholestatic liver disease to provide contrast [35]. This study did note that patients with CC suspected to be from NASH had an almost 100% chance of developing NAFLD in the post-transplant period compared to only 25% in the ALD and cholestatic groups. It should be noted that of the CC patients, most were included based upon histologic features concerning for NASH which as stated above may not be accurate once these patients progress to cirrhosis. In addition, they only included CC patients with suspicion for NAFLD and thus the near 100% recurrence rate post-transplant is somewhat confounding as these patients had a much higher pre-test probability to develop NAFLD than other CC patients. This design feature limits meaningful findings to only those CC patients with clinical and pathologic features of NASH rather than the entire population of CC patients. For a more complete assessment of the impact of CC on post-transplant NAFLD, it would be important to investigate all pre-transplant diagnoses and assess for post-transplant NAFLD in each group. For instance, one study noted that of six patients that developed fatty liver disease post-transplant they were evenly distributed among all the suspected etiologic groups suggesting that post-transplant pathology may not directly correlate with pre-transplant disease [15].

In addition, these studies assume that post-transplant disease is solely related to the recipient's pre-transplant disease, ignoring the potential impact of donor characteristics in the development of post-transplant liver disease. With the exception of viral hepatitis and ALD, which have a more recognizable influence on post-transplant liver dysfunction, it seems more feasible that a combination of recipient and donor factors lead to post-transplant NAFLD, autoimmune disease, and episodes of rejection. In fact, it has been theorized that donor graft steatosis may play a role in post-OLT development of NAFLD [39, 40]. This is further represented in the varying rates of disease recurrence from CC and NAFLD studies. Contos et al. note a rate of post-transplant NAFLD of nearly 100% while Ong et al. note a much lower rate of approximately 25% [34, 35]. Their definitions of CC clearly differ which contributes to their disparate results. Neither study adequately accounts for donor factors in their assessment of disease recurrence, a common flaw in CC studies [15, 36]. In an attempt to overcome some of these limitations Yalamanchili et al. compared distinct groups of patients with NASH cirrhosis at transplant to subjects with CC at transplant to assess differences in post-transplant outcomes. The authors note that the recurrence rate for NAFLD in the NASH cirrhosis group was approximately 45% but only 23% in the CC group. This may suggest that CC is not as closely related to NASH as previously thought, but more likely this represents our evolving understanding of NASH and its increased rate of diagnosis prior to transplant.

If we assume that NASH is a significant cause of CC, then as recognition and incidence of NASH cirrhosis increases over time, the prevalence of CC should

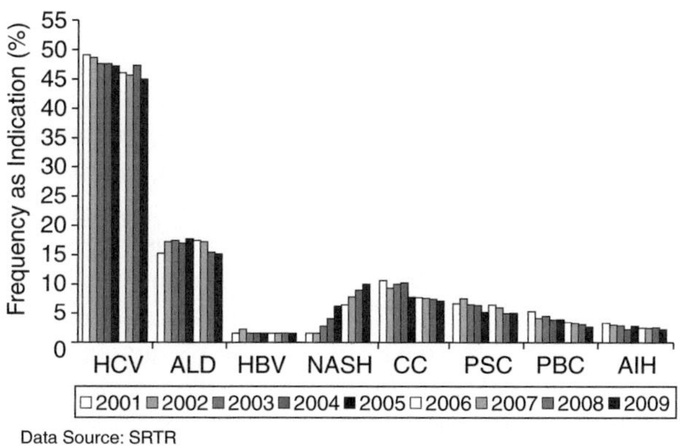

Fig. 18.1 The prevalence of specific indications for liver transplantation over time. *HCV* hepatitis C virus, *ALD* alcohol related liver disease, *HBV* hepatitis B virus, *NASH* non-alcoholic steatohepatitis, *CC* cryptogenic cirrhosis, *PSC* primary sclerosing cholangitis, *PBC* primary biliary cholangitis, *AIH* autoimmune hepatitis. Derived from Charlton MR, Burns JM, Pedersen RA, Watt KD, Heimbach JK, Dierkhising RA. Frequency and outcomes of liver transplantation for nonalcoholic steatohepatitis in the United States. Gastroenterology. 2011;141(4):1249–1253

decrease relatively. If the number of CC cases with previously unrecognized NASH decreases, then it is reasonable to conclude that post-transplant rates of NAFLD in the CC population will also decrease as NASH patients leave this group. This is supported by a recent analysis of Scientific Registry of Transplant Recipients (SRTR) data regarding the change in indication for liver transplantation from 2001 to 2009. In this study, the rates of NASH as an indication for OLT increased substantially while rates of CC decreased over the same time period [4]. According to this study NASH became the third leading indication for OLT behind HCV and ALD, and a more recent evaluation has shown that NASH continues to increase as an indication for transplant, overtaking ALD as the second leading indication for OLT (Fig. 18.1) [4, 5]. Epidemiologically this mirrors the increasing epidemic of NASH and obesity worldwide [19]. However, it should be noted that in both of the different databases used, NASH diagnosis was at least partially derived from CC patients who were obese. This assumption that obese CC patients actually had NASH as their underlying etiology biases these results in favor of increasing rates of NASH; thus, these studies should be interpreted cautiously. Large databases will in the future hopefully make a more concerted effort to differentiate between NASH and CC and therefore erase this type of overlap. Evolving terminology and nomenclature over time presents a significant limitation to use of these databases and must be acknowledged and accounted for in the analysis where feasible. Lastly, rare diseases such as lysosomal acid lipase deficiency as well as some drug-induced effects can mimic NAFLD/NASH on imaging as well as histology and may play a role in CC that has previously gone unquantified. (See Chapter 17 for a discussion of metabolic disorders that can lead to a diagnosis of CC when the correct diagnostic tests are not performed.)

18.2.2 CC and ALD

Alcohol related liver disease has been apparent for centuries and is easily one of the most recognized liver diseases worldwide [6, 7]. However, multiple issues arise when attempting to interpret the impact of ALD on CC. First, the definitions of alcohol-related liver injury have changed over time as we have gained better understanding of the amount of alcohol intake needed to cause significant liver injury, something which is likely affected by gender, genetics, and size [7]. This may result in subjects being misclassified into CC groups or other etiologies of liver disease due to an assumed inadequate alcohol intake. As the amount of alcohol intake required to cause ALD has decreased over the years the true prevalence of ALD has become clearer. Older studies have used a definition of 80 g or more per day of alcohol intake as significant enough to cause ALD [1]. They noted a slow rise in ALD over their study period and an overall slight decline in CC. While the exact number is unclear they report that up to one-fourth of the CC patients may have had some amount of alcohol intake, though less than 80 g/day [1]. Currently a much lower threshold has been suggested at which ALD may occur, approximately 40 g/day in men and 20 g/day in women [41, 42].

This discrepancy in definitions may have biased the authors' results toward the null; i.e., the increase in alcoholic cirrhosis may have actually been underreported if the patients in the CC group were drinking alcohol in excess of our modern standards for ALD [1]. In addition, there was no delineation between the intakes of men or women in this study, something that is now strongly suspected to have a significant impact on ALD [42]. Inherently, as more data is uncovered regarding chronic liver disease processes, better disease definitions will result in fewer unknown diagnoses with therefore reduced CC diagnoses over time.

Current recommendations in the United States regarding alcohol intake for ALD suggest a cutoff of 20 g/day for women and 40 g/day for men [7]. Using these numbers as representative of significant alcohol intake, ALD represents around 18% of the patients listed for liver transplantation with another 10% having ALD in conjunction with HCV infection [5]. This remains a significant burden while remaining significantly confounding. Despite current recommendations there is still incomplete data regarding the actual amount of alcohol intake necessary to cause ALD [42–44] and the role of genetic susceptibility is largely unclear [45–47]. For this reason, a more conservative interpretation of ALD when assessing etiologies of CC seems most reasonable. This approach reduces the risk of misclassifying an ALD patient as CC and improves assessment of NAFLD in CC but may lead to undercounting of CC patients. This approach was taken in a study by Caldwell et al. in which the authors were primarily trying to assess the potential impact of NAFLD, AIH, and viral hepatitis on the diagnosis of CC [27].

There may also be a component of overlap for some NASH patients. Obesity has been shown to increase risk for ALD and even lead to progression of cirrhosis without clinically apparent injury [48, 49]. However, moderate alcohol consumption may have no impact on obesity-related steatohepatitis and could possibly mitigate the injury [50–52]. This sort of overlap with NASH requires further investigation and opens the larger question of the interaction of alcohol intake with other previously diagnosed liver disease [20]. The overlap between ALD and HCV has been large enough that liver transplant databases separately report the combination of the two [5]. Fortunately, many of the studies of NASH and CC have gone to extreme lengths to exclude alcohol intake as much as possible, some including use of experimental lab testing [27, 29]. In a study by Ayata et al., up to 15% of patients had evidence, either clinically or histologically, of ALD, but the clear overlapping histologic features of ALD with NASH necessitates that this finding be interpreted with caution [23]. Depending on gender, genetics, and potentially recall bias, ALD may still play a significant part in development of CC, albeit probably less than other liver disease etiologies.

18.2.3 CC and Viral Hepatitis

Prior to the 1970s, viral hepatitis was primarily notable for an acute hepatitis with jaundice or a chronic mildly active hepatitis and was thought to be secondary to hepatitis B or hepatitis A. As hepatitis B was becoming better defined, there were notable cases of a transfusion related non-A, non-B hepatitis which was also noted in patients without transfusion exposure, eventually termed hepatitis C [12, 53]. The advent of widespread testing for hepatitis C infection in 1991 led to a whole class of patients with viral hepatitis being clearly defined [13]. To determine the impact of HCV on patients with chronic unknown hepatitis and CC many investigators began testing for HCV antibodies. Initially, using HCV antibody testing it was estimated that up to 50% of patients with CC in the United States were due to chronic HCV infection [54, 55].

In a subsequent study by the same group, evaluating patients with chronic hepatitis using HCV RNA detection, HCV infection accounted for 44% of the patients with chronic liver disease [2]. The authors overcame a large hurdle from their initial study in this more recent study by using the RNA test rather than the antibody test to detect true chronic infection rather than prior exposure without ongoing infection, but interestingly the overall number of CC cases did not change greatly [2, 55]. Only 5% were labelled as CC and almost half of this group had a history of blood transfusion suggesting that there could be another unnamed viral etiology involved, now coined non-A, non-B, non-C viral hepatitis. Unfortunately, the authors did not report rigorous testing for AIH or other metabolic disease that could have suggested NAFLD. They did note that histology was bland or nonspecific on many of the biopsies [15, 23, 29]. Subsequently, other investigators began looking into a viral etiology of CC. Many hypothesized that in the setting of immunosuppression after LT an occult viral infection would become more predominant and have clinical and histologic characteristics similar to other viral infections [56].

In a case-control manner, Maor-Kendler and colleagues assessed the post-OLT course of CC patients compared with other identified etiologies of cirrhosis and found a closer association with cholestatic liver disease and ALD as compared to HCV infection. While the authors could not identify a strong association with any particular etiology of cirrhosis, they did note a significant difference in post-OLT outcomes for CC and HCV, concluding that a viral etiology of CC was unlikely since it would be expected to follow a course similar to HCV in the setting of post-transplant immunosuppression [57].

Other viruses such as hepatitis G and TT virus were also assessed directly in studies of CC. Initial studies suggested there may be some association of these viruses with CC based upon a noted prevalence of up to 15% in CC patients and possible evidence of post-transplant hepatitis related to their presence [56, 58, 59]. These studies were observational studies related back to clinical outcomes and over time repeat studies determined that there actually was no significant impact on CC or post-transplant outcomes for these patients [27, 60–62]. This signifies the importance of repeating studies over time as previously noted associations may have been secondary to random chance or simply a biased sample rather than true association. Lastly, there has been some suggestion that occult or silent HBV infection may be implicated as a potential viral etiology for CC [63, 64]. In some of these studies the HBV core antibody positivity did not correlate with chronic hepatitis and its presence suggests prior exposure and natural progression of HBV rather than a true cause of CC [20, 65]. These patients were not prospectively followed through to liver transplantation and/or death due to liver failure which would have been very helpful as chronic HBV in the setting of immunosuppression is often severe and leads to a notable hepatitis [66, 67]. In more recent papers as well as a seminal paper in 1978, anti-HBc would have indicated persistent infection, the presence of cccDNA, occult HBV infection with blood and/or tissue positive for HBV by PCR, providing support for HBV as a cause of cryptogenic liver disease and cirrhosis. The additional data on HBV reactivation in patients with CLD and CC who flare and decompensate, need liver transplant or die further support that HBV can be a contributor to CC. With this new understanding of HBV being an incurable infection like other DNA viruses, it is plausible that HBV has had a significant impact on CC outside of its already recognized disease course in HBsAg positive patients.

18.2.4 CC and AIH

Autoimmune hepatitis was initially described in the context of lupoid hepatitis [14]. Over the years, discovery of particular auto-antibodies and biochemical as well as histological patterns of disease led to a diagnostic scoring system [14, 68–70]. Autoimmune hepatitis, when not presented in classical fashion, can be difficult to exclude as a cause of CC. While there is literature suggesting that cryptogenic chronic active hepatitis may be related to AIH, once cirrhosis is clearly present, it may become more difficult to discern the underlying etiology [71, 72]. In a study of type 1 autoimmune hepatitis patients almost 25% presented with cirrhosis despite an absence of prior clinically relevant disease [73]. Additionally, CC patients with suspected AIH may also have inactive cirrhosis histologically without significant features of AIH, further confounding diagnostic efforts [38]. This supports a similar hypothesis to the data in NAFLD patients that progression to cirrhosis may also lead to loss of classic histologic features. This may also suggest that patients previously suspected of having NASH related CC may have actually had AIH, with the only real separation being in clinical features of disease rather than histologic features. This can also be confusing when considering the impact of drug-induced autoimmune-related liver injury. These patients may have resolving inflammation with drug cessation but may still progress to advanced fibrosis or even cirrhosis [22].

Berg et al. showed that in their subset of patients with CC undergoing liver transplantation the group of patients with a hepatocellular pattern of injury (ALT predominant) had much higher median IAH scores as well as a higher number of positive HLA-B8-DR3 haplotypes suggesting a diagnosis of AIH [15]. These patients also had higher risk of post-transplant chronic hepatitis, which has also been noted in patients with diagnosed AIH-related cirrhosis [15, 74]. Ultimately, it should also be noted that a third of these patients had pre-transplant biopsies with bland cirrhosis again suggesting that once patients progress to cirrhosis, histologic features may not remain accurate for diagnostic purposes. The findings in this observational study of CC are telling in regards to AIH. The hepatocellular group of patients all had IAH scores of 10 or greater and had significantly increased risk of post-transplant chronic hepatitis suggesting burned out AIH as the underlying etiology [15]. These results are somewhat contrary to the study by Caldwell et al. that saw a more even distribution of AIH parameters among all subgroups of CC and could not adequately distinguish these patients from NAFLD patients [27]. Unfortunately, a control group of AIH cirrhosis patients was not included in the study by Berg et al. to confirm similarities between the hepatocellular subset of patients and true AIH patients. However a prior study with a control group of AIH cirrhosis subjects had different results suggesting no significant overlap between CC and AIH [38]. The benefit to this prior study is in the case-control design as this allows for direct comparison to an AIH control group. The disadvantage is that it is retrospective and makes it difficult to control for confounding variables. Unfortunately, these limited studies in U.S. populations present conflicting data in regards to the interaction of AIH with CC. While there does seem to be some degree of clinically inactive AIH that progresses to cirrhosis it is likely a small portion of CC overall, but further study should occur to better define this entity.

Similar to studies with NASH and CC, authors have attempted to assess the post-transplant course as a means to identify AIH in their CC patients as well [15, 24, 38]. The prior studies presented conflicting results in their determination of AIH as a cause of CC, at least partially due to differences in study design [15, 38]. European studies appear to suggest AIH as a more common cause of CC than their American counterparts [24, 75]. In the study by Duclos-Vallee the majority of CC cases were deemed to have been related to AIH, based upon IAH scores and also post-transplant findings of graft hepatitis as well as auto-antibodies. However, similar to our previous assertions with NAFLD in the post-transplant setting, it is unclear if AIH presenting post-transplant is relative to the recipient's pre-transplant disease or could be secondary to a donor specific factor, which would be more appropriately termed allo-immune hepatitis or, even more succinctly, rejection. In addition, AIH and acute cellular rejection frequently appear similar on post-transplant biopsy, thus making differentiation of these two entities difficult. The diagnoses of de novo or recurrent AIH are very difficult to make post-transplant, even in patients that had accurately diagnosed AIH in the pre-transplant setting.

Conclusion

In the United States CC accounts for up to 10% of patients listed for liver transplantation and is suspected to account for 5–10% of all patients with cirrhosis [2, 5, 76]. Previous studies note its prevalence to be much higher, but with better recognition of chronic liver diseases such as NAFLD, this has declined over time [1, 2, 4]. By its very nature as a diagnosis of exclusion, the epidemiologic study of CC relies heavily on advances in knowledge regarding diagnosis of other liver diseases rather than any direct diagnostic observation or finding, making it a difficult entity to investigate. The most direct example of this reductionist process has been the relationship between CC and viral infections, most specifically hepatitis C formerly known as non-A, non-B viral hepatitis. With the discovery of the hepatitis C virus and the advent of standardized testing, a substantial proportion of patients with previously described CC could be characterized correctly as HCV instead [2]. Since that discovery, the rising prevalence of correctly diagnosed NASH has been implicated in declining rates of CC, and the clinical overlap between these sets of patients is highly suggestive that NASH makes up most of the patients labelled with CC. However, as recognition of NASH becomes widespread in clinical practice, the prevalence of CC is expected to decline drastically granted the association between these two conditions is as strong as previously described.

There remain a number of key questions regarding CC. Does the descriptor ‘cryptogenic’ require histology or can this be a noninvasive diagnosis requiring careful serological and historical review? Clearly, despite many clinical diagnostic advances, there indeed remains a group of patients with advanced cirrhosis who lack NASH risk factors or an antecedent diagnosis of ‘fatty liver’, known history of high risk viral exposure such as blood transfusion or other blood exposure, associated autoimmune conditions, or significant ethanol exposure. However, studies based on even careful assessment of existing large databases are also subject to local practices, accepted diagnoses and evolving terminology and nomenclature. In such studies, extensive testing and thoughtful analysis for an individual patient invariably come down to accurate and informed data entry. This will inherently reflect local practices regarding institutional tenets such as acceptance of NASH as a cause of CC and local diagnostic tenets regarding advanced autoimmune- and alcohol-related liver disease. It seems likely to these authors that a residual core of patients will remain with true CC which warrants additional exploration of etiology.

Summary Table of Landmark Literature

Study title and authors	Study design	Summary results	Main limitations
Powell EE, et al. Hepatology. 1990;11(1):74–80	Retrospective cohort study of NAFLD patients to associate clinical outcomes and histologic changes over time	• First study to associate NASH with progression to CC—loss of histologic features of NASH • Weight loss may improve features of NASH	• Retrospective nature impedes ability to control for confounding factors
Caldwell SH, et al. Hepatology. 1999;29(3):664–669	Retrospective case-control study comparing patients with CC to patients with NASH, HCV cirrhosis, and PBC cirrhosis	• Metabolic features of NASH (obesity and T2DM) were significantly more prevalent in CC than HCV cirrhosis or PBC cirrhosis • NASH and CC groups had much more overlap than in clinical feature than other causes of cirrhosis	• Retrospective nature impedes ability to control for confounding factors • Absence of NASH cirrhosis or AIH cirrhosis control groups limit comparison
Poonawala A, et al. Hepatology. 2000;32(4):689–692	Retrospective case-control study of patients with CC at time of transplant listing compared to age-matched controls with other etiologies of cirrhosis	• Metabolic risk factors (obesity and type 2 diabetes mellitus) were significantly more common in CC and NASH than other causes of cirrhosis suggesting NASH as a major etiology of CC	• Retrospective in nature so could not control for all confounding factors • Selection bias introduced by using only patients listed for liver transplantation
Caldwell SH, et al. Ann Hepatol. 2009;8(4):346–352	Retrospective case-control study comparing histology findings in patients with NASH that has progressed to CC to patients with HCV cirrhosis	• NASH patients lose steatosis histologically once progressed to cirrhosis, but other features remain • Features of NASH are much less common in HCV cirrhosis biopsies	• Only a single comparison group of HCV cirrhosis patients—including other groups may have noted more overlap • Small sample size—only 7 NASH/CC patients
Charlton MR, et al. Gastroenterology. 2011;141(4):1249–1253	Retrospective cohort study of the scientific registry of transplant patients (SRTR) data	• NASH increased rapidly from 2001 to 2009 as an indication for LT • CC declined over the same period of time	• Selection bias from poor definitions of disease process in large, anonymous database

References

1. Saunders JB, Walters JR, Davies AP, Paton A. A 20-year prospective study of cirrhosis. Br Med J (Clin Res Ed). 1981;282(6260):263–6.
2. Kodali VP, Gordon SC, Silverman AL, McCray DG. Cryptogenic liver disease in the United States: further evidence for non-A, non-B, and non-C hepatitis. Am J Gastroenterol. 1994;89(10):1836–9.
3. Conn H, Atterbury C. Cirrhosis. In: Schiff L, Schiff E, editors. Disease of the liver. Philadelphia, PA: J.B. Lippincott; 1993. p. 875–934.
4. Charlton MR, Burns JM, Pedersen RA, Watt KD, Heimbach JK, Dierkhising RA. Frequency and outcomes of liver transplantation for nonalcoholic steatohepatitis in the United States. Gastroenterology. 2011;141(4):1249–53.
5. Wong RJ, Aguilar M, Cheung R, et al. Nonalcoholic steatohepatitis is the second leading etiology of liver disease among adults awaiting liver transplantation in the United States. Gastroenterology. 2015;148(3):547–55.
6. Patrick CH. Alcohol, culture and society. Durham, NC: Duke University Press; 1952.
7. O'Shea RS, Dasarathy S, McCullough AJ. Alcoholic liver disease. Hepatology. 2010;51(1):307–28.
8. Bloodworth J. Diabetes mellitus and cirrhosis of the liver. Arch Intern Med. 1961;108(5):695–701.
9. Ito K, Nakagawa J, Okimoto Y, Nakano H. Chronic hepatitis-migration inhibition of leukocytes in the presence of Australia antigen. N Engl J Med. 1972;286(18):1005.
10. Robinson WS, Clayton DA, Greenman RL. DNA of a human hepatitis B virus candidate. J Virol. 1974;14(2):384–91.
11. Alter HJ, Purcell RH, Shih JW, et al. Detection of antibody to hepatitis C virus in prospectively followed transfusion recipients with acute and chronic non-A, non-B hepatitis. N Engl J Med. 1989;321(22):1494–500.
12. Villarejos VM, Visona KA, Eduarte CA, Provost PJ, Hilleman MR. Evidence for viral hepatitis other than type A or type B among persons in Costa Rica. N Engl J Med. 1975;293(26):1350–2. https://doi.org/10.1056/NEJM197512252932606.
13. Garson J, Tedder R, Briggs M, et al. Detection of hepatitis C viral sequences in blood donations by. Lancet. 1990;335(8703):1419–22.
14. Mackay I, Taft L, Cowling D. Lupoid hepatitis. Lancet. 1956;268(6957):1323–6.
15. Berg T, Neuhaus R, Klein R, et al. Distinct enzyme profiles in patients with cryptogenic cirrhosis reflect heterogeneous causes with different outcomes after liver transplantation (OLT): a long-term documentation before and after OLT. Transplantation. 2002;74(6):792–8.
16. Ludwig J, Viggiano TR, McGill DB, Oh BJ. Nonalcoholic steatohepatitis: Mayo clinic experiences with a hitherto unnamed disease. Mayo Clin Proc. 1980;55(7):434–8.
17. Brunt EM, Janney CG, Di Bisceglie AM, Neuschwander-Tetri BA, Bacon BR. Nonalcoholic steatohepatitis: a proposal for grading and staging the histological lesions. Am J Gastroenterol. 1999;94(9):2467–74.
18. Matteoni CA, Younossi ZM, Gramlich T, Boparai N, Liu YC, McCullough AJ. Nonalcoholic fatty liver disease: a spectrum of clinical and pathological severity. Gastroenterology. 1999;116(6):1413–9.
19. Younossi ZM, Koenig AB, Abdelatif D, Fazel Y, Henry L, Wymer M. Global epidemiology of nonalcoholic fatty liver disease—meta-analytic assessment of prevalence, incidence, and outcomes. Hepatology. 2016;64(1):73–84.
20. Caldwell S. Cryptogenic cirrhosis: what are we missing? Curr Gastroenterol Rep. 2010;12(1):40–8.
21. Sharp JR, Ishak KG, Zimmerman HJ. Chronic active hepatitis and severe hepatic necrosis associated with nitrofurantoin. Ann Intern Med. 1980;92(1):14–9.
22. Stine JG, Northup PG. Autoimmune-like drug-induced liver injury: a review and update for the clinician. Expert Opin Drug Metab Toxicol. 2016;12(11):1291–301.

23. Ayata G, Gordon FD, Lewis WD, et al. Cryptogenic cirrhosis: clinicopathologic findings at and after liver transplantation. Hum Pathol. 2002;33(11):1098–104.
24. Duclos-Vallée J, Yilmaz F, Johanet C, et al. Could post-liver transplantation course be helpful for the diagnosis of so called cryptogenic cirrhosis? Clin Transpl. 2005;19(5):591–9.
25. Rothman KJ. Epidemiology: an introduction. New York, NY: Oxford University Press; 2012.
26. Singal AK, Hasanin M, Kaif M, Wiesner R, Kuo YF. Nonalcoholic steatohepatitis is the most rapidly growing indication for simultaneous liver kidney transplantation in the United States. Transplantation. 2016;100(3):607–12. https://doi.org/10.1097/TP.0000000000000945.
27. Caldwell SH, Oelsner DH, Iezzoni JC, Hespenheide EE, Battle EH, Driscoll CJ. Cryptogenic cirrhosis: clinical characterization and risk factors for underlying disease. Hepatology. 1999;29(3):664–9.
28. Henry ZH, Caldwell SH, Argo CK. Nonalcoholic fatty liver disease: prognosis and progression of disease. Curr Hepatol Rep. 2016;15(2):117–24.
29. Powell EE, Cooksley WGE, Hanson R, Searle J, Halliday JW, Powell W. The natural history of nonalcoholic steatohepatitis: a follow-up study of forty-two patients for up to 21 years. Hepatology. 1990;11(1):74–80.
30. Abdelmalek M, Ludwig J, Lindor KD. Two cases from the spectrum of nonalcoholic steatohepatitis. J Clin Gastroenterol. 1995;20(2):127–30.
31. Bacon BR, Farahvash MJ, Janney CG, Neuschwander-Tetri BA. Nonalcoholic steatohepatitis: an expanded clinical entity. Gastroenterology. 1994;107(4):1103–9.
32. Poonawala A, Nair SP, Thuluvath PJ. Prevalence of obesity and diabetes in patients with cryptogenic cirrhosis: a case-control study. Hepatology. 2000;32(4):689–92.
33. Ratziu V, Bonyhay L, Di Martino V, et al. Survival, liver failure, and hepatocellular carcinoma in obesity-related cryptogenic cirrhosis. Hepatology. 2002;35(6):1485–93.
34. Ong J, Younossi ZM, Reddy V, et al. Cryptogenic cirrhosis and posttransplantation nonalcoholic fatty liver disease. Liver Transpl. 2001;7(9):797–801.
35. Contos MJ, Cales W, Sterling RK, et al. Development of nonalcoholic fatty liver disease after orthotopic liver transplantation for cryptogenic cirrhosis. Liver Transpl. 2001;7(4):363–73.
36. Yalamanchili K, Saadeh S, Klintmalm GB, Jennings LW, Davis GL. Nonalcoholic fatty liver disease after liver transplantation for cryptogenic cirrhosis or nonalcoholic fatty liver disease. Liver Transpl. 2010;16(4):431–9.
37. Caldwell SH, Lee VD, Kleiner DE, et al. NASH and cryptogenic cirrhosis: a histological analysis. Diabetes. 2009;5:2.
38. Greeve M, Ferrell L, Kim M, et al. Cirrhosis of undefined pathogenesis: absence of evidence for unknown viruses or autoimmune processes. Hepatology. 1993;17(4):593–8.
39. Seo S, Maganti K, Khehra M, et al. De novo nonalcoholic fatty liver disease after liver transplantation. Liver Transpl. 2007;13(6):844–7.
40. Kim H, Lee K, Lee K, et al. Histologically proven non-alcoholic fatty liver disease and clinically related factors in recipients after liver transplantation. Clin Transpl. 2014;28(5):521–9.
41. Savolainen V, Perola M, Lalu K, Penttilä A, Virtanen I, Karhunen PJ. Early perivenular fibrogenesis-precirrhotic lesions among moderate alcohol consumers and chronic alcoholics. J Hepatol. 1995;23(5):524–31.
42. Day CP. Who gets alcoholic liver disease: nature or nurture? J R Coll Physicians Lond. 2000;34(6):557–62.
43. Becker U, Deis A, Sorensen T, et al. Prediction of risk of liver disease by alcohol intake, sex, and age: a prospective population study. Hepatology. 1996;23(5):1025–9.
44. Bellentani S, Saccoccio G, Costa G, et al. Drinking habits as cofactors of risk for alcohol induced liver damage. The Dionysos Study Group. Gut. 1997;41(6):845–50.
45. Day CP, Bassendine MF. Genetic predisposition to alcoholic liver disease. Gut. 1992;33(11):1444–7.
46. Brown K, Johnson DA, Cattau EL Jr. Alcohol hepatotoxicity: a genotypic predisposition? Am J Gastroenterol. 1992;87(5):677–8.
47. Monzoni A, Masutti F, Saccoccio G, Bellentani S, Tiribelli C, Giacca M. Genetic determinants of ethanol-induced liver damage. Mol Med. 2001;7(4):255–62.

48. Naveau S, Giraud V, Borotto E, Aubert A, Capron F, Chaput J. Excess weight risk factor for alcoholic liver disease. Hepatology. 1997;25(1):108–11.
49. Diehl AM. Obesity and alcoholic liver disease. Alcohol. 2004;34(1):81–7.
50. Davies MJ, Baer DJ, Judd JT, Brown ED, Campbell WS, Taylor PR. Effects of moderate alcohol intake on fasting insulin and glucose concentrations and insulin sensitivity in postmenopausal women: a randomized controlled trial. JAMA. 2002;287(19):2559–62.
51. Dunn W, Xu R, Schwimmer JB. Modest wine drinking and decreased prevalence of suspected nonalcoholic fatty liver disease. Hepatology. 2008;47(6):1947–54.
52. Cotrim HP, Freitas LA, Alves E, Almeida A, May DS, Caldwell S. Effects of light-to-moderate alcohol consumption on steatosis and steatohepatitis in severely obese patients. Eur J Gastroenterol Hepatol. 2009;21(9):969–72. https://doi.org/10.1097/MEG.0b013e328328f3ec.
53. Koretz RL, Abbey H, Coleman E, Gitnick G. Non-A, non-B post-transfusion hepatitis: looking back in the second decade. Ann Intern Med. 1993;119(2):110–5.
54. Jeffers LJ, Hasan F, De Medina M, et al. Prevalence of antibodies to hepatitis C virus among patients with cryptogenic chronic hepatitis and cirrhosis. Hepatology. 1992;15(2):187–90.
55. Barnes RE, Meyer RA, Gordon SC. Prevalence of anti-HCV in cryptogenic cirrhosis in a suburban Detroit community. Am J Gastroenterol. 1992;87(8):1001–4.
56. Charlton M, Brandhagen D, Wiesner RH, et al. Hepatitis G virus infection in patients transplanted for cryptogenic cirrhosis: red flag or red herring? Transplantation. 1998;65(1):73–6.
57. Maor-Kendler Y, Batts KP, Burgart LJ, et al. Comparative allograft histology after liver transplantation for cryptogenic cirrhosis, alcohol, hepatitis C, and cholestatic liver diseases. Transplantation. 2000;70(2):292–7.
58. Cleavinger PJ, Persing DH, Li H, et al. Prevalence of TT virus infection in blood donors with elevated ALT in the absence of known hepatitis markers. Am J Gastroenterol. 2000;95(3):772–6.
59. Charlton M, Adjei P, Poterucha J, et al. TT-virus infection in north American blood donors, patients with fulminant hepatic failure, and cryptogenic cirrhosis. Hepatology. 1998; 28(3):839–42.
60. Laskus T, Wang L, Radkowski M, et al. Hepatitis G virus infection in American patients with cryptogenic cirrhosis: no evidence for liver replication. J Infect Dis. 1997;176(6):1491–5.
61. Pessoa MG, Terrault NA, Ferrell LD, et al. Hepatitis G virus in patients with cryptogenic liver disease undergoing liver transplantation. Hepatology. 1997;25(5):1266–70.
62. Schiano TD, Fiel MI, Abe K, Thung SN, Bodenheimer HC. Absence of hepatitis g virus within liver tissue of patients undergoing liver transplantation for cryptogenic cirrhosis. Transplantation. 1999;67(8):1193–7.
63. BRechot C, Thiers V, Kremsdorf D, Nalpas B, Pol S, Paterlini-Bréchot P. Persistent hepatitis B virus infection in subjects without hepatitis B surface antigen: clinically significant or purely "occult"? Hepatology. 2001;34(1):194–203.
64. Chung H, Lai C, Lok AS. Pathogenic role of hepatitis B virus in hepatitis B surface antigen-negative decompensated cirrhosis. Hepatology. 1995;22(1):25–9.
65. Berg T, Nauman U, Heuft H. Serum and peripheral mononuclear cells (PBMC) as a source material for hepatitis B virus DNA detection by polymerase chain reaction in volunteer blood donors [abstract]. Hepatology. 1999;22(25).
66. Yeo W, Chan TC, Leung NW, et al. Hepatitis B virus reactivation in lymphoma patients with prior resolved hepatitis B undergoing anticancer therapy with or without rituximab. J Clin Oncol. 2008;27(4):605–11.
67. Cheng A, Hsiung CA, Su I, et al. Steroid-free chemotherapy decreases risk of hepatitis B virus (HBV) reactivation in HBV-carriers with lymphoma. Hepatology. 2003;37(6):1320–8.
68. Dawkins RL, Joske RA. Immunoglobulin deposition in liver of patients with active chronic hepatitis and antibody against smooth muscle. Br Med J. 1973;2(5867):643–5.
69. Johnson P, McFarlane IG. Meeting report: international autoimmune hepatitis group. Hepatology. 1993;18(4):998–1005.
70. Alvarez F, Berg P, Bianchi F, et al. International autoimmune hepatitis group report: review of criteria for diagnosis of autoimmune hepatitis. J Hepatol. 1999;31(5):929–38.

71. Czaja AJ, Hay JE, Rakela J. Clinical features and prognostic implications of severe corticosteroid-treated cryptogenic chronic active hepatitis. Mayo Clin Proc. 1990;65(1):23–30.
72. Czaja AJ, Carpenter HA, Santrach PJ, Moore SB, Homburger HA. The nature and prognosis of severe cryptogenic chronic active hepatitis. Gastroenterology. 1993;104(6):1755–61.
73. Roberts SK, Therneau TM, Czaja AJ. Prognosis of histological cirrhosis in type 1 autoimmune hepatitis. Gastroenterology. 1996;110(3):848–57.
74. Faust TW. Recurrent primary biliary cirrhosis, primary sclerosing cholangitis, and autoimmune hepatitis after transplantation. Liver Transpl. 2001;7(11B):S99–108.
75. Heneghan MA, Zolfino T, Muiesan P, et al. An evaluation of long-term outcomes after liver transplantation for cryptogenic cirrhosis. Liver Transpl. 2003;9(9):921–8.
76. Nair S, Verma S, Thuluvath PJ. Obesity and its effect on survival in patients undergoing orthotopic liver transplantation in the United States. Hepatology. 2002;35(1):105–9.

MIX
Papier aus verantwortungsvollen Quellen
Paper from responsible sources
FSC® C105338

If you have any concerns about our products,
you can contact us on
ProductSafety@springernature.com

In case Publisher is established outside the EU,
the EU authorized representative is:
Springer Nature Customer Service Center GmbH
Europaplatz 3, 69115 Heidelberg, Germany

Printed by Libri Plureos GmbH
in Hamburg, Germany